MW01029728

ALSO BY JERRY AVORN

Powerful Medicines: The Benefits, Risks, and Costs of Prescription Drugs

Up Against the Ivy Wall: A History of the Columbia Crisis (principal author)

Rethinking Medications

TRUTH, POWER, AND THE DRUGS YOU TAKE

Jerry Avorn, MD

Simon & Schuster

NEW YORK AMSTERDAM/ANTWERP LONDON
TORONTO SYDNEY/MELBOURNE NEW DELHI

Simon & Schuster
1230 Avenue of the Americas
New York, NY 10020

First Simon & Schuster hardcover edition April 2025

Interior design by Paul Dippolito

Manufactured in the United States of America

1 3 5 7 9 10 8 6 4 2

Library of Congress Cataloging-in-Publication Data has been applied for.

ISBN 978-1-6680-5284-6
ISBN 978-1-6680-5285-3 (ebook)

For Karen, who has made everything possible

Contents

Rethinking Medications

INTRODUCTION

A Friend of the Court

Where We're Going, and How I Got Here

This is a great moment for medical science. We understand biology with unprecedented insight, and we have figured out how to use that knowledge to create medicines to cure or prevent illness with a power that was impossible just a generation ago. It should be a glorious time to be a patient or a doctor, but most patients and doctors don't feel that way. Our remarkable scientific victories have not been accompanied by comparable advances in getting such discoveries to those who need them, or in doing enough to ensure the effectiveness, safety, and affordability of the medications that people take. In the pages that follow, we will explore what goes right and goes wrong after molecules leave the lab and make their journey into people's bodies. Sometimes the path is swift and direct and leads to excellent results. But other times it takes unexpected turns that can produce awful outcomes. Understanding this pathway can shed light on what drugs people should take or might want to question, and what needs to happen in the doctor's office, Washington, the states, and throughout all the layers of our struggling, complicated health-care system.

This matters a great deal to all of us who prescribe medications, and even more to everyone who takes them. If drugs are the hardware of the medication world, then everything that shapes how they are used—their testing, patenting, pricing, prescribing, and all the other "systems" issues that determine their place in health care—can be thought of as the all-important software. You can't think clearly about one without engaging with the other.

Millions of times each day, Americans open an amber medication container and ingest a pill from it or have something injected into their body, to make them healthier or keep them that way. Each act is a little like a sacrament embodying decades of research, transubstantiated into a chemical we incorporate, protecting us. But this quiet culmination of the therapeutic adventure follows many other steps: determining whether the medicine works or not, whether it's safe, what it should cost, and whether the doctor who prescribed it made the best choice. This crucial cascade of decisions isn't just a collection of interwoven stories from pharmacology, politics, medical education, economics, decision theory, and a dozen other disciplines, though that would be interesting enough. These processes also determine the health or sickness of millions of people, including the readers of this book. It is a tale of brilliant scientists, well-meaning but sometimes compromised government officials, single-minded corporations, and dedicated frontline clinicians trying to make sense of it all.

It's only been since the 1950s that we have had a solid understanding of how to create new medicines, how to test them rigorously, and how to get them safely into patients. We've made wonderful progress, and in the pages that follow we'll note these accomplishments with reverence and celebration. Every day, the world's basic scientists and clinical researchers make transformative discoveries about the fundamental mechanisms of life, how they can be perturbed by disease, and how we can undo or prevent that damage. After completing my training as an internist, in the 1980s I began a program of research that starts where that work leaves off. Over several decades, I built an interdisciplinary research team at Harvard Medical School to study the complicated journey of drugs from the lab to the patient, and what goes right or wrong along the way.

Our group takes those life-changing discoveries as the starting point and then focuses on the next steps: Once a new molecule is discovered, then what? How can we measure whether it makes a meaningful difference for patients? What are the best ways to identify its side effects early on, before it can sicken thousands? Why are so many people in the world's richest country unable to afford what we prescribe for them, and what can we do about that? How can we best communicate these complicated insights of effectiveness, risk, and cost to doctors and to patients to inform the millions of everyday decisions that shape what we prescribe and what our patients take? What is the effect of the training and socialization we offer our medical students in influencing the way they think about and prescribe drugs?

Finally and crucially, how do medications, our most common clinical intervention, fit into the larger health-care system in which they play such a central role? We have to grasp all these aspects of a drug's pre-consumer journey in order for medications to fully realize their enormous potential for good without causing awful new problems, either clinical or economic. Doing that requires us to examine processes rarely seen by patients and even by most doctors—taking a close look under the hood to learn how each of those steps can work well and why they sometimes don't. I delved into these processes in my last book, *Powerful Medicines: The Benefits, Risks, and Costs of Prescription Drugs*. Now, two decades later and with a few hundred more research papers under my belt, things have gotten even more interesting.

Two Tool Kits

Medicine makes use of two different kinds of tool kit: one for discovering new medicines and a second for evaluating, paying for, and disseminating those drugs once they've been discovered. Our health-care system has employed the first tool kit magnificently to invent new therapies for previously untreatable conditions, to improve the medicines we currently have, and to gain new insights into our very genetic makeup to attack disease. The second tool kit also works well, but many of its instruments—from the fields of policy, law, epidemiology, economics, education—are often wielded ineptly or not at all.

The questions we will pursue here start where biochemistry and pharmacology leave off. Medicines aren't just chemicals: the good they can do and how safe they are depend on how their use is shaped by human decision-making, policy, economics, and epidemiology along with many other non-biological inputs. A particular drug may work powerfully but isn't worth using because of its terrible side-effect profile. Or its effectiveness and safety are both good, but it's priced so high that people can't afford to take it. How many extra dollars should we pay for how much added efficacy and safety? How can doctors, patients, insurers, and regulators align these interacting factors optimally, fairly, and affordably? And whose job is it to put out balanced information about these conclusions? These post-discovery issues drive every prescription that is written and taken each day; if we could just be smarter about them, we'd have much more success translating the biomedical revolution into improved health outcomes.

- **How do we know if a drug actually works?** The randomized controlled clinical trial is the most powerful "truth detector" we have to determine whether or not a medicine is effective. But each year the nation has moved further away from that metric, relying more and more on simpler, less reliable measures that leave us doctors and our patients without the information we need to use new treatments well.
- **Is it safe enough?** For decades, the health-care system sometimes lost track of the side effects of widely used medications once they were initially approved, even when those harms might outweigh a drug's benefits. That started to change when several best-selling medicines turned out to cause unanticipated and dangerous problems. Those disasters led to implementing new ways to track the adverse events caused by commonly used prescriptions. These methods hold enormous promise, but remain underused.
- **What should it cost?** Drugmakers get to bypass the usual rules of economics when they are allowed to charge exorbitant prices for products well beyond their actual worth; this is even more concerning when such pricing is applied to drugs developed largely with public research funds. Americans pay medication prices that are twice those paid by citizens of other nations, and nearly one in four of our patients can't afford to take what we prescribe for them. We have good ideas on how to estimate what a drug's fair price should be, and many countries do just that, but federal and state lawmakers have taken the astonishing step of making it illegal to use such analyses to help shape American policy.

- **How do we get the word out on all this to patients and practitioners and students?** Drug companies are still a main source of what laypeople and doctors know about medications, and attempts to constrain their marketing now face opposition based on claims of corporations' free speech rights. But promoting only the costliest products distorts our understanding and often downplays the best evidence, leading to overuse of some drugs beyond reason and neglect of others that are excellent choices. And what is the effect of so much pharmaceutical financing coming into medical schools, where the doctors of tomorrow are trained and socialized? Some innovative educational programs have begun to address this.
- **How do all the pieces fit together?** Because drugs are the single most common intervention in all of medicine, how well the larger health-care system works determines patients' access to the doctors they need to prescribe their medications, as well as their ability to pay for them. Despite the innovative excellence of U.S. biomedical research, our care delivery is the least equitable and most overpriced in the industrialized world. As a result, despite our extremely high drug and health expenditures, the clinical outcomes we achieve are only about average compared to other wealthy countries, and sometimes below average—partly undercutting the successes we have achieved in devising new therapeutics. We'll see how one radical program in Massachusetts set out to fix the access problem and laid the groundwork for reforms that later rippled throughout the country.

As in clinical practice, getting the diagnosis right is the first step toward effective action; viewed clearly, all of these problems are addressable. We'll see how each of the pieces interacts with all the others and how they are intertwined, culminating in a single patient opening that amber-colored container and ingesting the final product—and everything that follows after that. The story will build on research I've done at Harvard with the multidisciplinary teams of colleagues I've been fortunate to put together over the last forty years. The work of over two dozen faculty in my research group along with talented programmers, trainees, and support staff have enabled us to develop new ways to diagnose problems in how we use medications, and to design innovative ways to address them. Unfortunately, each of these areas—measuring and communicating effectiveness thoughtfully, basing our understanding of risks on evidence and not ideology, and ensuring equitable access to new treatments for all—is deeply threatened by the policy and leadership changes that followed the 2024 U.S. elections. We will address these new challenges later in this book as they arise.

The discovery of a new drug is often heralded with great excitement, often through a press release from its manufacturer. But more thoughtful evaluation of its actual strengths and limitations may not come until much later, and generally gets far less attention. The initial discovery is a bit like an orgasm early in a relationship. It's dramatic and exciting and rewarding, but the most important assessment is more like a marriage: it requires thoughtful rethinking over years, with all the attendant ups and downs that come with experience. Ideally, that deepens the relationship with a medicine or with a partner, though sometimes the ongoing reassessment leads to divorce as the most sensible option; rarely is either trajectory evident at the moment of the first orgasm. Decision theory researcher and Nobelist Daniel Kahneman made a similar observation that could also apply to medications; he wrote that nearly every couple looks happy on their wedding day, though we know that half of those marriages will end in divorce. The probability of success is better for new drugs, but the illustration is sobering.

I'll bring to our discussion the perspective not just of a researcher but also that of a primary care doctor who spent years prescribing drugs to patients. Medicine is frequently taught through case studies, and we will use that tool as well to flesh out the challenges and possibilities we face:

- How did one of the most widely used drugs in the U.S. come to be taken by 20 million Americans for over five years before its manufacturer admitted that its product tripled the rate of heart attack and stroke?
- The opioid crisis is global, but how did the U.S. end up with the

highest prescribing rate for these addictive medicines, and the highest per capita toll of fatal drug overdoses?

- The breakthrough cancer drug Xtandi was developed at the University of California through years of research funded by American taxpayers. How did this lifesaving drug come to be privately owned, with its owners charging us two to five times what patients in other countries pay for it?
- Psychedelics from LSD to psilocybin and the club drug ecstasy (MDMA) hold the promise of impressive effectiveness in helping patients with many intractable kinds of mental distress. Why did the government criminalize research on them for over four decades before beginning to loosen its grip on these potentially transformative treatments?
- What lies behind the FDA's growing use of approval standards that allow new drugs for serious conditions like cancer, muscular dystrophy, and ALS onto the market even if they don't work?
- How does our health-care delivery system enable and even encourage some of our worst medication problems, and what can we change to fix that?

We'll zoom out from these case studies to look at the overall picture and consider how all the pieces—effectiveness, safety, cost, communication, and the system as a whole—interact with each other. Throughout, we'll consider how these issues affect consumers: whether the prescription drug you take tomorrow morning is likely to make you feel better or cause an unexpected side effect; whether the medicine the doctor prescribed for your mother has actually been proven to be effective or not; whether you or someone you know won't be able to take a lifesaving drug because it costs several thousand dollars out of pocket even if you have health insurance. Our rethinking will assume the perspective that clinical trialists refer to as "equipoise": the neutral belief that a new treatment may turn out to be much better than what we already have, or about the same, or worse. If we knew for sure which of these was true before starting a study, we wouldn't have to do the trial—and it could even be unethical to do so. That posture is useful for evaluating policy options as well. It's been said that the most important attribute of a scientist is the ability to hold two conflicting ideas in your head at the same time; I'll try to do that here.

We'll avoid medical self-congratulation, since there's plenty of that out there already. Instead, we'll analyze what we all need to do better: clinicians, patients, the drug industry, and government. My approach will be modeled on what people want in a visit with their doctor. On an all-too-brief encounter, you wouldn't want your clinician to focus on all the things you feel fine about: instead of discussing your robust appetite, acute vision, good balance, or refreshing sleep, it's much more useful to talk about the breast lump, the shortness of breath, the hip pain, or the bloody stools. In the exam room as in this book, dwelling on the positives isn't the most useful thing we can do together. It's more helpful to adopt a patient-facing posture of asking, "Where does it hurt?" and "How can I help?" rather than "Wow! Look at those abs!"

Sometimes we begin to understand a problem only after it brings about a crisis; that's why analyzing a plane's black box recorder following a crash can yield such valuable information. Loving something deeply and wanting to criticize it is an ambivalent sensation understood by anyone who's raised a child or has a pet; a similar tension informs much of the perspective in my group's research. In Boston, it can be daunting to take a critical view of these matters from within one of the most renowned and productive medical research centers on the planet, but also a place that is increasingly drawn into the business side of medicine and medicines. Some days I identify with the proverbial skunk at the garden party; others, I feel like I'm trying to set up a birth-control clinic at the Vatican.

My Own Pathway

The worldview that helped shape this book had its beginnings during my college days at Columbia at the height of the student activism of the late 1960s. In that era of civil rights struggle, protest against the Vietnam War and the ongoing disinformation about it that came from the government, I developed a healthy skepticism about authority and spent more time as a reporter and editor working on the student daily newspaper than I did on some of my pre-med courses. Our student-journalist work produced some excellent frontline reporting during a key moment in history; several of us came together to turn it into a widely read book on the 1968 student movement at Columbia called *Up Against the Ivy Wall*.

Despite this atypical background, I was nonetheless accepted to Harvard as a first-year medical student in 1969, and never left. My goal over the ensuing half century or so has been to figure out how to combine my interests in human health, biological science, and social justice. On finishing my clinical training in internal medicine in Harvard's teaching hospitals I was asked to join the faculty and launched an interdisciplinary research program to study the connections among medication effectiveness, risks, costs, communication, and policy. My interest in bringing a crosscutting perspective to our work probably had its roots in the interdisciplinary design of Columbia's intense core curriculum that I endured as an undergraduate. It required us to take two years of courses whose faculty had the *chutzpah* to try to teach us something about history, philosophy, sociology, economics, religion, political science, and several other fields, discussed in small seminar-like classes. (A companion course tried to do the same for art and music.) That ambitious approach can run the risk of superficiality; worse, in those days the definition of Western civilization comprised solely the writings of long-dead white males, and my courses had no readings about anything after World War I, or any culture east of Europe. But it still left me with the invigorating belief that a person could have at least some rudimentary understanding of several disciplines at once, and could begin to see how one field sheds light on another—a perspective that's harder to glimpse if you focus exclusively on just one department's offerings.

Once in Boston, following my internship and residency in Harvard's teaching hospitals, I began to assemble a team of physicians, epidemiologists, policy experts, statisticians, lawyers, and ethicists. Our research would focus on everything that needs to go right, but sometimes goes wrong after a new molecule is discovered, before it finds its way into routine use in patients: how its clinical trials are designed, how it's evaluated by the Food and Drug Administration (FDA) for approval, how we track its side effects before and after it enters the market, how the finished product is paid for, how we develop and transmit information about its benefits and risks to each other and to our patients. Combining clinical practice with research and teaching provided vital cross-pollination for me and our group as a whole. Some of the most important questions we've tackled stemmed from an issue that came up in my role as a primary care doctor and geriatrician in one of our teaching hospitals, or a question a bright medical student asked at the end of a class. And in the other direction, insights from our research have guided my care of patients as well as what I've tried to teach our trainees.

The Birth of DoPE

In 1997 our research group was granted the status of a clinical division in the Department of Medicine at one of Harvard's main teaching institutions, the Brigham and Women's Hospital, making it coequal (at least on the organizational chart) with more traditional groups that focus on cardiology, kidney disease, or infections. I named it the Division of Pharmacoepidemiology and Pharmacoeconomics, or DoPE for short (see chapter 17). It now includes over eighty of us with origins in a dozen countries and many kinds of training backgrounds. As we study all aspects of medicines' lab-to-patient trajectory, the clinicians have a lot to learn from the epidemiologists and vice versa, while the lawyers and ethicists talk to both groups about the policy implications related to medication use. Our trainees keep us all on our toes asking questions from their own perspectives, whether epidemiology or statistics or internal medicine or health services research or constitutional law. Some of our work draws on terabytes of data we've assembled on all the filled prescriptions and clinical outcomes of tens of millions of anonymized patients, drawn from coverage systems like Medicaid, Medicare, and commercial health insurers. My group was among the first to harvest such data on a very large scale to study drug use and outcomes; the same approach has proven to be a powerful way to "biopsy" the health-care system to understand what gets prescribed, how patients do or don't take those medications, and all the good and problematic real-world health outcomes that follow the use of hundreds of drugs in these very large populations.

Early on, I established a policy for our program that none of us would accept any personal payments as consultants to any drugmaker, an unusual (perhaps unique) policy in the world of Harvard medicine. We try hard to make sure that our work isn't seen as predictably pro-industry, as is the case with some units around the country, or anti-industry (ditto). DoPE has grown to become one of the most productive groups working in these areas, with several of us among the most highly cited researchers in the country. Our division's studies have generated 1,600 or so papers in the medical literature, numerous professorships, and about $20 million each year in research funding, mostly from the federal government; I set up a spin-off nonprofit organization in 2004 (see chapter 17) to disseminate the most current evidence on medications to health-care professionals all over the country. The goal of DoPE and of this book is to bring to a wider audience the insights that my colleagues and I have developed over many years of that never-dull work. The governmental transformations ushered in by the second Trump presidency will touch on all these topics, and run against the grain of most of the activities my colleagues and I engage in. That makes our work either far more important, or utterly hopeless. I spend part of each day wondering which of these is true.

A Maturing Profession

In the nineteenth century, the practice of medicine relied on received wisdom and reverence for authority. That gave us bloodletting, purgatives, arsenic, useless and often toxic herbal remedies, and the idea of drilling holes in people's skulls to treat seizures or mental illness. Those concepts had persisted for hundreds of years because Everyone Knew That Was the Right Thing to Do. Fortunately, there was far less adulation of received wisdom by the time I started medical school. Our training was based mostly on verified science, even if it was sometimes a narrow view of it. We learned in detail about then-cutting-edge experiments in biochemistry, physiology, and pharmacology, nearly all of it evidence-based. But we didn't hear much about how to question the clinical evidence, how to translate it into patient care, and how medicine fit into the larger society. To address those shortfalls, some classmates and I invented our own course to teach each other about all the unloved public health, political, and "soft science" issues that never made it into the official curriculum. That student-generated course more than fifty-five years ago laid the groundwork for my research since then, and in a way became the first draft of this book.

This orientation also led me to a decision to train as a general internist rather than as a cardiologist or psychiatrist or surgeon. A generalist approach seemed the best fit for me with the common human experience of illness: when we're sick, we may need specialists to consult on tough questions, but most of us also crave a well-trained all-around doctor to serve as our primary caregiver—someone who can see how the diabetes medication may relate to the falling problem, how the blood pressure drug may explain the chronic cough, how the depression and its treatment may be connected to the confusion and tremor. It felt right and I enjoyed it, even if this meant that I was choosing a field at the bottom of the scale for both pay and respect in American medicine. To move even lower on the scale of income and prestige, I developed an interest in the care of the elderly, especially the medications they took.

During my training as a junior doctor at Harvard's hospitals, some of our best conferences were the weekly "morbidity and mortality rounds," which we called M&M's. In each session, one of us would describe the case of a patient who had suffered an unexpected bad outcome and try to identify the key decisions and actions that may have led up to that event. The focus was to teach each other in a nonjudgmental way about what could have been done better, given the information available at the time. While those sessions were sometimes uncomfortable, they led to some of the best learning experiences we had. The attitude wasn't "This is a crappy hospital and these trainees are incompetent"; instead, the goal was to teach each other how to do our work better, together. Our colleagues across town at the Massachusetts General Hospital held similar weekly conferences in the Ether Dome, the picturesque amphitheater in which the use of that anesthetic in surgery was first demonstrated in 1846. In both these exercises the patient often died, but I've never heard anyone complain that the stories didn't have happy endings. Focusing on what goes well and has a pleasant outcome has its place, but analyzing what goes wrong is a much better way to teach, to learn, and to improve care.

In sessions like these, the final word often went to the pathologists—specialists we saw less often than our more clinically active colleagues. They'd emerge from their labs, which in those days sometimes reeked of formaldehyde, and present the autopsy findings that provided the definitive final answer; often it wasn't what anyone expected. (Those "disease-reveal" performances reminded me of the medical student joke that internists knew everything but couldn't do much, surgeons didn't know much but could do a lot, and pathologists knew everything—but too late.)

Early in my career I was attending a scientific meeting in San Diego and found I had a free afternoon. I used it to tour its famous lighthouse, still fitted out with the furnishings of a long-gone keeper: his little bed, his bookcase, his tiny kitchen, the tools he used to keep the light burning bright to warn ships away from the dangerous reefs below. A worthy kind of career, I realized: hard work, yes, and lonely. But you get to stay put and give people the information they need to keep them safe. . . . A person could even save some lives. I was engaged in patient care for much of my career, but that image of the lighthouse keeper still speaks to me. When my wife and I go traveling, if there's a lighthouse nearby we try to visit it. These days, many of them are just cute relics, as perhaps the two of us are becoming. The beacons have mostly been automated and depopulated, made less relevant by radar and GPS technology. But there's something about their spirit that still resonates deeply.

Celebration, Advocatus Diaboli, Whistle-Blowers, and Maggots

In thinking about how to best serve as a responsible internal critic in medicine, I've looked to some iconic precedents for guidance. One is the now-clichéd concept of the devil's advocate. We've all been in meetings when someone wants to shoot down a plan but still appear supportive and says, "Let me just play devil's advocate here"—and then goes on to eviscerate the idea. In fact, the role of *advocatus diaboli* was an official Church function created in the sixteenth century to sharpen the assessment of a person being considered for sainthood. The devil's advocate was tasked with uncovering flaws in the character of the nominated person, or the veracity of the miracles they were said to have performed. While the job title was formally terminated in 1983, the concept came back into prominence in 2003 when the Vatican asked the adamant atheist Christopher Hitchens to serve a similar contrarian role during the proposed beatification of Mother Teresa. He took on the task with snarky gusto, calling her "a fanatic, a fundamentalist, and a fraud." She was beatified anyway, but the debate was richer for his involvement.

Being an internal critic seems to work better outside the ecclesiastical world. Many institutions employ an ombudsperson—a neutral, confidential resource with whom an employee can talk about a struggle with the organization. Similarly, some newspapers created the role of "public editor" to serve as a reader-facing critic of its journalists' activities, though that function is scarcer each year, as are newspapers. In government, nearly all federal departments include an Office of the Inspector General to unearth and address problematic internal behavior; the office responsible for the FDA launched an inquiry after the agency approved an expensive drug for Alzheimer's disease that didn't work (see chapter 1). The executive branch also contains the Government Accountability Office, which used to have the more pedestrian title of Government Accounting Office; it made an important contribution to resetting the nation's course after the Vioxx tragedy (see chapter 9). I think of these units as performing a kind of "immunological surveillance" function for their organizations, akin to the cells that roam our bodies to detect and attack any cells that have gone rogue and become malignant; that is increasingly seen as one of the body's best defenses against the development of a cancer that could kill the whole organism. Although loathsome to think about, an analogous function is filled by the maggots that used to be common denizens of diseased flesh. Before antibiotics, physicians would sometimes intentionally place these creepy little creatures into wounds to feed on dead or dying tissue, keeping it clean and combating infection. Going after the bad stuff can serve a vital role in many different contexts.

Then there's the whistle-blower, a role that's become indispensable in illuminating transgressions related to medications as well as many other areas. The term dates to the nineteenth century, when police officers would blow a whistle to warn the public of a hazard or to summon help. It generalized to referees at sporting events, whose whistles called out an illegal play or a foul. In medicine, whistle-blowers have provided valuable evidence of once-hidden problems from within drug companies or government agencies or unscrupulous vendors—misdeeds that would have likely remained invisible otherwise. This works because many abuses or lapses can be detected only by the people inside a given system, whether it's a corporation, the government, or a university. A Freudian might see them as an organization's superego, there to limit the natural excesses of its id and its ego. People who lack a well-functioning superego are known as sociopaths; I know of no comparable term for organizations.

The most sophisticated instance of a useful give-and-take process to get to the truth is another reality-defining system, the peer-review process of scientific journals. The term is now heard refreshingly often in the media, as in "The paper hasn't yet been peer-reviewed, so its results aren't certain." The process is powerful and conceptually simple, and contrasts sharply with decision-making in the realms of religion, politics, or business. A scientific paper submitted to a journal isn't selected for publication solely by a group of editors, since no small cadre of people, however smart, can possibly have cutting-edge expertise in every area of medicine from molecular genetics to the economics of Medicare. Instead, the submission is sent out to a group of usually anonymous scholars in that field for a critical reading, a written assessment, and some recommendations—all done pro bono. It can take an hour or two to do each review, but it's how we keep the bad stuff out and let the good stuff in. In some ways it's like working at a neighborhood food pantry or as a volunteer firefighter. You don't get paid, but there's the reward of feeling that you're doing something for the community. I try to approach the task each time with a low-ego posture of equipoise: "I'm not assuming that this drug/paper is good or bad; let's subject it to evenhanded scrutiny without preconceptions or bias and see where that leads." This is the attitude I've tried to bring to the questions discussed here, because when that perspective works it's the best way we have of figuring out what's true.

Mortality rounds, investigative journalists, devil's advocates, inspectors general, peer reviewers, whistle-blowers, maggots—each serves a vital purpose in protecting the surrounding enterprise, as well as society at large. These roles often bring with them more than a little revulsion from the entities that house them, but they serve an irreplaceable function. In the chapters that follow, we will explore what goes wrong as well as what goes right as medicines make their bumpy way from lab to patient. The good news is that we get it right much of the time, and most of the problems we'll identify are fixable; practical solutions are offered at the end of each section. A companion website (www.RethinkMeds.info) will serve as a resource for concerned consumers, health-care professionals, and students to get involved further with these issues, and to connect with one another to build a movement that might carry some of these ideas forward. It will also be a place for updates and corrections of some of the topics below, given how fast-moving these fields have become.

The areas we'll explore are directly relevant to anyone who takes or prescribes a medicine or cares about someone who does, as well as to anyone who pays taxes or health insurance premiums. Other readers will take an interest in how our society grapples with some of its most important choices, and how the complex dimensions of effectiveness, risk, cost, communication, and policy interact to generate the therapeutic landscape that all of us live in. These issues both transcend and are shaped by different health-care delivery systems, variations in cross-national policies, and even political transformations such as the 2024 elections.

Awesome science underlies the medications we use—many of them developed by committed, brilliant researchers in universities and in industry, evaluated by smart, hardworking, and usually competent regulators at the FDA and its sister organizations worldwide, and deployed by health-care professionals with dedication and great skill most of the time. But we can't look away from the venality, arrogance, or incompetence that stain a small segment of drug development, regulation, promotion, and use. As medications become more and more impressive, our need to use them well and the downsides of failing to do that grow more intense each year. As Carl Jung wrote, "The brighter the light, the darker the shadow." These concerns have only become more interesting and acute since I wrote *Powerful Medicines*, which laid the foundation for many of the concepts here.

The content that follows is designed to serve as a "gateway drug" as well as an engaging book. Its final sections are designed to empower readers, whether consumers or health-care professionals and trainees, to get involved more deeply with these issues to promote their own health or education. Despite all the concerns we'll explore, there is reason for optimism: over the long haul, facts tend to win out even if it takes time, and the discordant messenger is often vindicated. I take comfort in this story of a nautical exchange on a foggy night:

Voice 1, through a loudspeaker, to a rapidly approaching ship: *Turn away! We are on a collision course and you are about to hit me!*

Voice 2, on a bullhorn from the ship: *I will not; you turn away!*

Voice 1: *You must change your course immediately or there will be a dangerous accident.*

Voice 2: *I refuse. I am an admiral in the United States Navy and am speaking to you from an American battleship. Why should I listen to you?*

Voice 1: *Because I am speaking to you from a lighthouse.*

– PART ONE –

Does It Work?

CHAPTER 1

How Do We Know?

> We have access to more information and evidence than ever, but facts seem to have lost their power.
>
> —*This Is Not Propaganda*, a book about the Soviet Union

In 2021, the Food and Drug Administration gave its approval to Aduhelm, a new drug for Alzheimer's disease that didn't work, could cause brain damage, and was poised to cost the nation each year a sum the size of NASA's annual budget. How did the world's once best prescription drug regulatory body fall so low? And how does this decline impact the medications that Americans take every day?

We need to start by considering how a drug is evaluated to determine whether it works, and what we even mean by "working." It took us over a century to learn how to rethink this question; knowing about that journey is key to understanding where we've ended up, and to contemplate the more primitive approach to which we may be returning. Before 1906 anybody could put anything they wanted in a bottle and call it a medicine, without even having to reveal what was in it. A manufacturer could then make any claims it wanted about the product's effectiveness for any condition. They were called "patent medicines," even though they were generally not patented. Many of them did no good at all, and some were downright dangerous. Pills and elixirs promoted to treat pain, depression, cancer, "female troubles," liver disease, and a host of other complaints filled store shelves and mail-order catalogues. Many were physiologically inert, but some contained hefty amounts of alcohol, opium, cocaine, or a combination of them. Yes, sick babies given narcotic or alcohol elixirs did seem to become more comfortable, stopped crying, and slept better. Many of them also stopped breathing. On the picker-upper side of the medicine cabinet, it's widely known that Coca-Cola got its name because the active ingredient in the original formulation was cocaine. Apart from its substantial addictive potential, this explains why so many people believed that things really did go better with Coke. That ingredient was removed in the early 1900s.

A Uniquely American Condition?

Around the same time, the Rexall company introduced its "Americanitis Elixir" to treat the ills caused by a rapidly industrializing society. The product was "as necessary as food and drink," its ads proclaimed, continuing,

> This unique medical discovery strengthens and tones the nerves. . . . It supplies to the body phosphorous in soluble form—a thing never before considered possible. Rexall Americanitis has accomplished wonderful results all over the country and its merits are now universally recognized.

The part about phosphorus was utterly meaningless; the product's real active ingredients appear to have been 15 percent alcohol and some chloroform, explaining the ad's tagline "Note how quickly that feeling of nervous strain disappears."

Companion advertisements for the product were directed at "nervous, over-worked, and run-down women," noting that the product "acts directly on the nerves." (Yes, alcohol and chloroform will do that.) The ad for women continued,

> Rexall Americanitis Elixir is the only remedy of its kind in existence. As its name implies, it's a specific for the peculiar exhausted nervous conditions resulting from the continuous rush and tension under which Americans live. This remedy fills an important gap in the line of medicines.

Other promotion in the early 1900s from the Bayer company touted its two recently invented compounds: Aspirin for fevers (that's worked out well over the years), and Heroin for cough (not so much). Both drugs had been created by the same chemist during the same period in 1897. Bayer's Aspirin found its way into nearly every home medicine cabinet, while Bayer's Heroin helped set the stage for a crippling epidemic of addiction, discussed more fully in chapter 20. This was before the invention of the categories of controlled substances or prescription-only drugs, so any doctor could recommend any substance to any patient. Nor was a doctor even needed: such substances could be bought directly by the consumer, with no requirement or guarantee that any of them be either safe or effective. It wasn't until the Progressive Era at the start of the twentieth century that the nation began to wonder whether government should do something about this chaotic abundance of sometimes-toxic choices.

The nation's first attempt at drug regulation simply proposed that manufacturers should be required to label what was in their products, which would be helpful for people trying to limit their inadvertent intake of opioids, cocaine, or alcohol. As modest as the requirement was, like all attempts to regulate medications over the decades it was met with charges of government overreach encroaching on the rights of citizens. But cooler if still timid heads prevailed, and in 1906 Congress passed the first Pure Food and Drug Act, creating the Food and Drug Administration. This small step did nothing to ensure that any of these products worked, or even were safe: manufacturers just needed to state what was inside the bottle or tablet.

The country still was not ready for something as modest as a law requiring that medicines not be poisonous; that didn't fall into place until over three decades later, in 1938 (see chapter 5). And then, for another quarter century after that, drugmakers still didn't have to prove that their products really worked. That revolutionary concept was proposed in legislation introduced in 1961 by Senator Estes Kefauver, a Democrat from Tennessee. Along with other proposed laws that dealt with the high prices of medicines—a recurring theme in American history—he introduced the radical idea that a manufacturer should be required to show that its product helped patients before it could be sold or promoted. No other country required that; at the time, this idea was seen as far too liberal, and the initiative seemed headed for certain defeat. The proposed reforms were met with the usual objections, this time put forward by an increasingly powerful pharmaceutical industry: the new rules would impose excessive government control, limiting the rights of doctors to prescribe whatever they chose and of patients to ingest anything they wanted. Furthermore, the argument went, it would harm the capacity of drugmakers to discover new products.

A Golden Era for Drug Evaluation

In one of those accidents of history that no one saw coming, the early-1960s Kefauver amendments were implausibly rescued at the last minute by the thalidomide tragedy, in which thousands of babies worldwide were born with congenital defects caused by a drug their mothers took during pregnancy (see chapter 5). Although a central goal of the Kefauver amendments was the containment of high drug prices and the thalidomide tragedy concerned drug safety, the birth defect debacle led to the passage of his legislative package and gave the government new powers in yet a third domain: medication effectiveness. The new 1962 law required a manufacturer to provide the FDA with credible evidence that a new product actually worked before it could be sold. Nothing like that had been put into place anywhere: it changed everything about how people think about and use medications, both in the U.S. and eventually around the world.

This evidence would have to come from what the law defined as "well-conducted studies"; that usually meant randomized controlled trials (RCTs) in patients. The logic behind the RCT is as powerful as it is simple. Many diseases wax and wane on their own. Enthusiastic doctors may attribute any improvement to something they had done, and patients often perceive benefit from ingesting compounds with no biologic effect at all. The RCT handles these problems elegantly through a remarkably simple approach: take a large group of patients with a given disease and randomly allocate some to get the drug being studied, and some to get a comparison treatment—often an inert substance, the placebo. The approach makes vivid use of the concept "all things being equal." If a large group is assigned to get treatment A or treatment B by the flip of a coin (or a computer random number generator), all things other than the treatment really *are* rendered equal across the two groups.

It's also important that neither the patient nor the doctor to know who got what. That key feature has traditionally been known as "double-blinding," but in deference to visually impaired people and their advocates, some now prefer the term "double-masking." At the end of the trial the data are unblinded (unmasked?); if the randomization worked well and the sample size is good enough to make a chance finding unlikely, then any differences that are seen in the group that got the drug are extremely likely to have been caused by the medication and nothing else. This simple approach, which wasn't in routine use until after World War II, utterly transformed our ability to know what works and what doesn't in medicine. For the same reasons, it also proved useful for understanding the frequency and severity of side effects, as described in chapter 6: patients sometimes develop symptoms they attribute to placebos, known as the "nocebo" effect, from the Latin root for "noxious." Randomization and double-blinding/masking help take care of that as well.

The RCT became the mainstay of drug evaluation relatively recently, in the second half of the twentieth century. Before that, respected authorities would decide what drugs worked based primarily on their own clinical experience (often an unreliable indicator), or assumptions about mechanisms of physiology and pharmacology predicting which drugs *ought to* work. For hundreds of years, medicine was under the sway of the utterly wrong precepts of the second-century Greek physician Galen, who taught that the body operated through a system of four "humors": black bile, yellow bile, blood, and phlegm; these had to be balanced to maintain or restore health. That gave us treatments like bloodletting and purgatives that created many side effects and occasionally death, but very little in the way of actual curing.

That is why the Kefauver amendments of 1962 were so important: they put the full force of law behind the potent idea of science-based evaluation through RCTs, empowering the government to mandate rigorous scientific assessment of new drugs for the first time. Comparisons with other progressive turning points of that era are hard to ignore: the right of every citizen to cast a vote is a good idea, but withers without congressional action that makes it a crime to deny it; the right of a woman to control her own fertility is just a theoretical construct without a Supreme Court decision that transforms it into a legal right. But just as with the Voting Rights Act that was passed a few years after the Kefauver amendments, and the *Roe v. Wade* Supreme Court decision of several years after that, the foes of these reforms didn't just accept defeat and go away quietly. Instead, in each case they spent the ensuing years laying the judicial and legislative foundations to undo each advance. To erode each of these reforms, the opposition built a well-funded, persistent, and highly organized counterattack. They elected sympathetic lawmakers and then applied relentless political and financial pressure on them; they amassed huge sums of money and deployed it in powerful lobbying efforts in Washington and the states; they designed creative legal onslaughts and employed novel constitutional arguments, presenting carefully chosen cases to sympathetic conservative judges appointed to key positions over years of disciplined political effort. This is what has happened to medication policy as well.

To put the degradation of our prescription drug-related policies into context, it helps to look at the legal and ideological arguments that were used to decimate those other now-crippled reforms. It wouldn't have gone over well to propose rolling back the Voting Rights Act to make it harder for Black people to vote. But arguments about states' rights and federal government overreach have the patina of judicial logic to them, just as the same doctrines were used to justify preserving slavery and segregation for so many years. Disenfranchisement was cloaked in the garb of redistricting, limitations on voting procedures, and other administrative maneuvers. Similarly, removing protections for abortion rights was redefined as a more faithful reading of the Constitution, protection of life and religious freedom, and restoring these decisions to the states, a level of government said to be closer to the people. We've seen where those arguments have gotten us. Similar retrenchments are happening to the legal structures that enabled the government to protect us from poorly effective prescription drugs, but those changes have been far less visible to the public.

The Compromise Begins

Criticism of our approach to drug assessment has come from all parts of the ideological spectrum. One of the most important transformations of the FDA's evaluation approach started out as a well-meaning program to help some of the nation's most vulnerable patients. The agency's fall from grace began a while ago, with the best of intentions.

Tony Fauci had a problem. The epidemic was advancing week by week, its death toll rising daily. Patients and potential future victims were panicking. Why wasn't the government doing more to address the crisis? The federal agency he headed, the National Institute of Allergy and Infectious Diseases (NIAID), was tasked with leading the country's research agenda for all communicable diseases; why did it seem to be dragging its feet so badly on this? And why were his colleagues at the FDA taking so long to approve new treatments that could save hundreds of thousands of people right now—people at risk of dying of this new fatal disease? Couldn't NIAID fund more research, and couldn't the FDA approve promising-looking new treatments faster to get them to the public? In the face of an unprecedented epidemic, many argued for the need to simply launch new treatments that might hold some promise and get them out there for patients to try, instead of watching so many people die of a lethal new disease while federal agencies slogged through their obsessive work as usual.

The angst, panic, and outrage weren't over Covid in 2020. They were about AIDS in the late 1980s—another new and potentially fatal infectious disease whose cause and transmission were not yet understood. A much younger Dr. Fauci was then at the start rather than the end of his forty-year career leading NIAID, his head still sporting a dense shock of black hair. Back then, as in 2020, Fauci was demonized as an unfeeling federal bureaucrat murdering innocent people. Larry Kramer, an outspoken leader of the growing AIDS activist movement, said as much. But instead of just focusing on the science and ignoring the public assaults on his motivation and character, young Dr. Fauci took the opposite approach. He met with his fiercest critics to understand their concerns about the government's rigidity and slowness in combating the AIDS epidemic, and to hear their demands about balancing rigorous review of new treatments with the urgent need to deal with a public health emergency. In the era of AIDS, he came to be seen as an ally trying to move the lumbering bureaucracy forward to help get new drugs out to the public.

The AIDS protesters of the late 1980s were enraged by what they saw as the sluggishness of Dr. Fauci's FDA colleagues in reviewing and approving promising new drugs. Their friends, their lovers, their whole community were dying. Even if new medications were developed to reduce the burden of this plague, they feared that the agency's cumbersome review process—a once-valued legacy of the Kefauver regulations—meant that many more people would succumb while the lengthy evaluation process trudged on. The crisis was personal and very urgent.

In October 1988, FDA employees coming to work were astonished to find the lobby of their headquarters in Rockville, Maryland, occupied by over a thousand furious AIDS protesters sitting and waving placards; one sign bore a red-stained palm print and read "THE GOVERNMENT HAS BLOOD ON ITS HANDS—ONE AIDS DEATH EVERY HALF HOUR." Another read "FDA—UNSAFE AT ANY DOSAGE." The activists chanted, "*Hey, hey, FDA! How many people did you kill today?*" and covered the lobby floor with a red liquid they said was blood. This was especially distressing for the FDA doctors, many of whom had chosen work at a government agency over the in-your-face stress of patient-facing jobs. The protesters used a clever strategy: contact with blood was known to be an effective means of transmitting AIDS, even though walking through it with shoes on was not a clear risk factor, especially if the liquid wasn't really infected blood.

The demonstrators were right that the FDA was acting slowly in approving drugs for AIDS. It was applying its standard meticulous review process mandated over twenty-five years earlier by the 1962 law requiring randomized controlled trials that could take a year or much more to evaluate new medicines, even those with particular promise. Cancer patients joined the AIDS activists and argued that, for them as well, new treatments that could reduce their own risk of imminent death seemed to be taking forever for the FDA to review as it lumbered through its seemingly endless assessment processes.

Until the AIDS crisis, the FDA appeared to be at the top of its game in evaluating new medications. After 1962, the world took admiring note of that productive marriage among science, government, and the pharmaceutical industry (probably better to call it a thruple). The nation's rigorous but fair drug evaluation system became the envy of the world as governments all over the globe sent representatives to the U.S. to study and then replicate its approach.

But that product of the progressive legislative era of the 1960s didn't fare well in the more combative 1980s. Ronald Reagan had been elected at the start of the decade on a platform of reducing federal involvement in the life of the nation. His first inaugural speech in 1981 set the tone for regulators' status in the coming decade when he announced that government could not solve the nation's problems because the government *was* the problem. As dark as it was, his formulation was gentler than that of Grover Norquist, the virulent antitax activist who said his goal was to "shrink government down to a size where you can drown it in a bathtub." An increasingly powerful Republican presence in Congress was eager to put its legislative muscle behind this vision. The AIDS problem may not have been too salient for President Reagan, who did not even utter the name of the disease in public during the first years of his presidency as the epidemic was growing and destroying more lives each day.

The fiscal stringencies that flowed from this conservative worldview took their toll on the nation's capacity to evaluate and approve medications, among many other things. Budgets for federal agencies were constrained, including that of the FDA. Beyond its culture of careful, sometimes obsessive scientific review (which its critics described as mere sluggishness), the agency was truly hampered by inadequate staffing. The 1962 Kefauver legislation had required it to apply an unprecedented level of scientific scrutiny to new drugs, and despite complaints by the drug industry that such evaluation would limit innovation, the productivity of the biomedical enterprise was increasing sharply year by year. A growing budget for the National Institutes of Health and new drug discoveries (many of them taxpayer-funded) laid the groundwork for more and more new medicines. And though the budget Congress allotted to the FDA increased, it didn't grow apace with this explosion of therapeutic discovery. A mandated follow-up program to evaluate scores of drugs that had been approved before the new efficacy criteria were in force had dragged on for two decades—which was fine with manufacturers, since the often-useless products couldn't be taken off the market until they were assessed.

By the late 1980s, when George H. W. Bush took the helm from Reagan and continued his anti–big government policies—enshrined in his menacing and ultimately self-destructive slogan "Read my lips, no new taxes!"—the FDA budget was simply inadequate to support enough scientists to review all those new drug applications efficiently. But such stinginess fit in well with the conservative ideology that was becoming more popular in Washington during those years. Conservative economist Milton Friedman had quipped that if the federal government were put in charge of the Sahara Desert, within five years there would be a shortage of sand. The second Bush president, George W., liked to call himself "the Decider," but when it came to government policies, he declared that "we don't believe in planners and deciders making decisions on behalf of Americans." In this climate, the most logical solution to the FDA's inability to get promising discoveries onto the market more quickly—giving it an adequate budget to hire enough scientists to review new drugs—was a political nonstarter.

Using Surrogates to Give Birth to Medicines

One regulatory response to the AIDS crisis was a new FDA program called Accelerated Approval, eventually made into law in 1992. It began as a plausible and well-intentioned attempt to address the concerns of the activists criticizing the FDA's slowness. A new social contract was offered: instead of the previous requirement of two or more randomized trials showing that a new drug improved patients' health, an innovative new pathway was created. For a serious condition with no satisfactory treatment, a pharmaceutical manufacturer could now get a product approved if the drug produced an encouraging change in a "surrogate measure"—a lab test such as an assessment of the viral load in the blood of an AIDS patient, or an improvement in an imaging study defining the size of a cancer patient's tumor—even if these weren't the same as showing an improvement in patients' health or survival. All that would be needed to win accelerated approval was to change a laboratory test or a scan result in a way that would be "reasonably expected" to predict future clinical improvement. The key second part of this social contract was that the manufacturer would then have to conduct follow-up studies once the drug was in use to measure actual clinical outcomes, such as how well patients functioned or how long they lived, to prove that the new treatment was truly beneficial. So far, so good. But the second part of that social contract—the follow-up confirmatory studies—were often neglected or delayed.

In the years that followed, under relentless pressure from the drug industry and its supporters in Congress, the FDA allowed this surrogate measure-accelerated approval system to expand so widely that it has begun to fray the agency's once-legendary drug review system. The current approach is similar to a car salesman whose dealership is located at the top of a hill suggesting that a prospective buyer take a vehicle out for a test drive and note its quick pickup and the strength of its engine; at the bottom of the hill, the salesman kindly offers to drive it back up to the office—the part of the trip on which those qualities aren't so evident.

Much of the work our group has done on FDA policies has been spearheaded by Aaron Kesselheim, a brilliant physician-lawyer who began working with me when he was still a resident; he now leads that effort in a very productive group we call the Program On Regulation, Therapeutics, And Law, or PORTAL. In 2016, Congress passed the "21st Century Cures Act" that many of us worried might further loosen approval standards; beyond accelerated approval, it created another expedited review process for so-called breakthrough drugs that seemed to many of us to be more hype than science. The term leads prescribers and patients to think that these are major new developments, but the designation just means a new drug is unusual—not that it actually works. For pharmaceutical companies, a lower evidentiary bar means shorter and less costly clinical trials, hastening their ability to get a drug to market much sooner. It also sharply raised the prospects that a new product would be approved: it's much easier to show a change in a lab test or a scan than to prove eventual patient benefit. A product could thus have more time to generate revenues before its patent expired, whether it really worked or not. The drugmakers' efforts were abetted by Congress and an administration marinating in funds from the pharmaceutical lobby, one of the most well-endowed pressure groups in Washington. Backup support came from vociferous concerned patient groups: many were utterly sincere, many were funded by those same companies, and many were both. With impressive synergy, the industry's enormous financial clout in Congress swayed key legislation; the pressure was transmitted in parallel to FDA officials through influence in the executive branch, whichever party was in power. More than half of new drugs are now evaluated through one or more expedited pathways that use lower standards of evidence.

These developments laid the groundwork for the 2021 approval of Aduhelm, the intravenous treatment for Alzheimer's disease that didn't work. A full autopsy of that drug is presented in the next chapter; for now, we'll consider more closely how the well-intentioned AIDS-era accelerated approval system was captured by special interests who have used it to weaken the evidence that doctors use to prescribe drugs, often the ones we give to our sickest patients.

Lowering the Bar

Even as the AIDS epidemic waned, the FDA was becoming more and more flexible about what surrogate measures might be "reasonably expected" to predict future benefit for an unproven drug. The accelerated approval pathway whizzed way past its original goal of green-lighting promising drugs for untreatable diseases and spun out of orbit, allowing companies to use lab tests, scans, or other findings of dubious relevance as a free pass to early marketing of treatments for many diseases. This was not a new idea. Goodhart's law is named after a British economist who observed that when a measure becomes a policy target, it stops being a good measure because people learn how to game it. In her book *Counting*, Deborah Stone provides other telling examples: Uzbek cotton pickers paid by weight soaked their harvest in water before bringing it to market; Soviet factories that were required to produce a certain number of meters of fabric each week adjusted their looms to make long narrow strips; railroad companies paid on the basis of how many miles of track they put down laid it out in winding paths. Daniel Kahneman wisely observed that people prefer to replace hard questions with easy ones. And we all know the classroom distortions that occur when educators start "teaching to the test." So we should not be surprised that the FDA's growing use of surrogate measures incentivizes the use of assessments that don't require showing that a new drug produces clear patient benefits.

Oncology has been an especially fertile field for such criterion-bending. In 2022, I was asked by *JAMA* (the publication formerly known as the *Journal of the American Medical Association*) to write a commentary on a study that examined cancer drugs approved on the basis of surrogate measures (there were many) and how many were then subjected to the required follow-up analyses to measure actual patient benefit (there were fewer). In virtually all cases, the medication remained in use even if the follow-up studies were not done, and even—amazingly—if they were performed and failed to confirm a benefit.

I titled the article "A Finger Pointing at the Moon," referring to a legend of the Buddha trying to teach a lesson to his students by showing them the moon. But the acolytes instead gathered in a circle and stared intently at his finger, totally missing the idea. The finger was the surrogate marker, of course, and the moon the more distant goal of making patients better. The use of surrogate measures has gone well past cancer and now constitutes a "Get Out of Jail Free" card for manufacturers of drugs for muscular dystrophy, ALS, Alzheimer's disease, and diabetes, among other conditions. All too often, companies take their accelerated approval, rush ahead marketing the product, and then don't get around to completing the mandated studies the law requires to determine whether the drug really helps patients. In a 2024 paper in *JAMA*, my PORTAL colleagues reported on over a hundred cases of cancer drugs granted accelerated approval based on surrogate measures. On follow-up, fewer than half had been shown to produce actual patient benefit, though they generally remained in use. Not much rethinking going on there.

Clinical and Ideological Justifications of Lower Standards

There is a legitimate policy argument here: We don't want to release a new drug into routine use before it's been adequately studied, but we also don't want to make that assessment so long and cumbersome that it keeps effective treatments from the patients who need them. How much evidence of effectiveness is enough for approval, and how much is too little? How much is too much? The AIDS activists' delay-causes-death case often comes up when drug manufacturers and patient groups advocate for quicker approvals, and sometimes it has merit. Hundreds of millions of dollars can also ride on this timing; a company that may have made a large investment in developing a drug (or didn't) cannot begin to make a profit until it can sell product. But arguments about speeding drugs to market don't go over well if they are justified primarily in terms of increasing industry revenue. It works much better to cite a clinical rationale that involves patients (see chapter 3). And sometimes those arguments make sense.

An important and laudable movement took hold in the 1990s in health care in general to rely more on well-collected evidence to guide everything we do in medicine. Before long, two clever but snarky satirical pieces appeared in the respected publication *BMJ* (formerly the *British Medical Journal*). *BMJ* has a time-honored tradition of running humorous articles in its Christmas issue each year, and two of these provide provocative challenges to our understanding of the role of randomized trials in medicine. The first purported to be a systematic review of all published clinical trials on the effectiveness of parachutes used when jumping from airplanes "in preventing major trauma related to gravitational challenge." Mimicking a critique often made by advocates of evidence-based medicine, the authors bemoaned the fact that even though parachutes are a very commonly used intervention, there was not a single published RCT documenting their effectiveness. They wryly concluded:

> Advocates of evidence-based medicine have criticised the adoption of interventions evaluated by using only observational data. We think that everyone might benefit if the most radical protagonists of evidence-based medicine organised and participated in a double blind, randomized, placebo controlled, crossover trial of the parachute.

My *Rethink* conclusion: you don't always need an RCT to know if something works.

A team of American doctors returned to the topic in the *BMJ* Christmas issue several years later. They actually conducted such a controlled trial, enrolling twenty-three volunteers to jump from a small plane or helicopter after being randomized to wear either a parachute or an empty backpack. Surprisingly, the authors reported no difference in the rate of injuries between the two groups. Illustrating the need to evaluate a paper's methodology carefully before inferring much about its findings, it took a dive into the study's design to figure out that the trial was conducted with the aircraft stationary on the ground. *Rethink* lesson: you have to read the details of any clinical trial carefully to understand how relevant its findings might be to actual practice.

Hunter and the Hunted

A more serious and compelling example of the RCT debate concerned the treatment of Hunter syndrome, a rare and devastating genetic disorder in which children can't make a key enzyme to break down large sugar molecules. Its victims suffer from delayed growth, hearing loss, and declining brain function, and die young. In the 1990s, researchers discovered how to partially replace the missing enzymes in Hunter syndrome and diseases like it. A new product, Elaprase, showed promise in early studies. Nothing like it had ever been seen for this condition; young patients given the new treatment in early evaluations did much better than expected. But the FDA declined to approve the new drug until those promising findings were confirmed in a yearlong randomized controlled trial in which some of the affected children would be assigned to get a placebo. Those requirements led to a long delay in its availability nationwide, and to further deterioration in the kids randomly allocated to the control group. In a compelling 2012 opinion piece in *National Affairs* magazine, a doctor pointed to that as an example of how excessive regulation kept a lifesaving medication out of the hands of Americans who needed it, for no good reason. That was true, even though it was an uncommon error in FDA judgment. The exception doesn't prove the rule; that's why it's called an exception. But it put flesh on the drug industry's favored argument that the FDA's too-strict evidence requirements were depriving the public of medicines that could save lives.

These clinical arguments were used to strengthen the case made by conservatives and drugmakers that the FDA was full of sluggish bureaucrats whose obsessiveness and stubbornness made the review process so slow and complicated that Americans couldn't get the drugs they need. But nothing could be further from the truth; most FDA reviewers are sharp, committed scientists who usually do their work astutely; when major gaffes occur, they are usually committed by FDA leadership, who sometimes have other priorities. The FDA's overall efficiency has been demonstrated clearly in studies by our group led by Kesselheim and by our Yale colleague, Joe Ross, and his colleagues. In a series of detailed papers, we've all found that the data show convincingly the FDA is as fast on average as any drug-regulatory body in the world, often approving new drugs before Europeans or Canadians have access to them. That period of review is now down to six months for urgent decisions, although the agency can move even faster in emergency situations: the first two vaccines against Covid-19 were approved remarkably quickly after the agency's receipt of their initial data on efficacy and safety. But the overly obsessive bureaucrat meme was a durable one, and is often used as a seemingly patient-friendly excuse to encourage Congress to lower the FDA's approval standards.

The author of the Hunter syndrome article in *National Affairs* was Dr. Scott Gottlieb, whom President Trump named FDA commissioner five years later. Trump then fired him in 2019 after just two years on the job, after Gottlieb tried to crack down on tobacco industry–backed vaping companies over their promoting their products to youngsters. Gottlieb landed on his feet, though: he joined the corporate board of Pfizer, where he earned $553,000 in 2022, and became a partner in New Enterprise Associates, one of the world's largest venture capital firms, advising them on new drug development and securing FDA approval. He also became a partner at the biotech firm Illumina, where he earns over $420,000 annually. More on that golden revolving door later.

Despite the very rare exceptions to the need for randomized trials, the bold Kefauver requirement that clinical effectiveness had to be shown before a drug could be approved has sometimes been watered down to an FDA message that in effect says this for many products: "You can market your drug if it makes a lab test look better in a short study, compared to a placebo. We won't be on your case too much about those confirmatory follow-up studies." Even apart from the accelerated approval pathway, this combination of surrogate outcomes and placebo controls means that a new drug for diabetes, for example, can be approved on the basis of a twelve-week trial showing it lowers blood sugar more than no treatment. But a main reason we want to lower blood sugar in people with diabetes is to prevent the damaging outcomes that patients and doctors really care about: heart attack, stroke, kidney failure, blindness, nerve damage. Yet demonstrating an effect on these important clinical outcomes isn't required for the FDA to approve a new diabetes drug. What matters for approval is lowering the blood sugar, even though we now know that some widely used diabetes drugs like Januvia (sitagliptin) do only that, while others like Jardiance (empagliflozin) or Ozempic (semaglutide) lower blood sugar *and* prevent heart attacks and kidney damage—a huge difference.

"Do Your Own Research"

Ideally, the approval of a new drug should be exclusively the province of science, but for a half-trillion-dollar-a-year industry, it couldn't possibly remain so. The same libertarian posture of the earlier twentieth century—the spirit that opposed government's right to require accurate labeling and prevent toxicity—lives on in the insistence by some advocates on the far right that the government shouldn't even be in the business of determining whether a drug works or not. Physicians and patients could determine which drugs work best and which don't, their argument goes, through decisions reflecting their individual clinical experiences.

This is such a bad idea that it's hard to know where to start in debunking it. Here are some basics:

Some of the detailed data the FDA receives from a drug's manufacturer is considered the company's private property and is kept secret, so any outside reviewer isn't playing with a full deck.

Furthermore, evaluating the results of a clinical trial can be tricky:

- Were the study groups truly comparable at the start of the trial?
- Were the randomization and blinding done appropriately?
- What statistical methods were used to compare outcomes?
- If the differences were statistically significant, were they also large enough to be *clinically meaningful*?
- Were the patients studied comparable to people a doctor is treating, or (as often occurs) healthier and younger?
- If the comparison drug was a placebo, how does the new drug stack up against all the evidence on other relevant treatment choices out there (perhaps including nondrug options) that weren't in the trial?

Beyond all that, the issue of selective publication of favorable results has bedeviled all of us who look to the peer-reviewed medical literature to guide our decisions about how well drugs work, a problem several researchers have documented. A worrisome analysis of this issue was published in the *New England Journal of Medicine* by

Erick Turner, a psychiatrist who had spent several years at the FDA reviewing new drug applications. While there, he noticed that the more favorable studies that crossed his desk were more likely to end up being published in medical journals than the less favorable ones. Once he left the agency, he and his colleagues followed up on the concern that drugmakers who sponsor studies have in the past published the results they liked and spent far less effort to get non-favorable trial findings into the medical literature. Turner et al. reviewed the raw data on seventy-four clinical trials submitted to the FDA evaluating twelve different antidepressants and found that almost a third of them had never been published. Virtually all those that depicted favorable outcomes made it into medical journals; but of the studies with negative or questionable results, nearly all were never published, or appeared with a positive spin on the results.

How are we clinicians or our patients supposed to independently rethink *that*, if the totality of the evidence never sees the light of day? Put differently, Turner's study found that if you looked at the then-extant medical literature you'd find that 91 percent of published trials of antidepressants found the drugs were effective; by contrast, only about half of all the original studies submitted to the FDA showed the medications worked. In response to problems like these, reforms were passed in 2007 to require public disclosure of plans for *all* clinical trials before they are launched. The less good news is that disclosure of their results is still far from complete (see chapter 9).

Still, many libertarians argue that Americans should just be able to do their own research to decide which drugs work and which don't. But going over the terabytes of data the FDA receives for a new drug submission takes large teams of smart, dedicated, specialized scientists months to get right. Over many years, we've found how hard it is to do this work well in our educational outreach programs when we try to synthesize such data to guide doctors toward better prescribing decisions (see chapter 17). So how could it make sense to let individual freedom decide what drugs are available for use? Surely no responsible government scientist would advocate for that, right?

One odd presentation of this anti–big government perspective was offered in an op-ed in the *Wall Street Journal* that argued for an approach in which the FDA wouldn't assess the effectiveness of new drugs. Instead, the author proposed, the agency should just make sure new products aren't terribly unsafe and then release them to the magic of the marketplace, so doctors and patients could figure out which ones work and which don't. This approach is reminiscent of a decision rule used in the Albigensian Crusade in thirteenth-century France: when an invading army was having trouble differentiating loyal Catholics from heretics among the townspeople, the monk leading the charge is said to have commanded, "*Novit enim Dominus qui sunt eius*," which roughly translates to "Kill them all and let God sort 'em out." That strange *WSJ* op-ed was written by Dr. Andrew von Eschenbach, appointed by George W. Bush in 2005 as FDA commissioner. While at the FDA Dr. von Eschenbach, whose clinical expertise was as a prostate surgeon, prolonged the agency's yearslong refusal to approve greater access to the morning-after contraceptive pill despite its proven safety and effectiveness. Apparently he felt there are some issues the marketplace shouldn't be allowed to decide on its own.

The same motif of *laissez-faire, caveat emptor* has inspired a nationwide "right to try" movement for unapproved medications, pursued aggressively in several states by conservative legislators seeking to enable patients to take unproven drugs. But this is a solution to a problem that doesn't really exist. For many years, to avoid being in the middle of this unwinnable debate, the FDA has allowed any physician to ask a company for access to an investigational drug that hasn't been approved by the FDA. The agency itself approves about 99 percent of such requests; when there is an access problem, it's usually the company that resists making the product available. But if a drug hasn't been determined to work, should such liberated patients expect their health insurer, or a government program, to pay for it? And if there is a dangerous side effect, would they expect society to cover the costs of caring for those consequences as well? When my colleagues and I wrote a paper for the *New England Journal of Medicine* about this issue, we used a common term to describe the policy: "compassionate use." The editors wisely made us change that to "expanded access," pointing out that there's not necessarily anything compassionate about helping people take an untested drug that may not work and could hurt them.

A Legacy of the AIDS Era

It's now well over three decades since the fraught days of those AIDS demonstrations in the FDA lobby in the late 1980s. Thanks to a wide variety of very effective drugs to treat HIV, many patients with that diagnosis are now living well into old age. A medical student working with me has even studied the interactions between drugs for geriatric conditions and the medications that aging HIV-positive patients take—a wonderful outcome few of us saw coming in those dark times. But world-changing events like the AIDS epidemic cast a long shadow, and interest groups of all stripes understood that a crisis should never go to waste. Changes in FDA policy put in place during the AIDS era—and extended several times in the years since—mean that now a large proportion of new drugs are rushed to market under one or another of the FDA's "expedited pathways": accelerated approval, fast-track review, breakthrough designation, priority review, orphan drug status, and others. In one recent year, fully 65 percent of new drugs were approved on one or more of these pathways. Drugmakers have become adept at linking up with patient advocacy groups to urge reliance on these tentative measures. Yet many drugs that received accelerated approval underwent "confirmatory trials" that were reported years later using the very same surrogate measures. And many of these products turn out not to work well—or at all—when subjected to more careful scrutiny. Worse, other speedily approved drugs never undergo the follow-up testing that was mandated following those quick approvals. One PORTAL paper found that only a fifth of new cancer drugs approved on the accelerated pathway were shown to prolong patients' overall survival. But sick people keep on taking them, and insurers and government programs are required to pay for them. For a company, foot-dragging on confirmatory studies makes sense: they can continue to charge full price for a drug approved on preliminary data; problematic follow-up trials can only derail that gravy train. We've allowed these evidentiary limitations to be omitted from the drug's official descriptions or advertising or price, so patients and doctors have no way of knowing about the problem—a lucrative omission we continue to permit. It's widely known that a vampire cannot enter your house unless you invite him to cross your threshold.

In late 2022, the inspector general of the Department of Health and Human Services issued a critical report noting that for more than a third of accelerated approval of drugs, a follow-up study had not been submitted on time, citing "ongoing concerns that sponsors of drug applications granted accelerated approval fail to complete their statutorily required confirmatory trials on schedule, and concerns that FDA's oversight of the trials is lax." The FDA announced new policies in 2023 to address these problems, but it isn't clear how effectively they will be implemented. The electoral victory of Donald Trump, combined with Republican ascendancy in Congress, make it far less likely that we will upgrade our evaluation of regulation of drugs anytime soon. Evidence for this can be found in Trump's enthusiastic advocacy of Robert F. Kennedy Jr. to head the federal Department of Health and Human Services, which oversees the FDA—a man with little scientific background who promoted drugs that don't work, such as ivermectin and hydroxychloroquine for Covid, and vehemently disputed the safety and usefulness of vaccines. Before November 2024, many of us thought the pressing policy goal would be to fine-tune the nation's drug review process. Now we are just hoping to save it.

Gregg Gonsalves was one of the AIDS activists in the demonstrations against the pace of the FDA's approval process in the late 1980s, when he feared that slowness could put his own life at risk. He's now on the faculty at Yale, and in 2023 wrote this:

> It thus deeply pains me to see patient groups today—not for AIDS, but for a host of other diseases—distort what we were fighting for, and use it for counter-productive purposes. Sometimes this stems from the sheer terror and desperation that I know so well, but it often emerges from thoughtlessness and outright collusion with drug companies. Their end goal appears to be to dismantle the FDA as we know it. As someone who fought alongside so many to change the way we develop and regulate drugs in the USA—including the role of the FDA—and who is only alive because of the fights that we won, I feel certain that these groups are making a terrible mistake.

CHAPTER 2

Decision-Making and Dementia

It is wrong always, everywhere, and for anyone, to believe anything upon insufficient evidence. . . . The danger to society is not merely that it should believe wrong things, though that is great enough; but that it should become credulous, and lose the habit of testing things and inquiring into them; for then it must sink back into savagery.

—William Kingdon Clifford, *The Ethics of Belief*, 1877

Not Thinking Clearly about a Drug for People Who Can't Think Clearly

Alzheimer's disease is a tragic affliction that affects millions of Americans and their families. How the FDA came to approve Aduhelm for that condition says a great deal about the deterioration of its decision-making. It can also point us to ways to get that process back on track.

Over years of caring for older patients with memory loss on the primary care or geriatrics services of three of Harvard's teaching institutions, I'd often see a daughter or son come in with an aging parent and report something like this: "Dr. Avorn, we're losing Mom bit by bit. First she forgot little things, then big things, then most of her words. Now on bad days she has a hard time even remembering who I am. She sits all day staring into space for hours, or watching anything that's on the TV, even cartoons. She's there, but she's not there." Patients with advanced disease may eventually lose the capacity to control their urine and stool; increasing confusion may make them hostile or paranoid. In the end, if another medical event doesn't end their lives (and patients with advanced Alzheimer's disease often live otherwise healthy lives for many years) they may spend their remaining days gazing around helplessly, unaware of where or who they are. A colleague once asked an elderly man why he kept visiting his severely demented wife in her nursing home, since she no longer had any idea who he was. "That's true," he answered. "But I know who she is."

It was even harder to hear such stories from the patients' own perspectives, at a point in the illness when they were impaired but intact enough to understand what was happening to them. One long-term patient told me: "Sometimes I don't recall anything that happened yesterday. I can't drive now because I get lost in my own neighborhood. People act like they know me, but I'm not always sure who they are. I think I'm losing my mind. Have we met before?" No plot from a brain-eating zombie movie could be more terrifying for loved ones, doctors, or the afflicted patients themselves.

For decades we had no new treatments to make a meaningful dent in this person-destroying disease; we didn't even really understand what caused it. For severe heart failure or end-stage kidney disease, at least we could offer treatments that could help even if the illness usually won in the end. Even cancer offered the possibility of surgery, chemotherapy, and in recent years remarkably effective and less toxic immunotherapy treatments. But not so for Alzheimer's disease. Nearly 7 million Americans have it, striking about one in ten of us over age sixty-five. And we've had no medications that are really useful in treating it.

In recent decades, much hope and billions of dollars of research funding have coalesced around the "amyloid hypothesis" concerning its cause: that the memory loss and other neurological deterioration of Alzheimer's disease are caused by buildup of that protein in the brain. At autopsy, such abnormal protein can be seen under the microscope as brown clumps or streaks in and among the neurons; it appears to be literally gumming up the works. With the development of immunology-based approaches to disease, many scientists hoped that if amyloid is the cause, then maybe we could combat the disease with an antibody designed in the lab to seek out and destroy it. Skeptics pointed out that many older people with normal memory are found at autopsy to have brain amyloid deposits, and some patients with what appears to be Alzheimer's disease die without much evidence of it. So is amyloid necessarily the cause, or is it the debris left behind as nerve cells degenerate? Or both? And even if it is the cause, might it do little good to get rid of amyloid deposits once they've formed? Moreover, amyloid-hunting antibodies would go after those deposits all over the brain, including in its arteries; destroying the sticky accumulations there could lead to cerebral swelling and bleeding. How large a benefit in memory function, if any occurred, would be worth risking those possible side effects?

Researchers developed several initial amyloid-eating antibody medications, but the first ones had no impact on the disease in clinical trials. Skeptics argued that this was evidence that the amyloid hypothesis was simply wrong; some of them used the snarky term "Amyloid Mafia" to describe the large group of scientists who had been receiving hundreds of millions of dollars from the National Institutes of Health to work on this theory and who advocated for it. But supporters of the approach argued that this often happens in drug development: the first few compounds based on a novel therapeutic approach might turn out to be ineffective, or to cause terrible side effects and have to be abandoned. Then eventually a new one works.

But to return to our question from the last chapter: Just what does it really mean for a medicine to "work"? Is it a yes/no determination, or a matter of degree? And what should be the measure of that "working"? An improved lab test, or imaging study like a brain MRI scan? Or how the patient actually functions over time?

The Rise of Aduhelm

In 2021, the Boston-area biotech company Biogen asked the Food and Drug Administration to approve its new drug for Alzheimer's disease. The company had invested heavily in its development, building on years of work all over the world and the enormous sums invested by the NIH and private philanthropies to advance amyloid-related research. The new medication had to be given by intravenous infusion every two weeks indefinitely, produced frequent infusion reactions, and could cause swelling and bleeding in the brain. Its clinical trials were not showing any clear patient benefit. Based on these results, Biogen's data-monitoring experts had convinced the company to give up on the drug as a lost cause, declaring "futility"—a statistician's fatal term meaning that a study's results were so disappointing that it was very unlikely the intervention could be shown to be effective even if the trial went on for another hundred years. That drug, which would eventually be called Aduhelm, started out with a harder-to-pronounce generic name, aducanumab. (Drugs based on monoclonal antibodies are usually given generic names that end in *-mab*, evoking Shakespeare's Queen Mab, "the fairies' midwife," a tiny mischievous creature that helps give birth to dreams.)

A team of investigative reporters for the Boston-based STAT news service later put together a disturbing timeline of what happened next. Biogen created a secret initiative to work with the FDA behind the scenes to bring its moribund drug back to life, an effort the company named "Project Onyx." (According to the reporters, it was originally going to be dubbed "Project Phoenix," but the lawyers wanted to avoid a rising-from-the-ashes image.) The STAT team recounted a March 2019 meeting in which the company's CEO and chief scientist met at Biogen headquarters in Cambridge, with its head of research phoning in from the Galápagos Islands, to receive the crushing news from the independent scientists who were monitoring the data coming from the drug's pivotal trial. Biogen had spent hundreds of millions of dollars on the study, but the evidence convincingly showed that the drug didn't work. When the executives shut down further development of the drug, the company's stock lost 30 percent of its value, a $16 billion hit.

Still, Alzheimer's disease represented a major unmet medical need and an enormous potential market. Within a few weeks of that meeting, some Biogen researchers found a different way to look at the same data that suggested that maybe the drug did have a small effect in reducing patients' rate of memory decline in one of the two studies conducted, at one of the doses. According to the STAT report, Biogen's executives set up an unofficial May 2019 meeting with Dr. Billy Dunn, the industry-friendly director of the FDA's Office of Neuroscience, who would have to be won over if the drug were to be brought back to life. Such unofficial meetings are prohibited by FDA policy.

Those encounters culminated in an unusual joint report prepared by the company and the FDA on the merits of the drug, a variance from the standard separation of such analyses. (Collaboration on the joint report also afforded Biogen a sneak preview of the issues FDA scientists would be raising with their outside advisers, and the chance to address them proactively.) By November 2020, two days before the agency's outside advisory committee would meet to give its opinions on the drug's evidence, the FDA announced there was a new way to look at the old trial data that could be seen as providing evidence for some clinical benefit. Biogen's stock went up by 45 percent on the news, for an instant gain of $17 billion. The nation really needed a treatment for Alzheimer's, and the company really needed to redeem itself in the eyes of its investors. Cynics reflected that "if you torture data enough, you can get it to say whatever you want."

The advisory committee meeting two days later did not go well for the company or its drug. Some FDA statisticians looked at the reworked data and concluded that it was still unconvincing. They were also concerned that a substantial portion of patients given the drug had evidence of bleeding or swelling in the brain, which could be a harbinger of stroke. About a quarter of the subjects had initial reactions to the every-other-week intravenous infusions of the drug that they would have to receive throughout the eighteen-month study. Even if these resolved, it would impose an additional clinical burden, and also raised the question of how the study could remain blinded if a quarter of subjects had an immediate reaction to the active drug. When the FDA's outside advisory committee met in November 2020 to review all the evidence, they were told the basis for approval would have to be significant clinical improvement, rather than assessing the drug on the "surrogate marker" criterion of brain amyloid levels alone.

The advisory committee agreed unanimously with the FDA's statisticians that the drug didn't help patients; not a single member voted for approval. Then Dr. Janet Woodcock, the senior FDA official responsible for making the decision, overruled them all. She acknowledged that there was scant evidence that the drug meaningfully affected patients' mental functioning, but then pivoted and focused instead on the reduction in brain amyloid levels. After the advisory committee made its decision she changed the evidentiary requirement and gave Aduhelm a green light under the accelerated approval surrogate-marker criteria based on a reduction in brain amyloid, bypassing the need to show a clinical benefit. As the STAT team reported, "Chastened after a decisively negative review from outside advisers, the Food and Drug Administration convened a series of internal meetings in March and April where top officials hammered out a plan to approve Biogen's Alzheimer's drug, Aduhelm. The meetings were revealed in a series of documents released Tuesday by the FDA to explain its decision to use a truncated pathway, called accelerated approval, to approve Aduhelm." (Policy experts pointed out that the accelerated approval pathway was never intended to be retroactively applied as a consolation prize *after* controlled trials had shown a drug didn't work.)

> A traveler to a remote part of rural America was surprised to find bull's-eyes painted on the sides of barns all over the countryside, with an arrow in the center of each one. "Who's the talented archer who did that?" he asked a local.
>
> "Oh, that's Old Clem," came the reply. "Some nights, he just rides around shooting at the barns with his bow and arrow."
>
> "What skill," said the visitor. "He must have great aim!"
>
> "Well, the real star is his son, Little Clem. He follows his dad and paints the bull's-eyes around where the arrows landed."

FDA commissioner Rob Califf deferred to the decision made by Woodcock, who then made another surprising decision: the agency would approve the drug for use in *all* people with Alzheimer's disease including those with severe dementia, even though the clinical trials had studied only people with early disease—the period when an amyloid-eating antibody might theoretically make a difference. As a commentator wrote in *Science*, "From the outside, it really looks now as if the FDA made it its mission to get this drug on the market one way or another." Many FDA frontline staff, who are generally smart, careful, responsible scientists, were appalled and demoralized. An outside statistician who analyzed the data for the FDA and disagreed vehemently with the agency's decision later spoke to our PORTAL group about the affair. "I get paid to be a skeptic," he explained. "I throw in the cynicism for free."

Once the approval was official, Biogen announced that it would price the drug at $56,000 per patient per year. The every-other-week IV infusion charges, doctor visits, and multiple necessary scans would be extra. Cost-effectiveness analysis seemed pointless to many of us, akin to calculating the right toll for accessing a poorly constructed bridge that led nowhere and sometimes dropped people into the ravine below. As is often the case in company-sponsored trials (as most are), Biogen had excluded sicker patients from the study; one assessment determined that over 90 percent of Medicare patients would not have qualified for inclusion in its trials. But that did not stop the FDA from authorizing the drug's use in a wide swath of patients. At that price, and with the FDA's excessively broad permission for use in all Alzheimer's patients, economists estimated that the new medication could cost the country annually as much as the budget for NASA.

Each year, the government actuary responsible for setting the monthly Medicare premiums adjusts them to match expected program expenditures. Once Aduhelm was approved, to spread its expected cost across the entire participating Medicare population, that charge rose from $148 to $170 per month for everyone enrolled in the Medicare Part B program—more than it had ever risen in the history of the program. The increased amount would be paid by nearly all the nation's elderly to cover the anticipated additional costs of this one drug, whether they used it or not; that's just how insurance works.

As the accelerated approval regulations required, the FDA informed Biogen that since the decision was based only on the surrogate measure of a change in a lab test, although they could begin selling the drug right away at full price, the company would have to follow up with a proper clinical trial to demonstrate an actual benefit in patients' mental functioning. But the agency gave the company a full *nine years* to do the study, during which time the drug would be widely available for sale with no restrictions—and with no clear clinical data. That time frame would make the eventual trial results virtually useless for doctors and patients, and ensure Biogen a massive revenue stream whether its product turned out to work or not. Shortly after Aduhelm's approval, the Alzheimer's Association, which receives substantial funding from pharmaceutical manufacturers including Biogen, took out a full-page ad in the *New York Times* announcing, "It's a new day in the fight against Alzheimer's."

Dementia Aftereffects

My colleague Kesselheim was a member of the overruled FDA advisory committee, and was distraught over the agency's bold abandonment of its own procedures and standards. He asked me whether I thought he should quit the committee in protest, as other members were considering doing. His question brought back similar conversations with fellow student activists at Columbia in the late 1960s. If the goal is to bring about social change, like fighting for civil rights or ending the Vietnam War, is it better to try and work inside the worn-out established channels or do something that might have a real impact, like abandoning The System and protesting more vigorously?

Resign from the committee, I told him. You guys shouldn't accept this affront to science. Make a bold statement.

He worried that then he would lose the chance to have an impact on what the FDA does.

You call this having an impact? I responded. If several of you quit, maybe *that* might have an impact on the way the FDA does business. Or not. As it is, they're just not listening to their advisory committees anyway.

Kesselheim publicly quit the advisory committee in June 2021 shortly after the approval was announced, along with two other prominent members, Drs. David Knopman of the Mayo Clinic and Joel Perlmutter of Washington University. Their resignations made headlines nationally, and raised questions about how sensibly the FDA was making its decisions. Kesselheim and I wrote an op-ed in the *New York Times* titled, "The FDA Has Reached a New Low." It would be better, we argued, to have no drug than one that didn't work and could put patients at risk. But it wasn't clear that anyone at the FDA was listening. Commissioner Califf later opined that in the future it might be preferable for the agency's advisory committees not to vote on questions, and instead just converse in public about the drugs they reviewed. The backlash to that zany plan was so intense that the change wasn't implemented. Yet.

In the end, Aduhelm was brought down not by the FDA coming to its senses, which it rarely does on its own, but by bold decisions in other parts of medicine. Doctors, health-care systems, and insurance companies around the country examined the Aduhelm trial evidence themselves and determined that the drug was so ineffective, so potentially dangerous, and so expensive that despite the FDA approval, they wouldn't use it or pay for it—a risky and unusual position to take. I joined several colleagues to write an article condemning the FDA approval. Riffing on the agency's abuse of its greased-skids pathway, we called for Aduhelm to undergo "accelerated withdrawal" from the market. (It was a term we made up, since the FDA hardly ever withdraws anything.)

Given the enormous impact the drug would have on funding for the nation's Medicare drug benefit, that program had its own scientists look at the trial data, assuming the role of the grown-up in the room. It made the nearly unprecedented decision not to cover the drug—virtually the only time Medicare refused to pay for an FDA-approved medication. That move put a rent in the fabric of a system that had always operated on the assumption that the FDA evaluates drugs for effectiveness and safety, and then Medicare pays for anything the FDA approves, at whatever price the drug's manufacturer has set.

That breach saved the day and effectively killed the drug.

The Medicare noncoverage decision meant that the nation's main funder of drug expenses could no longer trust FDA decisions. Were we now moving toward a new two-step procedure to assess drug coverage by federal programs like Medicare, Medicaid, the Veterans Health Administration, and others? Would there now be a first step in which the FDA makes its decision on whether a drug can enter the market, followed by a second step in which other parts of the government decide whether it's worth using at a given price? Many other advanced countries already have just such a system in place, in which a drug is assessed for efficacy and safety by one body and then a separate group determines whether to pay for it and at what price (see chapter 15). But for the U.S., that sensible new division of powers came as a shock. Former FDA commissioner Gottlieb decried the development, arguing that the government should be obliged to pay for any drug the FDA approved, no questions asked. But the credibility damage had been done.

One piece of evidence underlying the amyloid hypothesis had been a 2006 study published in *Nature* relating cognitive deterioration in laboratory mice to the buildup of amyloid in their brains; it had been cited by other researchers nearly 2,500 times. In June 2024 its authors said they were retracting the paper, admitting that key findings had been based on false data. An article in the *BMJ* noted problems with the FDA's approval of a third drug in this class, donanemab, related to its lack of meaningful effectiveness, financial conflicts of interest by the FDA's outside reviewers at the time of its approval, and the drugmaker's inadequate follow-up of patients who had suffered side effects in its pivotal clinical trial. The agency gave the company thirteen years to address that problem.

Won and Dunn: A Golden Revolving Door

After the Aduhelm debacle Dr. Billy Dunn, the director of the FDA's Office of Neuroscience who had been so deeply involved in the drug's approval, continued to oversee several other brain-related drug reviews. One was for Relyvrio, a proposed treatment for the terrible degenerative neurological disease ALS, also known as Lou Gehrig's disease. The product had been invented by a pair of undergraduates at Brown University, and began as a series of dorm-room conversations. The two speculated that combining two older medications might protect nerve cells from dying; a patent was secured on the idea and the two recent grads formed a company to sell it, with one of them its CEO. But there was no convincing data that the product worked. Despite that, when an FDA advisory committee met in 2022 to review the application, Dunn reprised the role that he had assumed at the Aduhelm meeting, arguing that it should be approved despite the lack of solid data behind it:

> Our underlying legal authority is clear in not only allowing, but also endorsing and encouraging the application of regulatory flexibility in the setting of serious and life-threatening diseases. [The drug's approval] is unquestionably relevant to ALS drug development in general. . . .

But the outside advisory committee recommended that Relyvrio be rejected, since there was virtually no convincing evidence it did any good. Under pressure, the FDA then took the unusual step of convening a second advisory committee meeting just a few months later to consider the question again. Dr. Richard Bedlack, head of the ALS center at Duke University, put the agency in a tough position, asking for a rethink based on the most challenging aspect of our "Does it work?" question:

> In your difficult job, there's always going to be a chance of making a mistake; it comes down to which mistake you would rather make. To approve [the drug] and find out in two years that it doesn't work—I doubt many are going to be very angry because people with A.L.S. got to try something that was safe and appeared promising in 2022. [But] can you imagine the mistake of saying no and then getting confirmatory evidence in two years that this really did work? And realizing all those patients were much more disabled or even dead when they didn't need to be? I don't know how you'll be able to live with yourself if you make that mistake.

Of course, that argument could be made for the approval of *any* treatment for any bad disease without exception whether it worked or not, as long as it wasn't yet known to be toxic. Dr. Bedlack, whose official photos feature him in a wild floral-print sport coat, reported in his publications that he served as a consultant for over twenty pharma-related companies, including the manufacturer of Relyvrio.

Despite continuing skepticism, the outside advisory committee relented at its second meeting. The FDA itself immediately concurred and allowed the drug to be marketed. The agency had fewer options than it did for Aduhelm; it couldn't use the accelerated approval route, since the new ALS drug didn't even produce any changes in a lab test to justify using that pathway. So it granted the drug full approval. The two young inventors made an unusual offer; to encourage an affirmative decision by the agency, they said that if a future confirmatory trial showed their drug didn't work, they would voluntarily take it off the market. Following approval, they also announced that they would charge $158,000 per year for this repurposed combination of two existing drugs. Wanting to offer a new treatment option to patients with an incurable degenerative disease may be a plausible position; charging that much for a combination of two old products that shows no evidence of effectiveness is not.

Across the Atlantic, European regulators evaluated the undergrad-invented combination product and rejected it because they saw no evidence it did any good. Several months later, the Europeans took another look at the drug and came to the same conclusion. If the FDA was supposed to be America's medication watchdog, it seemed to have been spayed.

In 2024, the results of a follow-up clinical trial showed the drug failed essentially all its performance measures; the price of the one-product company's stock fell 80 percent immediately, for a loss of about a billion dollars. True to their promise, the two young inventors agreed that they would take their product off the market, although the nation had already spent $381 million on it in 2023. The recent grads are now trying to determine whether Relyvrio might be useful to treat a rare inherited condition that causes diabetes, deafness, and loss of vision. The company reports that early results seem promising.

In early 2023, Dunn was overseeing the review of a drug for a different awful neurodegenerative disease, Friedreich's ataxia; the product would be given the optimistic brand name of Skyclarys. Dunn's advocacy was so pivotal that when he announced in February of that year that he would soon leave the FDA, the drug manufacturer's stock sank by more than a third. One industry observer remarked that the stock's move "isn't surprising given the nearly unanimous view on the street that [the drug] wouldn't stand a snowball's chance under the review of any other Officer/Director at FDA." That isn't something you'd expect to hear if one evidence-based scientist at the FDA were being replaced by another evidence-based scientist. The agency cleared the drug a few days later before Dunn left, and the company's stock price nearly tripled.

As a bonus, the FDA also awarded the company marketing Skyclarys a "priority review voucher," a strange additional prize with a sizable dollar value all its own. This is an odd economist-invented construct designed to incentivize companies to develop drugs for neglected conditions when doing so might not be profitable enough to attract their interest. If such a medication is eventually approved, the FDA also provides its manufacturer with a voucher that can be used to allow a different one of its products to jump the queue at the agency and get a faster, prioritized review even if it wouldn't normally qualify for that; that could reduce the review time for the second product from ten to six months. A few months of quicker approval can generate millions of dollars for a lucrative product like a new psoriasis medicine, even if it's no better than others on the market. But wait, there's more: if the company that wins such a golden ticket doesn't have a product of its own to put forward for a sped-up review, it can sell the priority review voucher to another company that does. Such vouchers have been sold by companies for up to $350 million; their street value is now about $100 million each.

A few months after Skyclarys was approved, its manufacturer was acquired by Biogen (maker of the failed Alzheimer's drug Aduhelm) for $7.3 billion.

His work at the agency done, Billy Dunn left and in less than three months joined the board of directors of Prothena, an American biotech company incorporated in Ireland (better for tax avoidance) that specializes in drugs for neurological diseases such as Alzheimer's and ALS. Dunn had been well paid at the FDA, with a salary listed at $322,000 in his last year there for a demanding full-time job, more than most physicians on the Harvard faculty make. (Senior directors at the FDA can earn as much as $400,000 annually.) But his deal at Prothena is likely much better: the average annual part-time pay for the company's directors recently was $350,000, in exchange for participating in a limited number of meetings per year.

> Plato's *Republic* tells of a shepherd named Gyges who comes upon a magical ring giving him the power to become invisible. Gyges secures a job as a messenger to the king, ostensibly to keep him informed about the condition of his flocks. Wearing the ring, he stealthily enters the monarch's castle, seduces the queen, conspires with her to kill the king, and takes over the realm.

The role of industry and its advocates in securing drug approvals isn't well understood by the public, doctors, or legislators. All that is evident to the naked eye is that the FDA evaluates data, hears from experts, has its own people review everything, and makes decisions—which have tended to be "yes" over 80 percent of the time for recent new drug applications.

"It Doesn't Not Work"

Less than two years after the final demise of Aduhelm, the same corporate partnership that created the drug, Biogen and Eisai, came back to the FDA for approval of a different amyloid-eating antibody product. This one was called Leqembi, whose generic name is lecanemab. It presented a tougher evaluation problem for the agency as well as for clinicians, patients, families, and those responsible for paying health-care bills: unlike its predecessor, it did achieve a slight change in cognitive function. On average, all subjects in the drug's large randomized clinical trial got somewhat worse—that is simply the inexorable nature of Alzheimer's disease and the impotence of our current drugs to treat it. But patients given intravenous Leqembi every two weeks over a year and a half deteriorated a very slight bit more slowly than those given intravenous placebo. By the end of the study, their decline was about a half point less on the eighteen-point scale that was used to measure cognitive function, compared to the decline seen in the patients given intravenous placebo for that period. Many Alzheimer's experts pointed to earlier studies defining the minimum change required for such scales to rise to the level of clinical detectability or importance, and argued that this slightly smaller deterioration after a year and a half might not even be noticeable to most patients, families, or doctors. On the downside, as with Aduhelm, a high proportion of patients had uncomfortable infusion reactions (about a quarter), and in the process of eating away at amyloid, Leqembi often caused areas of swelling or small bleeds in the brain, as did Aduhelm.

But according to the law and decades of precedent, if a drugmaker can show in an adequately conducted randomized trial that its product works better than placebo at a level that is statistically significant, even if it's not clinically meaningful, it's very hard for the FDA to reject it. This leaves a real problem for prescribers as well as insurers. While many argued that such a small reduction in deterioration might not even be noticeable to families, patients, or health-care professionals, others said it could be meaningful for some people, who should not be prevented from pursuing that possibility. In an early version of an op-ed for the *Washington Post* on Leqembi, I wrote that the problem with it was that "it doesn't not work." A copyeditor complained that the double negative was a grammatical error, but the sentence was correct. It was not utterly ineffective, just close to it.

Despite this very minimal effect, once the drug was FDA-approved the manufacturer listed its purchase price as $26,000 per patient per year. As with Aduhelm, that doesn't include the charges for the biweekly infusions, the required MRI and PET brain scans, and the extra doctor visits its use will entail. (The FDA is not empowered to take cost into consideration in approving a drug, and avidly embraces that limitation. In fact, a manufacturer will often not announce the price it will charge until just after a drug is approved.) Even if we ignore cost for the moment, which is hard to do at that price, how would its downsides stack up against that very slender benefit? Not too well.

In preparing educational materials for prescribers and patients about the drug (see chapter 18), I took the perspective of a primary care doctor or geriatrician, and added in a separate dimension we can think of as "burden." Not cost, not side effects, but the difficulty the drug would impose on people and their caregivers just to take it. Before qualifying for the medication, patients would have to undergo a potentially painful spinal tap or a PET (positron-emission tomography) scan to measure amyloid levels in their brain. And they'd also need to get a baseline MRI brain scan as well as repeat studies every few months to see if they were having brain bleeding or swelling. Then there are the burdens of the every-other-week intravenous infusions needed for at least a year and a half, each lasting an hour. I recalled how hard it was for some of my frail patients just to come in to see me every few months for their routine visits; trips to an infusion center every fourteen days would be substantially harder. Doing so to receive an effective cancer treatment could be lifesaving, but for a medication whose benefit might not even be noticeable? This dimension of patient burden is palpably clear to clinicians, patients, and their caregivers, but it doesn't appear anywhere in the benefit-risk calculations that form the sole basis of the FDA's decision-making. In its official evaluation, all that mattered for the "Does it work?" question was how subjects performed on a formal test of cognition, the CDR-SB (Clinical Dementia Rating Scale, Sum of Boxes)—a measure rarely used in routine practice.

Coincidentally, while I was developing our own educational outreach program on Leqembi, my doctor ordered an MRI scan of my knee to see if I needed another joint replacement. (I didn't; a steroid shot fixed it.) I had ordered scans of various body parts for patients for years, and had undergone a few myself (gallbladder, hip, the other knee). But I had never gone through a brain MRI. As I entered the MRI machine for my knee exam I pressed the radiology technician on an aspect of brain MRI I hadn't thought much about before—the patient's experience of being propelled into one of those sleek white tunnels, then lying immobile for twenty minutes during the scan wearing headphones that only partially block the extremely loud clacking noises the whirling magnet makes throughout the test.

"Do older patients have a problem going through this?"

"Some of them do. They don't like having their heads put inside the helmet." She pointed at a plastic cage used to hold a subject's head still during the duration of the scan.

"If a person has problems with confusion, does it make it harder for them to last the full twenty minutes?"

"Yes, some of them feel all closed in and try to bust out of the scanner. Sometimes we have to sedate them to get the test completed."

My own knee MRI went fine, but I thought about how much worse the claustrophobia, immobility, and clacking noise would be if it had been my head in a cage deep inside the machine—especially if I had cognitive impairment.

If Leqembi truly had no effect on cognitive performance, in a post-Aduhelm world it might have been easy for a chastened FDA to reject it—a no-brainer, you might say. But the fact that it technically "worked" in a statistically significant way to produce a tiny slowing of deterioration on formal cognitive testing made the idea of its "effectiveness" more complicated. In the *Post* op-ed, I suggested that companies should be paid less for drugs that barely work or that just make a small difference in a surrogate measure (see chapter 13). Our education nonprofit received some grants to present these concerns in a non-commercial outreach program designed to give doctors, patients, and families a more balanced understanding of the drug. In the materials for patients, I wanted to use the tagline "there's no 'you' in it!" but decided not to. Yet it illustrates how effectiveness is often not a simple yes/no property of a product, and how many nuances can be embedded in the question of whether a given medicine "works." For its part, the European drug regulatory authority simply rejected the drug.

In July 2024, the FDA granted full approval to yet another new amyloid-acting intravenous drug for Alzheimer's disease, Kisunla, with minimal effectiveness and substantial risks similar to Leqembi. A *New York Times* investigative report found that in clinical trials, both drugs' manufacturers tested subjects for a genetic trait that would render them more susceptible to brain bleeds from the medications, but did not tell them about their results.

The price of Kisunla is even higher than that of Leqembi, at $32,000 per year. I wondered anew how much an annual amount that large (again, not counting the costs of all those additional doctor visits and tests) could have provided if spent on home health aides for the older patients I've cared for with memory loss. Given the choice of a risky IV medication that may not produce a perceptible benefit, or $32,000 a year to spend on any kind of care they want, how many patients and families would opt for the chemical? But our system is optimally tuned to pay enormous sums to drugmakers who sell expensive products and to the doctors and medical centers that administer them—but always seems short of cash for covering low-tech frontline human-to-human services.

The passion to take a new drug to cope with a devastating degenerative disease is enormous and understandable. It's easy to see why an afflicted patient or family member will have little patience for careful assessment of clinical trial evidence if there aren't any good treatments available, and every month brings continuing, agonizing deterioration. But should that mean a return to Commissioner von Eschenbach's view that the FDA should just make sure a drug isn't dangerous, and then let anyone who wants it take it? (None of the amyloid-active drugs would pass the no-risk test in any case.) Surely that approach would lead to pharmacological chaos—even before we get to the question of who would pay for all those potentially useless and costly treatments. Why should the manufacturer of a drug that hasn't been shown to work—or one that has been shown to just barely work—be allowed to charge whatever they please for it? But for desperately ill patients and their families, all this obsessing about outcomes and statistical tests and insurance may seem beside the point.

After-Action Analyses

The FDA's disastrous approval of Aduhelm set in motion a series of investigations. Paradoxically, Dr. Woodcock herself called for an assessment of the process by the Office of the Inspector General (OIG) of the Department of Health and Human Services. Its harsh initial 2022 report focused on major problems in the FDA's implementation of its accelerated approval program, citing issues similar to those that had been documented by our research group and others. The report noted that since the pathway was created in 1992, the FDA had approved 278 drugs through it, at a growing annual rate. The OIG found that 40 percent didn't have their required confirmatory studies completed in a timely way: over a third of those had missed their agreed-upon due date, with some of them five to twelve years overdue. Yet the medications continued to be available, prescribed to patients, and billed—often with a very high price tag—to public and private health insurers.

Over a four-year period, the inspector general found, Medicare and Medicaid paid more than $18 billion for thirty-five accelerated-approval drugs that still lacked the required confirmatory trials. Worse, about 13 percent of drugs granted such approval later had to be withdrawn from the market. The inspector general concluded: "For a variety of reasons, sponsors do not always complete trials promptly. This can result in drugs staying on the market—and being administered to patients—for years without the predicted clinical benefit being verified. And insurers—including Medicare and Medicaid—paying billions for treatments that are not verified to have clinical benefit." A provision that a drug's official label would have to state that it was made available on the accelerated pathway—something you'd expect marketplace advocates to favor, to put more information out there to influence decision-making—was put into a 2022 bill, but then taken out under industry pressure.

A few months after the first OIG report, a congressional investigation released at the end of 2022 described at least 115 encounters between the agency and Biogen leading up to the advisory committee meeting, though the number is uncertain because the FDA didn't track all of them. It's useful and appropriate for a drug's manufacturer to be in contact with the FDA to review the details of a new drug submission, but frequent back-channel communications, some off the record, begin to look like shady meetings between a judge and one of the lawyers berfore the trial starts. In late 2022 a new law went into effect, the Food and Drug Omnibus Reform Act (known as FDORA, pronounced like the hat). It gave the FDA new powers to require better follow-up testing of drugs that had been quickly released for widespread use on the accelerated approval pathway. The long-awaited follow-up OIG report was finally released in the last few days of the Biden administration. It castigated the FDA for sloppy use of the accelerated approval process for three drugs, all considered here: Aduhelm for dementia, Makena to prevent preterm birth, and Sarepta's treatment for muscular dystrophy. The IG recommended that FDA get better outside consultation on several of these issues, but the FDA disagreed.

Skeptics questioned how aggressively the FDA would wield its new authority, arguing that the agency could have applied more pressure to manufacturers even before the law took effect, and didn't. Future enforcement will depend entirely on how FDA's new anti-regulatory leadership chooses to do its work.

Janet Woodcock retired from the FDA in February 2024 after nearly forty years at the agency. In an exit interview with STAT, she offered the following thoughts on the accelerated approval program:

> Some people might say . . . there were some that didn't work out. Well, that's how accelerated approval is set up. Is that wrong? What's the alternative? You hold back all of these until you have definitive evidence? Based on the results, you would have a lot of people who wouldn't be alive. Was that worth it to have all that certainty?
>
> . . . It's a tough dilemma. The families [of children with rare diseases] are like the HIV patients back in the day, if you recall, lying in the street, saying, "We don't care about the trials, we don't have anything, we're dying. We want to be able to try something." That's how a lot of families feel.

That simplistic analysis is troubling, coming from one of the FDA's most senior officials. As we will see in chapter 4, there are many better ways to rethink this issue more sensibly.

Many of these concerns about the complexities of assessing causal relationships faded into the background when Donald Trump announced his plan for Robert F. Kennedy Jr. to lead the enormous Department of Health and Human Services, to "go wild on health." Most Americans were aware of RFK Jr.'s strong advocacy of the disproven idea that childhood vaccines cause autism, and his position that many other vital vaccines—including those that combat Covid—are neither safe nor effective. Less well-known were his other health-related views that school shootings are caused by antidepressants, Wi-Fi signals and water fluoridation produce cancer, chemicals in the environment make children transgender, and the Covid virus has properties that spare Ashkenazi Jews and Chinese people. Becoming HHS chief would give Kennedy authority over all the programs of the FDA, CDC, NIH, and Medicare. He announced his intention to fire hundreds of scientists and other staff at these agencies, and "give infectious disease a break for about eight years." After Trump's endorsement, Kennedy sent this statement to FDA staffers: "FDA's war on public health is about to end. If you work for the FDA and are part of this corrupt system, I have two messages for you: 1. Preserve your records, and 2. Pack your bags."

If this was the sort of vision for drug evaluation that Trump favored for his second term, suddenly the accelerated approval program seemed like the least of our worries.

CHAPTER 3

Lowering the Bar

Even More Surrogates Give Birth to Even More New Drugs

Readers of a certain age, especially those from the New York area, may recall the holiday weekend telethons put on decades ago by comedian and actor Jerry Lewis to raise funds for research on muscular dystrophy (MD), a tragic genetic disease that strikes children soon after birth; it cripples them and then kills them at an early age. As I was growing up, watching these telethons was an annual tradition in our house. The host, exhausted and perspiring after many hours of nonstop appeals, surrounded by wheelchair-bound children, would beg viewers to send in money to help find a cure for the terrible disease. Millions of dollars were raised, but a cure remained elusive. Nearly sixty years later, MD-afflicted children of a new generation were wheeled out in support of a drug company to beg a different audience—the FDA—to end their suffering.

A common form of the disease is Duchenne muscular dystrophy (DMD), named after the nineteenth-century French neurologist who was among the first to describe it. The condition strikes boys primarily, initially affecting the legs in the first year or two of life, impairing the ability to walk and even to get up from a sitting or lying position. Then the arms and upper body become involved, and eventually most muscles in the body. Death often occurs in a patient's twenties or thirties. Over years, supported by the National Institutes of Health and private philanthropies funded in part by that telethon funding, scientists discovered that the disease is caused by a genetic defect that impairs the production of a key muscle protein, which they named dystrophin. Researchers sought to create a drug that could bypass the defect in the affected gene, to induce more production of that protein. The first product to attempt this elegant-seeming solution was called eteplirsen, made by Sarepta, a small Cambridge biotech firm based not far from our offices. Sarepta had conducted a study in only twelve boys, a remarkably small sample size; the company explained it was too poor to do a larger study. (Pharma giant Glaxo had previously completed a study of a similar drug for the disease in 186 patients, with placebo controls. It found no benefit.) Most of the Sarepta trial lacked a control group, so the company compared the boys' status to "historical controls" living in Italy and Belgium, a notoriously unreliable way to assess a new treatment.

Sarepta argued that the FDA should approve their product because although the boys in the study didn't show any clear improvement in function, they did have slightly higher dystrophin levels found on muscle biopsy, compared to other boys given placebo. Yet the company didn't have pretreatment levels of the protein to see if they actually rose with treatment, and there was no evidence that such minuscule increases in its level would produce any clinical benefit. An FDA reviewer reported that the agency had "consistently and strongly" urged the company to do a larger and better randomized study, but Sarepta hadn't followed that guidance. The agency's scientists had "expressed strong doubts" about the study design, but to no avail. If the drug were approved, it could then be far more difficult and perhaps even unethical to do an adequate placebo-controlled study later, since so many parents of the afflicted children would believe that the new drug worked. The clinical findings were unimpressive, but Sarepta urged the FDA to grant their product accelerated approval anyway, based on the surrogate measure of slightly increased dystrophin levels in muscle biopsy samples.

The agency convened a meeting of its Peripheral and Central Nervous System Drugs Advisory Committee—the same group that would review Aduhelm for Alzheimer's disease a few years later. Its public session in April 2016 was so heavily attended by patients, families, pharmaceutical company representatives, and members of the financial press that it had to be relocated to a large ballroom in a hotel in nearby Hyattsville, Maryland. The debate vividly illustrated the issues we're rethinking here:

- What does it mean for a drug to "work"?
- How can we know if an observed effect will actually help patients?
- What role should patient and family preferences play in drug approval decisions?

The head of the agency's office of neurological drugs, Dr. Ellis Unger, was struck with the massive presence of so many advocates at the hearing. "In my time at the FDA," he said, "it's unprecedented to have all these patients here." He urged the committee to focus on the trial data, since subjective patient and family perceptions about the waxing and waning of disability can be notoriously unreliable. His perspective was countered by his boss, Dr. Janet Woodcock, who five years later would push through the approval of Aduhelm. "We are instructed to take the views of the patient community into account as far as the benefits and the risks," she noted.

After discussions of the trial results, the audience was invited to comment on the data and give their perspective on the medication. (The costs of travel and accommodations for such representatives are often covered by a drug's manufacturer.) Among the large turnout of afflicted boys and their parents, many of the children wore bright orange T-shirts reading "n = 1," a term describing clinical observations based on just one subject. "I am afraid if you don't approve this drug I will become very weak," one fifteen-year-old boy told the committee. "FDA, please don't let me die early." A wheelchair-bound boy who had taken the drug said he was sure it had helped him. "It's time to listen to the real experts," he said. The head of an advocacy group told the committee, "The worst thing you can do is deny access to a drug and then find out it works—too late, after we have lost a generation of boys." Over forty DMD parents from Great Britain said they would move to the U.S. with their families to get the drug if the FDA approved it.

Other parents said it would be heartless to deny their sons the drug, since it was all that gave them any hope. One mother vividly described the deaths of two of her teenage sons from DMD. The disease had first made it difficult for them to walk, and then to stand, and then to move at all. She said that Sarepta's new treatment would have "significant, great impact" and a "positive incremental effect" on patients like these—despite the evidence of objective data from the clinical study.

The meeting lasted for hours. Committee members agreed that there was a major unmet need for a DMD treatment, but many said they feared that eteplirsen was not it, since the drug didn't produce a clear benefit. The law underlying the FDA's authority, dating back to 1962, calls for "substantial evidence from well conducted clinical trials" before a drug can be approved. The committee voted 7–3 that the single twelve-boy poorly controlled study did not provide that. On hearing the vote, many in the audience gasped. When committee members explained their decisions after the vote, one doctor who had said the data were inadequate to approve the drug said he hoped DMD families would participate in larger, better randomized placebo-controlled trials in the future. "How dare you!" a man in the audience called out. The consumer representative on the committee said he believed the drug was effective and voted yes; "Boys were getting better!" he exclaimed, and burst into tears. The assembled parents and families were enraged at the decision and some members of the advisory committee feared for their personal safety. ("They had to have security come and escort us out of the building," recalled my colleague Kesselheim, a committee member.)

Rewarding Mediocrity

FDA advisory committees are just that, and we've seen that the agency is free to accept or ignore their recommendations. When the furor after the meeting died down, Dr. Woodcock used the surrogate-measure/accelerated approval pathway to overrule the committee and approved the drug based on the minuscule differences in dystrophin levels, even though they were of no clear benefit to the afflicted children. In a surprising explanation of her controversial decision, she said that even though the drug was not a clinical success, Sarepta "needed to be capitalized," and FDA approval would help the company make enough money to continue its research on DMD and perhaps discover something that might work better. (Someone at the company had worried publicly before the meeting that it could go out of business if the agency didn't approve its product.) If drugs like eteplirsen were not approved, Woodcock explained, patients would abandon all hope and lapse into self-treatment, whatever that meant.

Her comment surprised all of us who thought the FDA's job was to evaluate the effectiveness of new medicines, not facilitate the cash flow of manufacturers. As we will see, the approval had precisely the opposite effect on useful innovation. A key FDA reviewer of the drug abruptly quit the agency that month. As required by the accelerated approval regulations, the FDA instructed Sarepta to perform a follow-up study to validate its initial finding. Its stock went up 90 percent on the news.

Once approval was granted, Sarepta gave its product the trade name of Exondys 51 and announced it would be priced at $300,000 a year. The cost would be heavily borne by state Medicaid programs; they are mandated to cover the health-care costs of the poor and other at-risk groups, and that cost could impoverish nearly any American. Many of these patients and families were forced to spend down their savings to qualify for Medicaid to pay for it, shifting the cost to each state as well as private insurers or even to Medicare, which covers the health-care costs of people who are totally disabled.

Our group looked at the paradoxical effects of this approval. In the years that followed, Exondys 51 brought in a huge windfall to Sarepta including net revenue of $1.1 billion in 2023, but the company didn't get around to conducting the follow-up studies that the accelerated approval required. To the contrary: the manufacturer learned from the approval decision that it could market a drug for DMD that didn't show any patient benefit as long as it had some effect on the surrogate measure of muscle dystrophin levels, however small and clinically irrelevant. So it went on to introduce two similar products that were variants of the same gene-skipping approach, called Amondys 45 and Vyondis 53, on the basis of modest changes in dystrophin levels without any meaningful clinical benefit. A Japanese drug company secured approval for its own similar treatment, Viltepso. Once the FDA had lowered the bar and set the precedent of accelerated approval based only on small changes in dystrophin levels, it could no longer say no. Each drug was granted accelerated approval.

Following its regulations, the FDA asked for post-approval follow-up studies for each drug to show that the surrogate-measure results led to actual benefits—in the case of eteplirsen, these findings were to be submitted by 2020. As of this writing no such studies have yet been submitted, eight years after the drug's approval. These drugs carry a list price of between $750,000 and $1.5 million per year. (In the U.S., companies can charge whatever they want for their products; we'll explore that further in chapters 5 and 6.) It's hard for payers to refuse to cover an FDA-approved drug, especially one for crippled children. Together, the group has cost public and private payers about $4 billion so far, and counting. As long as no follow-up studies were submitted showing the drug didn't work, Sarepta could keep selling its gene-skipping products as long as it wanted, and payors would have to pay for them. And if there were no countervailing results, until the passage of FDORA, the FDA has had no power to pull such drugs off the market. It doesn't take pathological cynicism to wonder whether that may have something to do with the company's failing year after year to submit the follow-up findings that the accelerated approval regulations require. As we reported in a series of papers from PORTAL, Woodcock's decision did succeed in capitalizing Sarepta, but it didn't produce innovation. Quite the opposite: it produced imitative mediocrity, enormous unjustified costs, and an economic windfall for the drugs' manufacturers.

(The Japanese company selling its own mutation-skipping drug for DMD did perform the required follow-up studies. In May 2024, it announced that its product turned out to have no significant advantage over placebo. It is not clear yet what if anything the FDA will do about those results. At the time of this writing, it is still on the U.S. market at a price of over $730,000 per year.)

Apart from raising Sarepta's stock price (it rose fivefold after Woodcock's approval decision), some of that money also underwrote the company's development costs for a new approach to DMD it was developing—gene therapy. The new approach was not just to skip the nonfunctional part of a patient's gene, but to replace it altogether. The idea was that the inserted gene could make enough of a new kind of muscle protein, to be called "micro-dystrophin," to enable patients to function more normally. The new product, called Elevidys, had the unmemorable generic name of delandistrogene moxeparvovec-rokl. Despite unimpressive initial clinical data and the resistance of FDA scientists, in June 2023 Peter Marks, Dr. Woodcock's counterpart on the gene-therapy side of the FDA, intervened and awarded it conditional approval because it slightly increased levels of micro-dystrophin, which thus became a new surrogate outcome—even though it didn't convincingly demonstrate patient improvement. Upon that initial approval, Sarepta announced an even bigger price tag for its newest product—$3.2 million per patient for a one-time treatment, making it the second-most expensive medication in history, second only to a new gene therapy treatment for hemophilia that actually worked.

The FDA said it would reassess its initial approval once the company completed a new randomized clinical trial to see if the gene therapy really helped patients; its much-anticipated results were announced in October 2023. The main clinical end point to be measured had been agreed upon in advance; it was a widely used gold-standard seventeen-item measure of clinical function in DMD patients that assesses how well these kids can walk, stand, and perform other basic muscle-based activities. Because of its wide acceptance by doctors who treat these patients, it's named the North Star Ambulatory Assessment. But the new gene therapy product failed on that primary outcome measure, showing no statistically significant advantage over placebo. It did enable the patients to produce small levels of micro-dystrophin, of no known clinical importance.

Study subjects did have slight improvement on some secondary clinical measures, though such findings usually don't outweigh a failure on the main comprehensive outcome studied. The more secondary tests you look at, the higher the possibility that one or more of them will happen to come out "positive" just because of chance. We measure that probability with a study's *p*-value: the likelihood that a particular finding could have occurred randomly, like flipping a coin four times and having it come up heads all four times. That doesn't mean it's a special coin—only that things sometimes happen by chance, and not always perfectly predictably. Flip that same coin a hundred times, and I guarantee it will come up heads quite close to half the time. The *p*-value for a given study simply tells us the likelihood that a given finding could have occurred by chance alone. The generally agreed-upon level for *p* of .05, or 5 percent, means that such a finding would have occurred randomly just one in twenty times that you ran the study; we can live with that. Similarly, if we look at enough secondary outcomes when testing a drug, it's likely that one in twenty will show a "significant" benefit at this level, even if the drug is inert. It's just probability. Sarepta's gene therapy flunked this time-honored metric for its main outcome measure.

Probabilities and Profits

Why be so tough about this criterion? After all, kids with DMD are doomed to a progressive downhill course of disability ending in death at an early age. Why not give a pass to the new gene therapy, since there are no good alternative treatments out there? As with Sarepta's prior products, anguished parents of DMD patients argued that their own instincts and hopes should prevail over the data about the failed gene therapy study. One mother wrote a *New York Times* op-ed that carried the headline "Why Can't More Children Get the Treatment That Saved My Son's Life?" (There is no evidence that Sarepta's DMD gene therapy ever saved anyone's life.) She objected to the FDA's pickiness about data, criticizing

> the roadblocks that prevent more families from gaining access to these new treatments—[including] dissent over how flexible regulators should be in interpreting clinical trial results and tak-

> ing qualitative improvements into account. . . . [The government should] make the wheels of regulatory approval for these drugs less onerous. . . . [A] narrow focus on numbers ignores the real quality-of-life benefits doctors, patients, and their families see from these treatments. . . . [The FDA experts] seemed unable to see the forest for the trees as they focused on statistics versus real-life examples.

The author hoped that after FDA approval, pressure would be applied on insurance companies to pay for this $3.2 million treatment, and/or the government would subsidize patients to cover their costs.

No, no, no. “A narrow focus on numbers”?! Numbers are all we have in figuring out which drugs work and which drugs don’t, as long as we’re measuring the right things, including level of disability. I empathize with the plight of parents forced to watch their sons become ever more crippled with every passing month, moving inexorably through years of increasing paralysis toward an early death. But we can’t return to the primitive days of assessing drugs by having patients or families decide whether a new treatment works or not based only on their subjective impressions, which we know are so prone to the placebo effect. The DMD gene therapy flunked an agreed-upon, well-established measure of functional status specific to that disease; that can’t be ignored in favor of those subjective n=1 observations. And who is supposed to pay Sarepta’s $3.2 million charge for a treatment that appears not to work? The problem here isn’t inflexible regulators, or experts who don’t understand quality-of-life considerations, or obsessive statisticians, or stingy insurance companies. The problem was the drug’s poor performance.

Once the novel DMD gene therapy trial showed no benefit in its main outcome measure, the nation waited expectantly for the FDA’s final decision—not just in relation to this devastating disease, but as a sign of where the agency would set its evidentiary bar following so much controversy about its poor recent calls. In June 2024, Dr. Marks overruled three review committees and two senior scientists at the agency and gave full final approval to the new treatment, as well as extending its initially narrow authorization to an even wider population of DMD patients who had not been studied in the trials. Doing so sidestepped the new powers that had so recently been granted to the FDA under FDORA. If Marks had kept the new gene therapy in the category of accelerated approval, Sarepta would have been required to conduct the follow-up studies it had so effectively ignored for years on its previous DMD drugs. But now public and private insurers would be under considerable pressure to pay over $3 million per patient for yet another one of the company's treatments for DMD that demonstrated unconvincing effectiveness.

Worse, the FDA decision lowered the bar for all other new gene therapies, signaling to the industry that the government would greenlight new treatments in this burgeoning class even if they failed to achieve agreed-upon end points in their pivotal clinical trials. And then, of course, manufacturers could charge whatever they wanted for them. My PORTAL colleagues wrote a compelling op-ed in the *Washington Post* calling attention to the travesty under the headline: "This gene therapy may not work. So why did the FDA fully approve it?" Dr. Luciana Borio, formerly the FDA's chief scientist, told STAT: "Peter Marks makes a mockery of scientific reasoning and approval standards that have served patients well over decades. This type of action also promotes the growing mistrust in scientific institutions like the FDA."

Bad approval standards can poison the well of drug research in other ways as well. Recruiting patients to any future placebo-controlled studies becomes much more difficult once the FDA has approved a drug, even a bad one. For a debilitating condition like DMD, once the FDA has allowed an approved treatment onto the market, who would want their child to be given placebo in a randomized trial of a new, perhaps better product? Poorly effective gene therapies carry an additional burden beyond the dumbing down of standards. Once a patient's genetic endowment is changed forever by a gene transplant, even one that yields mediocre results, a child who has undergone such treatment makes a poor candidate for future studies of both genetic and nongenetic therapies, since his chromosomal identity has been changed forever. Worse, he could have a subsequent dangerous reaction to the virus vehicles that are an integral part of these treatments, likely to be used in a newer and perhaps better gene therapy. So much for "compassionate use" of unproven treatments. A smarter approach would be for the FDA to get beyond its common yes/no posture of "It works, it's approved, it should be paid for in full" or "It doesn't work, it can't be sold." A nonbinary rethink, which would have made much more sense here, is described later on.

A few days after Dr. Marks's ill-advised full approval of the new gene therapy, the main DMD patient advocacy group held a meeting in Orlando, heavily subsidized by Sarepta. Attendees were allowed to question a company executive after his presentation; as reported by STAT, the mother of an eighteen-year-old patient confronted him over how little evidence the company had provided about its trial:

> "You haven't delivered any of this evidence you're supposed to have for your $3.2 million drug," she said. "You don't see how we are all pissed off, and at a certain point we're going to turn on you. We're the people who give you the millions of dollars but you're not giving us anything back, which is facts, data, and science. You're just taking the money."

The meeting was videotaped and the proceedings were to be posted on the patient advocacy group's website. But under pressure from Sarepta, the group deleted that interchange.

Cancer Cures That Don't Cure Cancer

Problematic as the surrogate measure problem is in muscular dystrophy, the approach is used most often in oncology, with a growing number of cancer treatments approved every year on that basis. The surrogate markers used may be stability or a change in tumor size as seen on an MRI or CAT scan, or a reduction in a chemical marker in a lab test. That's understandable as a starting point, and we can all relate to the perspective of researchers, patients, doctors, regulators, and manufacturers eager to get a new cancer drug into people as rapidly as possible, whatever the completeness of the evidence that supports it, each for their own reasons. But such changes don't always predict what patients care about the most: whether a treatment enables them to survive longer or feel better. One concerning example was the cancer drug Avastin (bevacizumab). It's a great medication that has proven extremely useful in many types of malignancy, so its manufacturer persuaded the FDA to give it permission to promote it for the treatment of metastatic breast cancer even though it hadn't been studied rigorously for that purpose. The FDA did so because the drug worked well in other malignancies and it seemed to slow tumor growth on imaging studies in patients with metastatic breast cancer, resulting in greater "progression-free survival" (PFS) than a comparison treatment. That term, which sounds innocent but can be problematic, refers to how long a tumor appears not to be increasing in size.

That seemed plausible enough. But PFS has a surprisingly variable relation to actual survival, which is the real goal that cancer patients and doctors care about most. When more careful studies were done, it turned out that while Avastin made the imaging studies look better than the comparator drug, it did not keep breast cancer patients alive any longer. While leaving Avastin on the market for the other purposes for which it worked so well, the FDA moved to withdraw authorization for its specific use in metastatic breast cancer. Vociferous objection to this came from the manufacturer (predictably) and patients (harder to justify), delaying the change in the official recommendation for many months.

The surrogate measure of progression-free survival is sometimes a predictor of overall survival, and sometimes not. Yet it remains a common standard for FDA approval of cancer drugs. That would be less of a problem if the agency went on to require follow-up studies to figure this out, and if the manufacturers complied with that requirement—but they often don't. But it's worse than that. In several studies of this process from our group, Kesselheim and colleagues have found that in many of those "confirmatory" studies manufacturers simply used the same surrogate measure that initially won the drug's approval, instead of conducting a proper clinical trial to see if there is really an effect on actual patient outcomes.

Worse still: we've followed up on those "required" post-approval studies and found that they are often begun late, done slowly, never completed, or never even started. A 2024 study from our group looked at 129 cancer diagnoses for which drugs were approved on the basis of such stand-in measures. Among trials of products with five years or more of follow-up, fewer than half of the medications were shown to enable patients to live longer or have a better quality of life.

Could the situation be any worse than that? Yes. Not only do imaging-based measures like progression-free survival fail to predict long-term benefit consistently, in some clinical trials patients with "improved" PFS actually died sooner than control patients. In a remarkable 2023 paper published in the respected *Journal of Clinical Oncology*, five of the FDA's own scientists reported on studies in which patients randomized to get a new cancer drug did better in their so-called progression-free survival based on imaging studies, but actually lived less long than patients given the comparison treatment. Tellingly, they titled their paper "Irreconcilable Differences: The Divorce between Response Rates, Progression-Free Survival, and Overall Survival." Making the same argument the other way around, the FDA researchers also described studies of drugs that really did prolong actual survival, but had flunked their measures of PFS.

Might cancer drugs benefit people if they made them feel better, even if they didn't prolong their lives? That would be an important kind of benefit, but evidence shows that a longer PFS may not produce any quality-of-life improvement benefit, either—often, quite the opposite. An international team of researchers reviewed fifty-two trials that measured both progression-free survival and quality of life; they found no significant evidence that the former improved the latter. A commentary in the medical journal *Lancet* noted that the word "survival" in PFS can be misleading; better to use the more neutral term "progression-free interval," the authors proposed, to avoid giving such drugs more respectability than they deserve.

In sum, as a result of what the FDA likes to call its regulatory flexibility, every day cancer patients are prescribed medications to treat their disease—often at great cost—that haven't been shown to offer any survival benefit to them and are never adequately reassessed. The treatments often make them feel sicker, and sometimes even shorten their lives. This is particularly upsetting in light of all the excellent new cancer treatments that can benefit patients enormously. Our approval system, and the information it provides to doctors and consumers, doesn't do well in distinguishing these great new therapies from others that are not nearly as effective.

Gaming the System

The FDA has often claimed that once a drug is approved, it lacks the clout to force companies to do what it asks, though many have argued that one cause of this regulatory dysfunction syndrome is the agency's insufficient institutional virility. The 2023 FDORA legislation was designed to fix that; time will tell how well that works. So where does this leave us? The FDA's weakening approach to drug approval standards means that people with many different diseases, from cancer to Alzheimer's disease to muscular dystrophy, can't really know whether the drug a doctor prescribed for their condition will actually help them. Even more troubling, the doctors prescribing these medicines may not even know what we don't know.

The deterioration of the FDA's approach to evidence is one of the best-kept secrets in health care today. It is exacerbated by the proliferation of a number of expedited pathways to facilitate drug evaluation and acceptance, powerfully encouraged by pressure from the pharmaceutical industry and its allies in Congress. By 2022, more than half of all new drugs evaluated by the FDA were in one of these expedited review pathways, and about 80 to 90 percent of new drug submissions were approved: nearly every contestant wins a prize. The studies used to garner approval have been getting shorter, include fewer patients, and may not even have adequate control groups. The FDA has been calling upon outside advisory committees less and less, and seems more and more willing to disregard their advice if it's negative.

But isn't it better to get new drugs out to patients more quickly before full testing is complete, even if they don't all work? Actually, no. All medications can have side effects, since all the ones that work have them. If we have good data on actual clinical benefits, we can compare that with adverse effects and we and our patients can make an informed benefit-risk assessment. But if all we have on the positive side of the ledger is an improvement in a lab test, it's hard to know how many cases of an adverse immune reaction or liver failure are worth incurring to achieve—what? And if the approval is granted on the basis of a shortened one-night-stand kind of assessment, we're certain to miss problems that come up with longer use. (I've called this analytic dysfunction "premature extrapolation." It's more common than many people think.)

And given the very high cost of many of these hastily approved new drugs, how much should we ask patients or insurers to pay for incompletely evaluated products, either directly or through their (and everyone's) health insurance premiums? Or society, since taxpayers cover nearly half of all drug expenditures through government programs? This *de minimis* approach also doesn't provide enough to work with for researchers like my colleagues and me who try to compare the true clinical benefit (not to mention the relative cost-effectiveness) of several competing drugs a doctor or patient might choose for a given condition. That's hard to do if all we know is the effect of each of them on a lab test or imaging study—especially if manufacturers' studies of different drugs use different end points. It's not just apples and oranges, it's apples and aardvarks. The FDA's current policies end up making needed clinical trials more difficult at the same time they make them less necessary to win approval.

Finally, there's the negative impact these low-bar approvals have on the pharmaceutical ecosystem. When the FDA approves a drug that may not provide clinical benefit, it doesn't "encourage innovation" by attracting payments to companies working on tough problems—quite the opposite. Once companies learn they can bring partially tested and poorly effective drugs to the agency and win approval, they will continue to do so, rather than being required by government or the marketplace to keep working at the problem until they come up with a medication that actually helps patients.

He Who Pays the Piper

Sensible drug evaluation and approval require finding the sweet spot on a continuum running from the silly libertarian idea that nearly all drugs should be approved, through the other extreme of obsessive and unreasonably demanding regulatory requirements that can delay treatment and cost lives. Observing that the FDA's shortage of scientific reviewers during the AIDS crisis was hurting all participants in the system, in the early 1990s—the same time the accelerated approval pathway was introduced—the pharmaceutical industry came up with a friendly suggestion: "*We can help you with that!* Just let us pay 'user fees' to help cover the cost of evaluating each drug application we submit. You can use all that money to hire the staff you need to review our products quickly, if Congress won't provide it."

The approach would be just like entry fees in the national parks, advocates argued. After all, those were government operations, too, but it's only fair that the people who use them should help shoulder the burden for their maintenance. For drugs, there would be a different kind of quid pro quo: in exchange for accepting user fees, the FDA would agree to speed up its decisions to comply with certain deadlines; those are now set at six months to review a drug on a priority track, and ten months for the others. In 1992, with the penurious Bush administration aligned with an increasingly conservative force in Congress, industry-sponsored user fees began to look like the only way to get the FDA the budget it needed to do its work. The program grew, and by 2022 user fees accounted for about two-thirds of the agency's salary costs for the staff reviewing conventional drugs, or $1.4 billion a year, and 40 percent of the paychecks of the scientists who review biologics—the more complex molecules like the amyloid-eating drugs for Alzheimer's disease. What could possibly go wrong?

The national park analogy, of course, missed the point. National parks don't regulate vacationers the same way that the FDA has jurisdiction over the pharmaceutical industry; there was a predictable shift in the balance of power once a regulated industry started to pay the salaries of its regulators. Some FDA reviewers reported feeling that the user fee–imposed deadlines limited their ability to thoroughly evaluate some drugs. My colleague Dan Carpenter of the Harvard Government Department and I analyzed reviewers' decisions that were made right up against the deadline compared to those made in a less constrained way. As we reported in *NEJM*, drugs approved close to the deadline were significantly more likely to have safety problems arise later on.

The original 1992 user fee legislation has continued to reverberate twice each decade, and will continue to do so. It was designed to sunset after five years, but additional budgetary support for the FDA was still not forthcoming from Congress. So by 1997 the agency had to come to a renewed agreement with the drugmakers over the terms under which they would continue to pay those fees. Failure was not an option: if the FDA and industry didn't agree on a plan to continue that system, the agency's budget would shrink dramatically. Ever since, the user fee reauthorization has been renegotiated every five years to enable the FDA to keep the lights on, and each new version has gotten its own name. The original 1992 law was named the Prescription Drug User Fee Act, or PDUFA (rhymes with "Palooka"). Over time, requirements were loosened: the expectation that more than one pivotal trial was needed to win approval was replaced with the rule that just one study can be acceptable. Having patients in those studies randomly allocated to get a new drug or a comparator—was that really necessary? Kesselheim and I found that, more and more, drugs for rare diseases were being approved without the same kind of rigorous study designs that had been mandated before. That trend has broadened to other kinds of approvals, and intensified.

Doing a Complete End Run around Science for Some Products

In the 1990s, the FDA tried to rein in a unique category of bogus drugs: those marketed as "dietary supplements." Many were merely silly, including simple elements like magnesium or selenium that are totally unnecessary in the average American diet. But others were potentially dangerous: the stimulant ephedra caused heart attacks, strokes, seizures, and psychotic reactions and is now banned; Hydroxycut, a weight-loss supplement, produced liver and muscle damage; and some vitamins can lead to dangerous overdose. Many over-the-counter "supplements," especially those sold for weight loss, sexual potency, or muscle building, have been found to contain active ingredients like stimulants, Viagra, or steroids.

During his impressive tenure as FDA commissioner (1990–1997), David Kessler sought to rein in these unregulated nostrums by bringing them within the FDA's purview and requiring a manufacturer to demonstrate safety and effectiveness, as for prescription medications—some of which are much less potent and dangerous. But the supplement industry is powerful, well organized, and very lucrative: its sales are estimated at $40 to $50 billion annually in the U.S., and at least four times that globally. Its ingredients are trivially cheap, and there is hardly any meaningful research and development process to pay for.

Kessler's attempts to bring some rationality to the market led the industry to mount a fierce response with the help of Senator Orrin Hatch of Utah, since many of these companies are based in that state. Instead of tighter oversight, the FDA's plan backfired: a new law enabled those products to officially escape that agency's purview altogether and come under separate, more trivial government regulation. The 1994 law that codified this protection was called the Dietary Supplement Health and Education Act, known as DSHEA, pronounced as if it were a French-Irish surname, deShay. Rather than bringing supplements into the orbit of modern regulation, DSHEA effectively castrated the FDA's oversight role, eliminating its authority to require demonstration of safety or effectiveness for these products; the agency can now only step in after the fact to investigate a serious safety problem once it has been documented. Efficacy? Forget about it, said the new law. All that a supplement manufacturer has to do is to put wording on its claims that says, paradoxically, "This product is not intended to diagnose, treat, cure, or prevent any disease. These statements have not been evaluated by the Food and Drug Administration." Sometimes these disclaimers are in print so small they are nearly invisible; other times, that language is omitted altogether, but enforcement of this requirement is virtually nonexistent. DSHEA did for medications what Marcel Duchamp did in 1917 for sculpture when he took a porcelain urinal, turned it on its side, and declared it to be a piece of art because he was an artist. But apparently the health-care system of today has an even lower bar than the art world of the early twentieth century. The exhibit to which Duchamp submitted his urinal usually accepted anything at all for display, but rejected his submission.

Surveys indicate that most people think that the supplements they see advertised so widely have been evaluated and approved by the government, and some of these ads look like those for prescription drugs. One of the most egregious campaigns is for Prevagen, "made from jellyfish," which claims to reduce cognitive problems in older people, but lacks compelling clinical evidence that it does anything. Previously, supplement makers would use weasel words in their ads like "supports immune function" or "restores joint health." Prevagen, too, promotes itself as "supporting brain function," but also makes the audacious and indefensible claim that it "improves memory." This is perfectly legal. Neuriva, a similar product, includes obscure ingredients such as "whole coffee cherry extract." It was studied by the manufacturer and its consultants, who administered a battery of tests to 128 people in their fifties. The study used an unconventional data analysis approach and reported that after six weeks, the subjects given Neuriva improved on some tests but not others, and acknowledged that up to 100 percent of their findings may have been attributable to the placebo effect. Given the large number of tests administered in this cherry extract study, it's possible that there may have been some cherry-picking of the data in extracting it. No scientific review is required for supplements, and it's not reasonable to expect consumers to go back to the medical literature and check it out themselves. Other heavily advertised "supplements" for dieting make audacious claims about weight loss that are absurdly inaccurate. And thanks to DSHEA, no one can stop them. This has worked out well for Dr. Mehmet Oz, made famous by his television appearances promoting a variety of dubious supplement products. Following the 2024 elections, he was put forward by President Trump to run the Medicare and Medicaid programs.

These useless and misleading products fit well with arguments made by some extreme conservatives. They begin with contempt for traditional scientific methods and federal standards. "Doing your own research" is seen as just as useful as anything the government or scientists might determine. More ominous is the role some companies play in fueling zany data-free political statements. The conspiracy theorist and media celebrity Alex Jones, who denied that the mass shooting of children at Sandy Hook Elementary School happened, funded his toxic operation by selling a line of dietary supplements as groundless as his political statements. The Centers for Disease Control has estimated that over half of all Americans use one or more of such nostrums. Besides wasting people's money, this can also prevent them from getting real medicines from actual health-care professionals that could really do them some good. I can think of many ways that patients and the American health-care system could spend that $50 billion a year more effectively.

Different disciplines have their own truth-seeking approaches. In his book *The Constitution of Knowledge*, Jonathan Rauch describes an "epistemic crisis" infecting many aspects of contemporary life, making it harder to know what's really true and what isn't; these problems are not unique to drugs. In medicine, for less than a century our North Star has been the randomized controlled trial—the unparalleled truth-seeking device that has such amazing powers to reveal what works and what doesn't. It's one of the best inventions of the last hundred years, but it's fallen on hard times in some places. RFK Jr., President Trump's choice to head the government department that oversees virtually all of the nation's health-related agencies, has long expressed his disdain for scientific evidence about the benefits of medical products (such as his advocacy for Covid treatments proven not to work) and their risks (such as his arguing despite many studies that childhood vaccines cause autism). Ignoring decades of evidence involving thousands of patients, Kennedy also claimed that the polio vaccine causes cancer and does not really prevent polio; one of his key aides petitioned the FDA to have it withdrawn from the market. Seventy-five Nobel Prize winners signed a statement objecting to Kennedy's appointment to such a powerful post, but that did not diminish Trump's support. In other moves that stunned medical scientists, the re-elected president proposed doctors to head the NIH, the CDC, and the FDA who gained notoriety during the pandemic by questioning the usefulness and safety of widespread vaccination and social distancing to limit spread of the disease.

The venerable and increasingly vulnerable RCT is just a concept, of course, but I sometimes imagine it as a machine, like the clock in Greenwich, England, that once enabled millions of people to share the same reality by transmitting the official time all over Great Britain (and, via undersea cable, to Harvard). Maybe if my imaginary "RCT machine" had gears and bells and whistles, it would get more of the respect it deserves. I once envisioned such a device enshrined behind glass in a mythical place of honor at the FDA, with smaller versions housed in each of its divisions. In that vision, I saw some of the smaller models humming along well in several of the agency's offices. But now I think of the original prototype in the FDA's headquarters covered in dust, its glass case cracked. The lights don't blink as brightly anymore, the smooth whirring sound now grates and stalls. Vandals covered it with graffiti after the guard on duty was laid off because of budget cuts. There are rumors that the second Trump administration has plans to lock it in the basement, or smash it with sledgehammers. But it's still a worthy device, and many of us are ready to roll up our sleeves and put it back in working order if they'd just let us in the building.

CHAPTER 4

Standards That Matter to Patients

We've seen how complicated it can be to determine whether a new medication "works," and even to agree on what we mean by that. However, patients, doctors, and those who pay for drugs do not have to cede to the pharmaceutical industry the authority to design, pay for, and run so many of the key clinical trials on which our knowledge depends. Many of the researchers who work at these companies are honest and as sharp as any I know in academia. Likewise, the reviewers at the FDA are generally dedicated, astute scientists who do an excellent job trying to get their recommendations right. So why do things sometimes go off the rails in both settings? If the people doing the frontline work are so smart and conscientious, where does the mischief start?

The golem is a creature from Jewish folklore dating back to the Middle Ages; stories about it gave me nightmares as a child. It's a figure fashioned from an inert substance like clay; when magical words or letters are inserted into its mouth, the golem takes on extraordinary powers to act on whatever commands it is given. Sometimes its actions were benevolent: in sixteenth-century Europe at a time of widespread anti-Semitic violence, the golem was imagined as a protector. But a golem could also wreak havoc, transforming from a strong ally into a mindless, destructive hulk. That could happen when the golem followed its instructions too literally, leading to disaster.

Golem stories circulated widely in Europe in the late eighteenth century when Goethe envisioned his "Sorcerer's Apprentice," and in the early nineteenth century when Mary Shelley wrote *Frankenstein*.

Both authors invented golem-like figures endowed with awesome strength—powers called forth with good intentions, but which then got horribly out of control and created chaos. Because none of these creatures had any insight or internal restraints, they sometimes went way too far in acting on their programmed instructions. So, in an ethical sense, the damage they did wasn't completely their fault.

Similar moral ambiguity is built into tales dating back to Aesop in the sixth century BCE. In one, "The Farmer and the Viper," a man takes pity on a snake he finds freezing in the cold and puts it under his coat. As the viper warms up it fatally stings the farmer, explaining, in essence, "It's what I do." Similar ancient stories recount various pairs of prey and predator. In one, a scorpion asks a frog to ferry it across a river.

"Why should I?" asks the frog. "You could bite me and I'd drown."

"Don't be silly," responds the scorpion. "If I did that, we'd both go under."

The frog accepts this logic and invites the scorpion to hop on its back. Halfway across the river the scorpion stings the frog.

"Why did you do that?" the frog demands as they sink. "Now we're both going to die."

"It's what I do," replied the scorpion as they drowned.

In some ways, these stories are exculpatory: the creatures are just doing what they are designed to do. Putting aside the venom and the havoc can help us to think more clearly about the behavior of corporations, including those that make drugs. (Similar arguments can be made about government agencies whose leadership falls under the sway of the industry they're tasked with regulating, and even about nominally nonprofit health-care systems that act like the enormous corporations many have become.) In the case of for-profit corporations, people entrust them with their money to grow their investments; as the economist Milton Friedman reminded us, that's the only reason those corporations exist. In fact, you could argue that a company whose officers and employees don't do everything in their power to increase shareholders' return on investment isn't doing its job right. Failing to fulfill that fiduciary responsibility as fully as possible would represent a breach of legal and ethical responsibilities to investors.

We know that drug companies, like the FDA, employ thousands of smart and honorable scientists. But the actions of corporations (including nonprofits) and federal agencies are shaped by leaders seeking to fulfill their missions as they see them, and that's where problems can start. Agendas and priorities get defined at the top, and can lead organizations to engage in golem-like behavior. It's just what they do.

For companies, the duty to generate profits is supposed to stop short of breaking the law. But if there's a way to *modify* the law—about approval standards or pricing rules or influencing regulators, for example—and tens of millions of dollars of lobbying clout are available to leadership for that purpose, then that becomes part of a company's job as well. Nothing personal, it's just business. The problem isn't that corporations do what they have to do to fulfill their legal responsibility to maximize profit; we aren't likely to change that. The problem comes from having unfounded expectations that they will do otherwise, and failing to properly regulate those inherent, inevitable urges. In other parts of the economy, if sellers and buyers both have adequate information about the worth of the goods and services they buy and sell, and regulators act as effective umpires to enforce the rules, those countervailing pressures might work reasonably well. But in our complex $4.5-trillion-dollar health-care system, where arcane specialized knowledge plays such a key role in decision-making and government agencies sometimes forget whom they're working for, the internal checks and balances of the marketplace are often ineffective, and we shouldn't be surprised at that.

Free Research Isn't Cheap

This brings us back to the societal bargain in which drug manufacturers offer to bear the expense of designing and conducting the clinical trials on which their products' fates depend. That's not a good deal for the country: delegating clinical trial design and funding to manufacturers isn't a smart money-saving plan. We've spent billions on a suite of unimpressive muscular dystrophy treatments; similar economics apply to dozens of poorly effective cancer drugs, as well as the failed painkiller Vioxx (see chapter 6). Wouldn't it make more sense and cost us far less to rethink the process and have a group of clinicians, vetted to rule out conflict of interest, design those studies and oversee their conduct and interpretation? Running the trials could be accomplished by any one of dozens of contract research organizations (CROs) whose business is doing just that; in fact, many drug companies hire them to run the trials they've designed. The task requires careful management and obsessive quality control, but it's not rocket science (or molecular genetics, for that matter).

One remarkable success story of a similar approach came early in the Covid pandemic. Researchers at Oxford University wanted to find out whether the steroid dexamethasone might blunt the extreme inflammatory response that often provided the lethal *coup de grace* that killed so many of these patients. No treatment had been shown to lower the disease's terrible death rate, but since the steroid had been generic for decades, no pharmaceutical company was eager to study it. So the Oxford researchers used the universal coverage and data management systems of the British National Health Service to rapidly enroll more than 11,500 patients in 175 NHS hospitals in a randomized controlled trial of the drug compared to usual care. They launched the ambitious study in March 2020, early in the pandemic, and announced its impressive results in June, just three months later: dexamethasone reduced the death rate of seriously ill Covid patients by up to a third. The results immediately changed the way the world treated Covid, and saved countless lives. The study is an example of the "pragmatic clinical trials" that could answer so many pressing questions if we just did more of them.

Compared to What?

Studies designed primarily to meet patients' needs rather than to ensure quick product approval would also require that one study arm in a trial would represent the best available treatment for the disease under consideration and not just an inert placebo, as is often the case. Drug company lawyers will argue that all they are legally required to demonstrate is that a new drug is "effective," and traditionally it's often been acceptable for that to mean a product is better than nothing, unless ethical considerations make such a comparison unthinkable. But there's no law against also including a study arm of patients who get an active comparator drug alongside the placebo group—especially if a publicly funded entity were conducting the trial. Being better than nothing might still be good enough legally to get the drug approved by the FDA; but the active comparator arm would tell prescribers, patients, and payers what we really care about—whether a treatment is truly an improvement over what we already have. Would that make the clinical trial more expensive? Sure, but it would still be far cheaper than having the government, private insurers, and patients spend hundreds of millions of dollars a year paying for new drugs that are no better than less costly alternatives.

Doing this isn't within the FDA's legal authority nor its orientation, and the agency doesn't have the resources or inclination to take on these tougher questions. But we need assessments like these to guide the decisions made every day by physicians and patients and insurers. Since many people can't afford their medicines, it would also be very useful to define a new drug's benefits and risks in light of its costs (see chapter 13). Since the FDA can't and won't do this, the best way to yield the most relevant science and save the most money would be to stand up a separate organization inside or outside government, as many nations already have done.

Rethinking Secret Findings

The scandals of the early 2000s pushed us to overcome much of the problem of companies hiding trial results they don't like. Another problem is less widely known: if a drug doesn't win FDA approval, the details of its clinical trials can be kept secret as private corporate property by the drugmaker that paid for (i.e., owns) those studies. This is bad for the public good: What if an important side effect was discovered in the suppressed trial findings? No one in the public might ever hear about it. The FDA has those data, but cannot reveal them to the public; that's also true for some of the information companies give to the FDA for drugs that are approved—another hit to the libertarian argument that doctors and patients can just do their own research to decide if a drug works. So valuable is this proprietary information to companies that the penalties for its release by FDA staff can be more draconian than those that other government employees face. We discussed transparency options with FDA commissioner Rob Califf when he visited PORTAL, and he became exercised at the prospect of releasing some of those vital data: "My people could literally go to jail for doing that!" he exclaimed.

Even if Califf's depiction seemed dramatic, any such secrecy is an abuse of the generosity of the study subjects—almost always unpaid—who devote their time and put themselves at risk to help evaluate an untested chemical. A public-minded Congress could pass a law that no medical data about the clinical effects of drugs can be considered to be private property, just as it's not legal to sell embryos or people's organs. Having more drug trials publicly funded would also help address this issue.

Who's Using Whom?

Another bargain that needs a second look are those industry-paid user fees now essential for the FDA to pay its scientists' salaries. As with companies' offers to cover the costs of clinical trials, we need to rethink this apparent windfall. Shouldn't a government agency that regulates 20 percent of all dollars Americans spend have a budget big enough to get its work done? Just as we wouldn't allow one side in a courtroom to pay the judge, we need to see the FDA's work as a public good that must be supported publicly. That would save the nation far more than it would cost, but it isn't compatible with plans for slashing the federal budget.

The scathing critiques of the FDA's management of its accelerated approval program that appeared in reports by Congress and the Health and Human Services inspector general led to the FDORA legislation giving the agency more authority to monitor that pathway, and to require timely follow-up studies and act on their findings sensibly and rapidly. It also will need to be more thoughtful about problems with its additional greased-skids expedited pathways, such as the "breakthrough" designation, orphan drug status, priority review vouchers, and others.

Becoming Nonbinary

Paradoxically, a medication can at the same time be both "effective" (when a test difference is statistically significantly different from zero), and "ineffective" (in the sense that this difference won't do much good for the patients who take it). This violates what philosophers call the "law of the excluded middle," and it has ancient origins. Aristotle started the problem nearly 2,400 years ago in his *Metaphysics* when he declared that every statement must either be affirmed or denied, with no intermediate position allowed. (Interestingly, he chose a gender example to illustrate this, noting that it is impossible for a person to "be a man" and "not be a man" at the same time. It's hard to understand how he could have come up with that narrow-minded contention in ancient Greece; maybe he needed to get out more.)

The difficulty of seeing something as having two different contrasting properties at the same time has confounded conventional logic for millennia, just as it haunts our official determinations of drug effectiveness. It took until the twentieth century for formal counterexamples to sink into Western culture. In quantum physics, Erwin Schrödinger tried to explain how an electron could simultaneously be someplace and yet not be there. He created a thought experiment in which a cat could be understood to be both alive and dead at the same instant; "Schrödinger's cat" has become a staple of undergraduate physics courses. In utter seriousness, and with the utmost respect, I can recall caring for patients on life support who had the same property.

A few decades after Schrödinger, psychedelic drugs smashed the life-death duality paradigm in a totally different way (see chapter 19). Similarly, our views of masculinity and femininity have also evolved in their sophistication. But the FDA remains stuck in a rigid either-or mode in its approval decisions; it often has a hard time getting beyond the old-fashioned rule that says, "This drug has been proven to work, and can be prescribed by any doctor," or "This drug is ineffective and cannot be used in clinical practice."

Several rethinking options can lead us out of this confusion about the nature of effectiveness and get us to a much better place. Take cancer: initially, we might want to facilitate access to drugs that lead to improvements in imaging studies or reduce levels of apparent tumor markers on blood tests. We also know that these encouraging findings can sometimes be illusory. Yet we don't want to keep these medicines off the market for many more years until we're totally sure how all those longer-term studies come out. There is an obvious and workable policy fix here that's been discussed far more than it's been implemented: an initial category of conditional approval can be assigned as further testing is conducted. A medication could be made available to patients who desperately need it, while requiring a plan to carefully study its effects before it is authorized for unrestrained prescribing to anyone. Such rethinking would restrict its use to a limited number of research centers in which doctors could prescribe the drug while collecting rigorous data on real patient outcomes, like overall survival for cancer patients, or functional status for patients with Alzheimer's disease or muscular dystrophy. Medicare calls this "coverage with evidence development," but the practice is used all too rarely for drugs, and when it's tried it's often done poorly. The whole accelerated approval pathway was designed with this approach in mind, but its enforcement has been tragically lax. And we've seen how the FDA initially decided to grant provisional approval to Sarepta's $3 million gene therapy for muscular dystrophy pending successful completion of a more careful clinical trial, only to grant full approval when that study failed to show clear benefit. Similarly, the government tried to demand ongoing evaluation of the new Alzheimer's drug

Leqembi by requiring that all patients be entered into a registry, but the data collection required will be so minimal that it will be of very limited use.

Alternatively, the powerful methods of observational studies using modern pharmacoepidemiology approaches (see chapter 9) to analyze the medication use and outcomes of patients in routine care could enable us to rigorously track the outcomes of people given the drug in the real-world near-randomness of clinical practice, carefully controlling for differences in those who got the medicine compared to those who received another treatment. Modern approaches to such data make this an increasingly useful way to measure comparative effectiveness, if done rigorously. After a period of three or so years a drug could be formally reassessed and either promoted to the status of full widespread use, or studied further in a limited setting, or taken off the market. Our pharmacoepidemiology group in DoPE is actively exploring this approach.

In a separate survey of a sample of over five hundred randomly chosen internists, only two in five said they actually understood how the FDA evaluates drugs, and nearly all said that if confirmatory studies didn't prove the benefit of an accelerated approval medication, it should be taken off the market, which hardly ever happens.

A more threatening suggestion was made by FDA commissioner Rob Califf, normally quite friendly to manufacturers, who told attendees at a large convention of biotechnology companies in Boston that maybe they should charge less for drugs that were approved only on the basis of a surrogate measure, with the price going up only after the drugmaker proved its product helps patients. He explained the idea with a graphic if homespun analogy: "If I had a basketball that's probably going to stay inflated and it looks pretty good in the store but we don't really know, you wouldn't really pay the same as you would for a first-rate basketball" that you were sure would stay inflated. It was brazen to use a partially-deflated-ball analogy in our town, and his sensible idea was greeted with alarm by the audience. Their unease was tempered by relief that although Califf was the FDA commissioner, he had no jurisdiction over how much companies get paid for their products (see part 3, on drug prices).

Getting Rid of the Bad Stuff

Our understanding of medications keeps evolving—that's how science works. But the system is much better at adding products than removing them, even when evidence emerges that they're ineffective. One striking example was Makena, a drug designed to help women at risk of preterm delivery carry their pregnancies to term. It had been granted accelerated approval in 2011 on the basis of a surrogate marker. As usual, the FDA told the manufacturer to perform follow-up studies to see if affecting that marker actually improved patient outcomes. Years passed and the company failed to submit any evidence that it was really effective. The FDA began trying to take Makena off the market beginning in 2020, but for years couldn't get it done. Reports were issued. Hearings were held. It wasn't until 2023, twelve years after approval, that the FDA was able to stop sales of the useless drug. No other medications can reliably prevent preterm birth in high-risk women, who are disproportionately Black. But allowing use of a drug that doesn't work isn't offering them any help at all.

Another example has been ubiquitous in the medicine cabinets of millions of Americans: phenylephrine, sold widely as an over-the-counter (OTC) decongestant. It had replaced pseudoephedrine, which worked well to stop runny noses and was widely marketed under the brand name Sudafed. But then underground chemists figured out a way to use it to make methamphetamine, so it was taken out of the standard OTC product and replaced with phenylephrine. To maintain sales at the price of some confusion, the manufacturer kept the name of the new product as Sudafed.

The problem is that phenylephrine doesn't work as a decongestant—or as much else, for that matter. Pharmacologists have been pointing that out for years, but it remained available as one of the most widely used OTC products in the country, selling briskly but providing no relief to patients. For years the FDA couldn't get manufacturers to stop selling it. The best reason for keeping it available seemed to be "At least you can't use it to make meth!" It was only in 2023 that the agency's yearslong efforts led to the announcement that phenylephrine would be removed from store shelves . . . at some point in the future, an aspiration repeated in 2024. Many other OTC medications work well to treat nasal congestion; continued use of the ineffective phenylephrine actually crowds out their use. It's also staggering to think how many millions of dollars were wasted over such a long period by American families on yet another useless OTC product. Despite the plan to withdraw it, phenylephrine is still on the market, both as a generic and as the still-confusingly-named Sudafed. (Consumer tip: The real pseudoephedrine is still stocked in drugstores *behind* the pharmacist's counter. You just have to ask for it by name and provide some identification. Tell them Jerry sent you.)

We now know more than enough to make some obvious evidence-based recommendations to help us rethink our approach to understanding the effectiveness of drugs:

- Reduce the overuse of accelerated approval of new drugs based only on changes in lab tests or imaging studies that may or may not predict a real benefit to patients. Return whenever possible to the FDA's legal standard of requiring that a drug must be shown to actually help patients before it can be sold.
- Some new medications will truly merit accelerated approval, such as treatments for awful diseases for which the surrogate marker is a clear predictor of patient benefit.
- FDORA may have strengthened the FDA's hand, but the agency will have to do a better job of using that enforcement power to require companies to complete timely follow-up studies showing their drugs work. The sale of products that can't do this should be suspended until such proof is in hand.
- The FDA ought to move to wide use of a category of conditional approval for drugs that cause promising changes in surrogate markers but haven't yet shown patient benefits, so they can be prescribed on a limited basis (and paid for on a limited basis as well) as they are studied further.

- Support far more publicly supported pragmatic clinical trials like the Oxford Covid study to answer pressing medication-related questions, rather than waiting for an interested drug company to offer to design and pay for medication research.
- Given the enormous political pressure on all branches of government to please the pharmaceutical lobby, we need a new body that can put recently approved products into an evidence-based context for prescribers, payers, and patients. This could be akin to the health technology assessment (HTA) organizations of other countries (see chapter 13). The U.S. version could be created without congressional action through philanthropic and other private funding, as is currently the case with the respected Boston nonprofit Institute for Clinical and Economic Review (ICER), though it focuses heavily on drug pricing rather than on prescribing advice or comparing choices within a class. The recommendations of such a new advisory group wouldn't have the force of law, a major advantage for HTA groups in other wealthy countries. But they would have a respected provenance and could take on the enormously important role of putting new treatments into clinical perspective—something the FDA has neither the mandate, the skill set, nor the appetite to do.
- As these reforms come into place, we will also need to develop communications channels to push out those findings to clinicians and patients so that their main source of information about new drug products isn't predominantly the sellers of those products. This area is discussed more fully in chapter 18, "Better Signals."

We've learned a lot over the years about what goes well and what goes badly in measuring the effectiveness of the medicines we prescribe or ingest. Although political pressure has distorted our application of that knowledge in the last decade or two, finding our way back up that evidentiary mountain could be easier than when we had to scale it for the first time—unless politics once again undercuts that effort.

– PART TWO –

Is It Safe?

CHAPTER 5

How Do We Find Out about Drug Risks?

> I want a new drug
> One that won't make me sick
> One that won't make me crash my car
> Or make me feel three feet thick.
>
> —Huey Lewis and the News, "I Want a New Drug," 1983

A few clinical tragedies had stutteringly propelled the field of medication evaluation forward by the start of the twenty-first century:

> 1906: A drug's contents should be listed on the container, and not kept secret.
> 1938: It should not be poisonous.
> 1962: It should actually work.

But as late as 2007, we still weren't able to meet this standard:

> If it triples the risk of a dangerous side effect, we should know that before it's been on the market for five years.

Any medication that works will also carry with it the chance of side effects. We cannot discover, prescribe, and take medicines with no risks—that's impossible. Instead, we need to define the nature and magnitude of those side effects well enough to enable us to decide whether the good a drug can do will make it worth taking those risks. Merck's blockbuster product Vioxx, an anti-inflammatory drug that was the best-selling medicine in the world before it turned into one of the biggest drug safety problems ever, taught us a lot about how to rethink the risks of medications, why we sometimes get that wrong, and what we can do to manage things better. It became a veritable textbook of lessons on what can go awry in assessing side effects and brought about major changes in the way we approach prescription drug risks and policies to this day.

A Test Case

In 1967 Mike Humeston, a few years older than me, was serving combat duty as a Marine in Vietnam when a mortar round pierced his left knee with shrapnel. He was awarded two Purple Hearts, but the wound left him in chronic pain for the rest of his life. That year, I was a premed college kid protesting the war and writing exposés for the student newspaper about the university's involvement in military research. About four decades would pass before Humeston's path and mine would cross.

By the 1990s, the research unit I was building at Harvard Medical School had gathered momentum. We were creating new ways to teach doctors about the risks and benefits of prescription drugs and developing an innovative method to study medication use and side effects: using powerful computers to scan the prescriptions of drugs taken by millions of patients and link that to the clinical events that appeared in their medical records. In 1991, I wrote a paper, "Epidemiology in Plato's Cave: Claims Data and Clinical Reality," arguing that the "shadows" cast by billing data could be a useful way to track the filled prescriptions and medical outcomes of large populations of people. I collected scores of nine-track reels of tape holding anonymized data on the medication use and clinical events of tens of thousands of patients in Medicaid, Medicare, and any other programs that would send them to me.

During those years, Mike Humeston was working at the U.S. postal facility in Boise, moving heavy sacks of mail from trucks and carrying them across the warehouse floor, making his chronic knee symptoms worse. In 2001, his doctor suggested a relatively new medication made by Merck, called Vioxx. It was seen as a major advance in pain treatment, and Humeston began taking it.

In September 2001 Humeston, then fifty-six, was watching the evening news when he felt a pressing, crushing pain in his chest. The symptoms of a heart attack are sometimes subtle or even absent. But when they're classic, they can point to the diagnosis like a laser. "If a patient ever tells you they feel like an elephant is sitting on their chest," a teacher told me when I was a medical student, "or makes a clenched fist in front of his thorax to describe the pain, admit him right away and work him up; he's probably having an MI." (Myocardial infarction is the medical term for heart attack, two words Humeston would hear often over the next six years.) As his cardiogram tracing spooled out in the emergency room, it was clear: he was having a heart attack.

As data began to emerge linking Vioxx to cardiac events, he sued Merck on the grounds that Vioxx was the cause. The company said it wasn't. Who was right?

How can we know which bad clinical events are drug side effects, and which would have happened anyway? Sometimes that's pretty clear. In 1937, a drug company chemist took an early antimicrobial, sulfanilamide, and dissolved it in a new solvent to make a syrup that would be tastier for children to ingest. We now know the solvent, diethylene glycol, as the main ingredient in antifreeze. It was understood at the time to be poisonous, but checking for lethality was not yet a requirement for producing medicines; the elixir was distributed widely across the country. The story was well described in an FDA publication; here is the account of A. S. Calhoun, one physician who prescribed it:

> Any doctor who has practiced more than a quarter of a century has seen his share of death. But to realize that six human beings, all of them my patients, one of them my best friend, are dead because they took medicine that I prescribed for them innocently, and to realize that that medicine which I had used for years in

> such cases suddenly had become a deadly poison in its newest and most modern form, as recommended by a great and reputable pharmaceutical firm in Tennessee: well, that realization has given me such days and nights of mental and spiritual agony as I did not believe a human being could undergo and survive. I have known hours when death for me would be a welcome relief from this agony.

The mother of a young victim of the toxicity disaster wrote to President Franklin Roosevelt and pleaded with him to put better drug safeguards in place:

> The first time I ever had occasion to call in a doctor for [Joan] and she was given Elixir of Sulfanilamide. All that is left to us is the caring for her little grave. Even the memory of her is mixed with sorrow for we can see her little body tossing to and fro and hear that little voice screaming with pain and it seems as though it would drive me insane. . . . It is my plea that you will take steps to prevent such sales of drugs that will take little lives and leave such suffering behind and such a bleak outlook on the future as I have tonight.

The product had been made by the Massengill Company. Dr. Samuel Massengill, the firm's owner, responded by noting:

> My chemists and I deeply regret the fatal results, but there was no error in the manufacture of the product. We have been supplying a legitimate professional demand and not once could have foreseen the unlooked-for results. I do not feel that there was any responsibility on our part.

The tragedy came to be known as the Massengill Massacre. The name of the company survives today as a widely selling feminine hygiene product. The owner lives on in another way: the Urban Dictionary defines "Massengill" as "A slang term for someone who can be correctly classified as a douche."

Over a hundred people, mostly children, died after taking the sulfanilamide elixir before it could be recalled. So did the chemist who made the formulation change; he did not adopt Dr. Massengill's posture of innocence, and took his own life. The FDA commissioner of the day, Walter Campbell, noted how easily these events could have been prevented by requiring simple toxicology testing, and how inevitable future tragedies would be if new laws were not put in place:

> These unfortunate occurrences may be expected to continue because new and relatively untried drug preparations are being manufactured almost daily at the whim of the individual manufacturer, and the damage to public health cannot accurately be estimated. The only remedy for such a situation is the enactment by Congress of an adequate and comprehensive national Food and Drugs Act which will require that all medicines placed upon the market shall be safe to use under the directions for use.

The tragedy led to a new and radical-seeming requirement in 1938 that modified the thirty-two-year-old federal Food and Drug law of 1906: henceforth, a manufacturer would have to test its products to ensure that they were not poisonous.

A Heroic Government Employee

Years later another side-effect scandal, this one involving birth defects, led to the next transformation of our drug regulatory apparatus. In 1960 Frances Kelsey, a young Canadian doctor with a PhD in pharmacology joined the FDA as one of only eleven physicians reviewing drugs there. One of her first assignments was the evaluation of Kevadon, a medicine widely used around the world as a sedative and antinauseant, especially in pregnant women; its manufacturer sought permission to market it in the U.S. The drug had been touted overseas for its lack of adverse effects, since an older category of sedatives, the barbiturates, could lead to overdose or addiction. In fact, a 1960 ad in Britain for Distaval (another brand name for the same product) promoted its safety by showing an adorable toddler snatching pill bottles from an open medicine cabinet; the ad warned that competing products like barbiturates were a common cause of accidental poisoning. Distaval, the ad pointed out, didn't pose that risk.

The drug's manufacturer expected quick approval in the U.S., but Dr. Kelsey was concerned that she hadn't seen adequate studies of its safety. Instead, she was sent testimonials from happy pregnant women in other countries who lauded the drug's effects in relieving their nausea, helping them get a good night's sleep, or both. Dr. Kelsey explained to her supervisor that this was not the same as actual facts and figures, and asked for more safety information. The manufacturer objected, and the request was depicted as yet another example of an inefficient government bureaucrat keeping a needed treatment from the American public. But as the back-and-forth wore on, disturbing individual case reports began to appear in Australia, Great Britain, and other countries. Doctors wrote to medical journals that they were seeing babies with phocomelia—a very rare fetal malformation in which a child is born with stubby flippers instead of normally formed limbs. The reports identified various drugs taken by the mothers during pregnancy, but initially no clear pattern emerged, since the drug was being sold under many different names all over the world.

No systematic international system was in place for detecting drug side effects, so it took a while to put the pieces together. The drug was thalidomide, and Kevadon was one of its many international trade names. Dr. Kelsey's demand to see more safety data kept it off the market in the U.S. Elsewhere, thousands of babies with phocomelia were born to mothers who had taken it during the first trimester of pregnancy. But thanks to Dr. Kelsey's efforts, there were very few cases in the U.S. The few that did occur here were the children of women who had obtained the drug from overseas or had participated in manufacturer-sponsored "seeding trials," in which a company would distribute an unapproved drug to doctors as part of so-called studies whose main purpose was to open the way to market introduction after FDA approval. Dr. Kelsey was declared a hero, and John Kennedy awarded her the President's Award for Distinguished Federal Civilian Service in a White House ceremony. But a more enduring legacy of her work was the way it prodded the nation to rethink drug regulation, spurring the passage of the Kefauver amendments in 1962, requiring companies for the first time ever to provide the government with clinical trial evidence that their drugs worked and were safe before they could be sold.

Hundreds of years ago, Indigenous people discovered that scraping the bark of the willow tree yielded a substance that could relieve pain and swelling; it became a mainstay of prescientific medicine and home remedies. From the time Bayer introduced its own synthetic version of that substance and named it "Aspirin" around the turn of the twentieth century, these compounds became ubiquitous in medicine. Aspirin was the world's first multipotent wonder drug: it relieved pain, it lowered fevers, it reduced inflammation. The 1982 Nobel Prize in Medicine was awarded to three academic researchers—two Swedes and one Englishman—for explaining that the action of such compounds was mediated through a class of hormone-like substances known as prostaglandins, so named because they were first found in seminal fluid.

By the 1990s, researchers came up with a variant of aspirin they hoped would work even better: ibuprofen, now marketed widely as Advil and Motrin. It was the first entrant in the new class of NSAIDs—nonsteroidal anti-inflammatory drugs. (They were called that because they reduced inflammation as steroids do, but weren't steroids. Aspirin itself is an NSAID, but the new term added some cachet for ibuprofen and its cousins that followed in rapid succession.) All these drugs had a common property: they worked by inhibiting the effect of the enzyme cyclooxygenase, or Cox for short, that mediated the production of those key prostaglandins and related compounds. The Cox enzyme was partly responsible for the pain, inflammation, and fever that patients and doctors seek to reduce. But the years of basic pharmacology research that led up to the 1982 Nobel made it clear that Cox also did some very good things, including protecting the lining of the stomach and intestine and preventing bleeding. Inhibiting those good effects could cause gastrointestinal hemorrhage, a common and worrisome side effect of all these drugs. Aspirin and the other NSAIDs tuned down *all* the prostaglandins made by the Cox enzymes; that reduced pain and inflammation, but it also lowered the ability of the GI tract to protect itself, a problem for all drugs in that class.

Researchers sought ways to inhibit the bad functions of Cox while leaving alone its good ones, especially the protection of the stomach and intestines. During the 1990s, several research teams, primarily in academic medical centers and funded by the National Institutes of Health, tried to separate out those good and bad Cox functions. A scientist at Brigham Young University (BYU) discovered the Cox-2 variant of the enzyme. A team at the University of Rochester further clarified that Cox-1 was responsible for its good effects, and Cox-2 was the cause of the gastrointestinal bleeding. The Rochester researchers even devised a way to determine the extent to which new NSAIDs could selectively inhibit Cox-2 vs. Cox-1.

Drug companies immediately saw the enormous clinical and commercial advantage of a *selective* Cox inhibitor that could block the pain and inflammation effects of one of the Cox enzymes while sparing the protective effects of the other. By the late 1990s, almost exactly a hundred years after Bayer first marketed aspirin, the Cox-2 competition came down to two companies: the U.S. pharmaceutical giant Merck, which was developing Vioxx, and G. D. Searle, which was developing Celebrex. Searle was later bought by Pharmacia, which was then acquired by Pfizer. (For simplicity, we'll just refer to Celebrex as Pfizer's drug.) The companies raced to market drugs that could selectively inhibit the Cox-2 enzyme discovered at BYU; the assay designed at Rochester helped to predict which new compounds would be able to do that. BYU had signed a royalty agreement to help develop the drug that became Celebrex, but had trouble collecting. It had to sue Pfizer to get paid, with the drugmaker delaying that settlement for years, until 2012. The Rochester scientists also asked for royalties on the medications based on their research, but the companies said their claim was invalid. That refusal was held up by the courts, which ruled that while the Rochester research on identifying Cox-selective compounds was crucial to the development of these drugs, the companies had patented the actual drug molecules, not the university researchers.

Once Pfizer came to own the drug discovered by Searle, they and Merck went on to conduct the cumbersome and expensive randomized controlled trials necessary to show that their drugs were effective in reducing pain and inflammation. Celebrex was approved by the FDA on the last day of 1998; Merck's Vioxx was approved five months later. The race for market share was on.

But by the early 2000s, some studies had begun to raise the question of whether selective inhibition of Cox-2 might also have a downside. Cox-2 also mediated the production of the "good" prostaglandin prostacyclin, which helped keep arteries dilated and inhibited blood clotting. It was in constant equilibrium with another prostaglandin-related substance, thromboxane, which had opposite effects. In theory, blocking the beneficial effects of prostacyclin could increase the risk of blood clots, causing heart attacks and strokes. But in the enthusiasm over the GI benefits of blocking just Cox-2, the risks of these other effects were minimized. Early research on Vioxx in animals and humans did reveal some possible signals of this clotting risk, with a few more heart attacks and strokes than expected in dogs and people given the new drug. These signals weren't judged to be important, and defenders of the drug argued that the expected reduction in gastrointestinal hemorrhage would outweigh these risks even if they were real. Vioxx and Celebrex quickly became two of the best-selling drugs in the world. Reports of cardiac damage continued to emerge as the drugs came into extremely wide use in the early 2000s.

A Causal Association, or a Casual One?

In denying any connection between cardiovascular problems and its product, Merck made this case: Millions of people take Vioxx. Many of them are old or have high cholesterol or high blood pressure—known risk factors for heart attacks and strokes. And millions of people suffer those events every day. In any given patient, how could you prove that this drug caused their particular heart attack? This might be described as the "shit happens" defense. At fifty-six, Mike Humeston was not particularly old, didn't smoke, and wasn't overweight; he did have elevated cholesterol, as tens of millions of Americans do. The company argued that this made it impossible to attribute his heart attack to Vioxx. How could anyone ever know whether the drug caused the cardiac event? The question was a vital one for doctors, patients and, increasingly, lawyers.

By 2000, nearly forty years after the Kefauver amendments ensured that prescription drugs actually worked, physicians and patients had hundreds of effective new medications at our disposal. But not much had changed in how we learned about their safety once they were in widespread use. An increasingly powerful pharmaceutical industry resisted additional regulation or oversight; it would take another national crisis to bring about change: Vioxx would become the sulfanilamide and the thalidomide of our time.

Shotguns, Not Lasers

"Every drug you prescribe will have at least two effects," a wise old clinician once told me. "The one you expect, and the one you don't." Most patients think we know all about drug risks or can access that information readily, but neither is true. Ideally, company-run trials or FDA requirements would reveal much of what we need to know about this in some detail, but they don't. Several steps in the development of a prescription drug can provide vital evidence about where those unexpected effects might turn up, and in the case of Vioxx, Merck managed to misinterpret the data, or misrepresent it, at every point. First is the *biology* of how the molecule does what it does—what biochemical pathways in the body it affects. Second are the *tests in animals* required before a new drug can even be studied in humans. Inevitably, many drugs don't emerge from these stages with a totally clean bill of health. Sometimes early problems can kill a promising new product—one reason why drug discovery is so expensive. Or an abnormal finding will turn up that bears watching. If it's mild or very rare, it may not be enough to block further evaluation; if that happened, we'd have hardly any new drugs. Rather, these signals can flag issues to keep a close eye on as the medicine progresses further through its testing and eventual use.

Next come the *clinical trials* that a drug must undergo to determine if it actually works. Were some adverse events more common in patients given the new product, compared to controls? The accurate and timely *reporting of these results* is a vital part of this stage of drug development. That sounds embarrassingly obvious, but it's sometimes done incompletely, late, in a distorted way, or not at all. Last comes the *systematic follow-up of huge numbers of typical patients* who take the drug once it's been approved for widespread use. That didn't start being done routinely and on a large scale until after 2007—an advance we owe to the Vioxx crisis.

Building the Franchise

Initially, the FDA approved Celebrex and Vioxx as garden-variety NSAIDs just like ibuprofen (Advil, Motrin) and naproxen (Naprosyn, Aleve) to treat pain and inflammation in arthritis and other conditions. But in light of their more elegant capacity to selectively inhibit just the bad Cox-2 enzyme, each company sought FDA permission to promote their new product as safer than existing NSAIDs because they would be less likely to cause gastrointestinal bleeding. Merck had done a study of volunteers, many of them medical students, who were given the new drug or a comparison product and then had an endoscope passed into their stomachs to look for bleeding. Sure enough, those given Vioxx had fewer small bleeding points than the controls. But the FDA, to its credit, said that wasn't enough to warrant a promotional claim that these drugs would reduce the risk of clinically important GI hemorrhage. The agency stood firm on the principle that for both Vioxx and Celebrex, that claim would have to be proven in a randomized trial evaluating actual GI bleeding, and not rest simply on an elegant pharmacological hypothesis and the view from inside medical students' stomachs. (Today, given the agency's much greater willingnesss to accept surrogate measures, it might have been satisfied with that and not have required a large clinical trial—with disastrous results.)

The FDA took the position that for either company to claim its drug was gentler on the GI tract, it would have to conduct large clinical trials randomizing patients to take the newer drug or an older NSAID, and then follow them to see how many in each group developed a clinically important GI bleed; both firms rushed to begin these studies. In the end each trial became a notorious example of dishonest reporting of findings; their infamy has persisted for over two decades as cautionary tales of scientific misconduct.

What the COX-2 Drugs Revealed about Clinical Trial Reports

Drugmakers like to give catchy acronyms to high-profile clinical studies, so the makers of Celebrex named their study CLASS, for Celecoxib Long-term Arthritis Safety Study, and Merck named its study VIGOR, for Vioxx Gastrointestinal Outcomes Research. Other industry-funded trials around that time were named ACCORD (Action to Control Cardiovascular Risk in Diabetes), CHARISMA (Clopidogrel for High Atherothrombotic Risk, Ischemic Stabilization, Management, and Avoidance), and one of my favorites, CRASH (Corticosteroid Randomization After Significant Head Injury)—and that's just a few from *A* through *C*. By contrast, during the same years a vitally important federal trial enrolled over 68,000 women to determine whether estrogen treatment reduced the risk of heart disease (it didn't), or increased the risk of breast cancer (it did); it was named WHI, for Women's Health Initiative, which I guess would be pronounced "Why?"—much less catchy.

A CLASS Act

With billions of dollars at stake, the Celebrex-Vioxx rivalry brought out the worst in each manufacturer. Pharmacia/Pfizer was eager to take advantage of its first-mover status. In September 2000, *JAMA* published a striking paper describing the findings of a trial the manufacturer had conducted in which patients were randomly assigned to take either Celebrex or older NSAIDs. The paper's authors included academic researchers from medical centers throughout the country, along with six employees of the sponsoring company; the second author was the former head of post-approval drug safety research for the FDA, who had become a private consultant.

CLASS followed over eight thousand volunteers to see who developed gastrointestinal hemorrhage. Physicians, patients, and Wall Street were impressed to learn that when evaluated six months after the trial began, people randomized to take Celebrex had a substantially lower rate of GI bleeding than those randomized to take an older NSAID. The difference was clinically impressive as well as statistically significant; the study seemed to vindicate the benefits of selectively inhibiting the Cox-2 receptor, with enormous implications for patient care as well as for Pfizer's economic success.

But just over a year later, it turned out that the paper published in *JAMA* reflected selective inhibition of the study's findings, not just of cellular receptors. The six-month data did look impressive, but the trial had been designed as a twelve-month comparison, and the full results did not confirm the findings of the first half. Worse, the full twelve months of data were already available when the original paper was written, but the authors chose to report only the more favorable findings of the first six months. Following the debacle, in a virtually unprecedented move the editors of most of the major medical journals coauthored a statement, "Sponsorship, Authorship, and Accountability," which they published concurrently in twelve high-profile journals, decrying the contamination of clinical research findings by industry funding. But the deceptions surrounding Merck's parallel study of Vioxx turned out to be even greater.

Vigorous Deception

In VIGOR, a costly and difficult trial, Merck identified thousands of people with rheumatoid arthritis who required hefty doses of an NSAID, and randomly assigned them to take either Vioxx or an older NSAID, naproxen (marketed as Naprosyn, and now over-the-counter as Aleve). The idea was that naproxen, like nearly all other widely used NSAIDs, indiscriminately blocked both Cox-1 and Cox-2, while Vioxx would block primarily the "bad" Cox-2 enzyme. The company recruited about 8,000 patients from 301 centers in 22 countries around the world—a massive and expensive undertaking—and randomly assigned them to take Vioxx or naproxen. The research subjects were then followed for an average of nine months to see how many in each group developed a GI bleed.

About ten weeks after the problematic CLASS trial came out in *JAMA*, in November 2000 the *New England Journal of Medicine* published the VIGOR trial on Thanksgiving Day. At first, it looked like the study would give Merck a lot to be thankful for. The paper, appearing in the most prestigious medical journal in the world, showed that Vioxx provided pain relief as good as that seen with naproxen, *and* also reduced the incidence of gastrointestinal bleeding. The findings would soon enable the company to make that claim officially in its communication materials to doctors and patients. The FDA would allow Merck to widely expand its marketing to both audiences, and Vioxx became the most heavily promoted product in the country's direct-to-consumer advertising of prescription drugs. The company's budget for promoting Vioxx to patients reached $161 million the year after VIGOR was published, more than PepsiCo spent to promote Pepsi, or Budweiser spent to advertise its beer. Along with an aggressive selling campaign to doctors, this quadrupled the drug's annual sales to $1.5 billion by the end of 2001—a substantial part of the record $20 billion increase in sales of all drugs in the U.S. that year.

I recall the excitement that the VIGOR paper generated among practitioners like me when it came out. The study seemed to elegantly show how an insight from basic pharmacology could lead to a new drug that proved the initial concept and offered an important advance for patients. But in passing in the results section of the *NEJM* VIGOR paper, its authors wrote this: "Myocardial infarctions were less common in the naproxen group than in the rofecoxib [Vioxx] group." That meant that in the patients randomized to receive naproxen, the authors explained, only a quarter as many had a heart attack as those given Vioxx. And the difference met the high bar of statistical significance, uncommon for side-effect comparisons. At first, this elegant bit of verbal jiujitsu didn't attract a lot of attention. But normally, if researchers find a higher rate of a side effect for a new medication, it's described as an *increase* in risk in patients who took that drug, not as a *protective effect* of the comparison drug. But Merck was known to take a particularly heavy-handed role in writing up the results of the trials it funded, as we later learned in our own research. And this was the heyday of the belief that the oldest NSAID, aspirin, could prevent cardiac events, a concept put forward in a major study by physicians in another part of our own Department of Medicine at the Brigham. (That idea has since fallen out of favor as a general rule: for people who haven't had a prior cardiovascular event a daily aspirin will lower that risk, but the increased bleeding it causes outweighs the benefit. This is another example of the old adage "Use the new discoveries as soon as you can, while they still work." Daily low-dose aspirin is now recommended only for people who have already had a heart attack or stroke. Otherwise, the benefit-risk trade-off isn't worth it.)

Dr. Lou Sherwood, Merck's senior vice president for research, visited the Brigham after the publication of VIGOR and I asked him about the difference in heart attack rates. His answer was dismissive: "That's just because naproxen seems to prevent MIs. Like aspirin. It's an interesting side observation." But that explanation didn't take into account the fact that if naproxen produced a *three- or fourfold* lowering of heart attack risk, that would mean it reduced the risk of heart attack *by 75 percent*, which would be a clinical miracle unprecedented in the annals of preventive medicine, and a boon for disease prevention. But it wasn't being used that way. Which interpretation was right?

A Power Struggle

I used to give a lecture to Harvard medical students that I called "Pharmaco-epistemology," but the title scared away a lot of them. Yet all of us—prescribers, patients, policymakers—need to understand where the drug information we use comes from and what it's based on, so we can know what to do with it. Many people, including many doctors, apparently believe that the FDA itself tests drugs before they're allowed on the market. They don't. As we've seen, the nation has long preferred to outsource the design, funding, and conduct of those vital studies to the companies seeking to market a drug. Discussions occur between FDA staff and the manufacturer about study design and what kind of data would be needed to win approval, but in the end the conduct and literally the ownership of those pivotal trials and their data traditionally remained in the hands of the drugmaker sponsoring the product. There are potentially dozens of ways to structure a clinical trial: what kinds of patients are included or excluded, what outcomes are measured and how, even how long the trial lasts. Each can tip the scales in an often-predictable direction, as occurred in the key studies of Vioxx. These pivotal clinical trials can cost hundreds of millions of dollars to conduct, and then shape the use of drugs that can generate even larger amounts in potential sales each year, sometimes into the billions. That's why drugmakers like to perform and pay for these studies themselves.

The occasional distortion of findings from company-funded clinical trials also poisons the well of trust in all such sponsorship. Concerned that this mistrust might inhibit the uptake of important findings from solid industry-sponsored research, Kesselheim and I published a study in *NEJM* in which we presented over five hundred internists with the results of hypothetical studies of three new drugs. Telling them the study was sponsored by a drugmaker sharply reduced readers' willingness to believe the results and their interest in prescribing the new product. Sometimes skepticism can go too far.

2001: Things Begin to Unravel, and Our Team Gets Involved

If the "naproxen is good for you" talking point was wrong and Vioxx tripled or quadrupled the risk of heart attack, would its gentler-on-the-stomach advantage still be worth it? After all, most GI bleeds caused by NSAIDs aren't lethal. While catastrophic hemorrhages do occur, most of the problems can be detected early and their worst consequences usually prevented by stopping the drug and implementing other measures. But heart attacks cause permanent damage: not all patients survive them, and if they do it's often with a piece of dead tissue replacing some of their cardiac muscle.

Unfortunately, the FDA generally doesn't weigh in with much nuance on such risk-benefit trade-offs. It lists the adverse effects reported by the manufacturer, but usually doesn't quantify them very well in comparison with a drug's benefits, and it doesn't deal with the most important issue we doctors and our patients face: *Are this drug's benefits worth its risks, compared with other alternatives?*

Merck's answer to this question when it came to Vioxx was more about promotion than benefit-vs.-harm considerations. *It works as well as existing NSAIDs!* (There was never any credible evidence that the drug was actually better at reducing pain or inflammation.) *And it's better for your GI tract!* TV ads starred Olympians Dorothy Hamill swooshing around on the ice and decathelete Bruce Jenner (before he transitioned to Caitlyn Jenner), along with testimonials from both athletes.

FDA rules concerning those annoying drug ads to consumers require the manufacturer to describe side effects and risks in any commercial that promotes a medication for a particular condition, even if that description is done at breakneck speed while distracting visual images fly by. But that's not required for an ad that just mentions the disease but not the drug, or the drug name without any reference to a disease. To evade the requirement of discussing risks, Merck ran two Hamill mini-commercials: one with her skating around that named Vioxx but didn't mention pain or arthritis, and another with her skating around that mentioned arthritis but not Vioxx. The latter contained the familiar tag line "Ask your doctor . . ." about available treatments for arthritis, along with a 1-888-MERCK phone number.

Despite the enduring questions, the company got what it needed from the VIGOR trial. It was now taking in over a billion dollars a year on Vioxx, but the difference in heart attack risk seen in VIGOR was still not resolved. Fueled by heavy promotion, the product's use kept increasing along with its revenues. Like many physicians in the early 2000s, I prescribed Vioxx selectively, for patients who needed an NSAID but were at increased risk of gastrointestinal bleeding. But with every prescription I wrote, I wondered: Is the good I'm doing in lowering their bleeding risk worth the possibility of increasing their chance of heart attack? Without any new clinical trials likely to be done, could we learn something from the extensive experience of the millions of people who were now taking the drug? Were they having strokes or heart attacks at a higher rate than similar people prescribed other NSAIDs? This seemed like an ideal question to answer by mining the hundreds of thousands of records we had amassed of "real-world" patient experience, using the tools of pharmacoepidemiology that my group and others were developing.

Is the Signal Real?

Pharmacoepidemiologists like those in our research group can scan the medication use and clinical outcomes of millions of people to help figure out how they might be connected. But in doing so we have to deal with the same problem faced for millennia by sentries patrolling the edge of a city, or more recently by radar technicians scanning blips on a screen. For the former, was that a wolf or an enemy attacker? For the latter, is that a foreign missile, or a Chinese spy balloon, or a flock of geese? Getting these calls wrong in either direction can be catastrophic. And the chance of making such an error when you work for a company that has billions of dollars riding on that call makes difficult decision-making even more challenging.

For decades, the FDA had a kind of attention deficit disorder concerning drugs it has already approved. Despite the millions of dollars that flow to it annually from user fees paid by industry, the agency continues to see itself (sometimes plausibly) as chronically understaffed and overwhelmed. One way it has historically dealt with this is by limiting its focus primarily to paying obsessive attention to all details of new submissions. To its credit, unlike drug-regulatory bodies elsewhere, it rereviews all the clinical trial results that companies send in, at a patient-by-patient level if needed, setting a standard for rigor unparalleled elsewhere. But after approval, the agency was traditionally in the habit of paying much less attention to outcomes of the drugs it had already okayed.

Until the Vioxx debacle, the FDA relied for that information primarily on spontaneous reports concerning individual patients that were submitted by doctors, pharmacists, drug companies, or patients themselves. The idea was that people would voluntarily fill out and send in forms (generally by fax, in those days) describing anything suspicious that happened to a patient taking a particular drug. It's easy to see all the ways this could go wrong, and it did go wrong in all those ways. No doctor or pharmacist is eager to have a new set of official forms to fill out; there are also the unappealing professional and legal problems that could be caused by sending the government a report that says, in essence, "I prescribed this drug to a patient and then something bad happened to them." Not surprisingly, it's been estimated that well over 90 percent of drug-induced side effects are never reported to the FDA.

For common events like heart attacks, it's also hard for any individual doctor caring for a single patient to conclude much about causation—whether the drug precipitated the problem or not. Once these forms arrived at the inboxes of harried FDA workers—at a rate of about a thousand a day in the Vioxx era—staffers would examine each, sometimes seek some additional information from the reporting source, and tabulate what was submitted. The "rates" thus estimated weren't really rates at all, given their very sketchy numerators and often-unknown denominators. Most of us in this field don't take such analyses too seriously. As a wise epidemiologist once noted, the plural of "anecdote" is not "data." The absence of any decent external numbers enabled Merck to deny that any of the Vioxx plaintiffs' heart attacks were caused by the drug. After all, many of these people were old, or had heart disease, or risk factors like hypertension or diabetes. The FDA hadn't initially made any effective demands on Merck to start a systematic surveillance program of its drug for that problem, even after the suggestive signal in VIGOR came out.

Every major drug trial empanels a separate Data and Safety Monitoring Board (DSMB) charged with arm's-length oversight of trial results as they come in. Such committees conduct confidential rolling assessments of clinical findings as they emerge, and can unblind the results if such ethical issues seem to be developing—in either direction. In December 1999, the safety committee for the VIGOR study was shown unblinded data indicating that more heart attacks and deaths might be occurring in patients randomized to Vioxx rather than naproxen. The committee told Merck to establish a new plan to follow cardiac events in trial patients; the company was at first reluctant to do so, but eventually agreed to an interim analysis. The DSMB was led by a smart and affable rheumatologist with considerable clinical trial experience, the kind of talented expert clinician to whom you'd send your mother. Awkwardly, later media accounts reported that his family had significant holdings of Merck stock, and that while his discussions with the company were going on he signed a new consulting agreement with them for future work at the rate of $5,000 per day.

During 2001, the VIGOR advantage continued to unravel. As the trial wound down, Merck continued to count the outcomes favoring their product (fewer GI bleeds), even after it stopped counting the bad study outcome, heart attacks—a violation of the most basic rule of evenhanded treatment of trial data. Worse, it later emerged that the VIGOR data submitted for publication had omitted some heart attacks that had occurred in the Vioxx group. The company reported the missing events to the FDA, as it was legally obliged to do. But it didn't correct the paper before *NEJM* published it.

Tensions increased further when a team of cardiologists from the Cleveland Clinic published a paper in *JAMA* reanalyzing the heart disease findings from Cox-2 trials including VIGOR, adding back in the additional heart attacks Merck had left out; it confirmed the increased risk of cardiac events and cast further doubt on the idea that the VIGOR findings were the result of some protective effect of naproxen. As additional improprieties piled up, the editors of *NEJM* published not one but two unusual "Expressions of Concern" on their editorial pages, accusing the company and the VIGOR authors of misleading analytical practices. The company claimed there was no problem and the drug remained on the market, with sales eventually reaching $2.5 billion a year in the U.S. alone.

By 2003, the stage was set for a historic drug scandal that would force the nation to rethink a number of issues—problems that were well known to many of us in the drug research community, but until then had been largely ignored by the wider medical and regulatory worlds:

- relying on spontaneous reports of individual cases of suspected side effects is a totally inadequate way for the FDA to track drug safety;
- allowing drug manufacturers to have unfettered control over the design and conduct of their clinical trials can produce dangerously skewed results;
- keeping study data secret can lead to distorted reporting of both benefits and harms;
- when billions of dollars of product sales are at stake, people sometimes do bad things.

CHAPTER 6

Downfall of a Giant

> We try never to forget that medicine is for the people. It is not for the profits. The profits follow, and if we have remembered that, they have never failed to appear.
>
> —George W. Merck, president, Merck & Co., 1929

In Boston, my colleagues and I had been expanding our racks and racks of magnetic tapes describing all filled prescriptions and clinical encounters for thousands of anonymized patients, to fuel our research on medication use and outcomes. We realized we could explore the Vioxx–heart disease question by analyzing the millions of data points we had accumulated on the patients who took the drug versus another NSAID, and what happened to them. We'd have to control for multiple factors, including the age, gender, diagnoses, and underlying cardiac risk of each patient, as well as all the other drugs they were taking. But our emerging field of pharmacoepidemiology was developing powerful tools to adjust for those differences.

Here is how the approach works: every time a patient fills a prescription at a pharmacy or sees a doctor or is admitted to a hospital, detailed information about each event is entered into a computer—not to help academics like me with our research, but simply to process the payments. All this information, generated automatically each day all over the country, offered an enormous collection of very rich data to work with. Since the early 1980s, I had been collecting such paid claims data from entities like Medicaid, Medicare, other state drug benefit programs, and the health insurance companies that pay drugstores, doctors, and hospitals. After removing personal identifiers to protect patients' privacy, we assembled the data into huge databases that enabled us to analyze patterns of medication use and outcomes for hundreds of thousands of people. No doctors, patients, or pharmacists had to fill out any forms or make any judgments about what might have caused what. We just let the payment system do its thing, and then harvested the copious data that flowed from it.

In those early days of the field, our developing approach reminded me of the development of the microscope by Antoine van Leeuwenhoek, the Dutchman who perfected that tool in the late 1600s. It enabled him to study everyday objects in a way that made it possible to see for the first time a universe of structures and creatures that had been there all along, but were now suddenly visible. Another common thread with our work was that his day job was in the textile industry; he started out using his new tool to assess the quality of the fabric he was buying and selling, just as our work with billing data records rested on the commercial rather than the biological side of health care.

Our work in this area was strengthened considerably by recruiting Sebastian Schneeweiss, a German-trained physician who joined our program while he was doing his doctoral work in epidemiology at the Harvard School of Public Health, and many years later succeeded me as chief of our division. With other DoPE faculty, he developed innovative methods to address the key "Compared to what?" question—though here it was really "Compared to whom?" As we've seen, since observational studies lack the awesome power of being able to randomize people to get one treatment versus another, we have to deal with the world as we find it, with people taking whatever their doctors prescribed to them. But what if a new drug (like Vioxx) were being used in routine care preferentially on just the sicker patients? Or older ones? Or those with more cardiac risk? Or less? Sebastian and our colleagues used increasingly powerful computers and methods to examine all the characteristics of each of the people who took one drug in a class versus another, and employed that information to adjust for all those differences, so that any differences we saw in their outcomes could be attributed to the medication they took, rather than to their underlying differences at the outset. Would it have been cleaner to just do a new clinical trial that randomized thousands of patients to get one drug versus another? Sure. But randomized trials take years to arrange and conduct, cost tens or hundreds of millions of dollars, and may still not give us the answers we need—just look at VIGOR. By contrast, observational studies of the kind we could do in our increasingly large and detailed databases could include tens of thousands of typical patients getting routine care, assess any outcomes we want, and be completed in a tiny fraction of that time and at much lower cost. All the filled prescriptions and clinical outcomes we wanted to look at had already occurred and were sitting in the bowels of our computers just waiting to be studied.

There was another way our growing field of pharmacoepidemiology could produce results even better than those of a randomized clinical study: understanding the outcomes of medications in populations that are often underrepresented in clinical trials, like the elderly or racial and ethnic minorities, or that are usually omitted altogether, like pregnant women. It's ethically problematic to include the latter group in drug trials, unless a medication is designed to treat pregnancy-related problems. So for routine drugs like antidepressants, seizure medications, cardiac treatments, and scores of others, doctors just don't have clear answers about their safety in these patients. This is an area where observational studies can shine. In the course of regular care, some doctors caring for pregnant women will stop some of these drugs, while others will continue them. If one could study the records of hundreds of thousands of pregnant women along with those of their offspring, and adjust for all measurable differences between those who took certain drugs during pregnancy and those who didn't, you could do some powerful analyses of any links that might exist between that drug use and the course of their pregnancies—including effects on the fetus or newborn. That research in our program was led by Krista Huybrechts, a Belgian-born epidemiologist who started her work in DoPE, as Sebastian did, when she was a graduate student, as did Niteesh Choudhry, a Canadian-trained internist. Krista's collaborator in our division was Brian Bateman, who began working with me when he was still a resident studying anesthesia. Sebastian, Krista, and Niteesh are now professors of medicine at Harvard; after years of collaboration in DoPE, Brian became chair of the Anesthesiology Department at Stanford. Another multi-year collaborator at DoPE was Til Stürmer, who went on to become chair of epidemiology at the University of North Carolina. One of the joys of building and running our program has been the ability to work with smart researchers from the very start of their careers and see them develop so well. I described the early evolution of this aspect of DoPE's research in more detail in *Powerful Medicines.*

Back to our Vioxx question: If the selective Cox-2 inhibitors like Vioxx did cause heart attacks and strokes, then our databases of filled prescriptions and clinical events could enable us to figure that out by examining the detailed medication use and clinical histories of the people taking them: we could try to see whether cardiac problems were more common in patients who used Vioxx compared to similar people taking other NSAIDs. My colleague Dan Solomon had begun work with me when he was a medical resident at the Brigham and continued through his fellowship there in rheumatology; I then asked him to join the DoPE faculty. After the VIGOR study came out, he and I asked some of the smartest senior doctors we knew whether they thought Vioxx caused heart attacks, and their answers were split down the middle. Yes, it probably could, based on the Cox-1/Cox-2 imbalance issue. No, it probably couldn't, since it was an aspirin-like drug, and Everybody Knew that aspirin prevented heart attacks. It was becoming clear that a large-scale observational study of people taking the drug in routine care might help answer the question. And we could make it more inclusive than VIGOR had been, since we didn't have Merck's incentive to exclude sicker subjects.

The team for the project included Solomon, who led it, epidemiologists Schneeweiss and Rhonda Bohn, statistician Bob Glynn, a Japanese physician-trainee named Yuka Kiyota, and a group of talented programmers who had joined our program after fleeing Russia during the Save Soviet Jewry emigrations of the 1980s. Together, we had built a database of hundreds of thousands of people for whom we had complete records of every filled prescription and clinical encounter. By 2002, we were ready to probe that data to see whether older people who had heart attacks were more likely to have taken Vioxx than similar drugs, after we adjusted for every discernable difference among them. To accomplish this we would use what then seemed like very big computers; I recall the excitement of one of our programmers in the early days that he'd get to use a machine with a whole gigabyte of memory.

Doing Our Own Research

All we needed was some funding to pay for programming, update the database, and cover the costs of our time. (Faculty in the clinical departments at Harvard have to generate their own salaries—a common arrangement in many teaching hospitals. Our program receives essentially no fiscal support from Harvard or the Brigham.) I approached the National Institutes of Health, but was told that it preferred to support research on the fundamental mechanisms of disease. "We don't fund Coke-versus-Pepsi studies," my contact there said, completely dismissing the fields of epidemiology and comparative effectiveness research with a snarky junk food metaphor. The Food and Drug Administration explained that it didn't have much of a budget for such external research, explaining helpfully, "We usually ask the companies to do that kind of work." Private foundations were a long shot, and I couldn't find any that would support this research with a rapid turnaround. Colleagues suggested that I ask Merck itself to fund the study. I was initially skeptical, knowing that billions of dollars might ride on the results. But with no other support available, I ran the question by Dr. Harry Guess, the company's head of epidemiology. A courtly, gentle southerner trained in pediatrics as well as epidemiology, he was an anomaly, working part-time as a faculty member at the University of North Carolina while overseeing post-approval drug surveillance at one of the world's largest pharmaceutical companies. The field of pharmacoepidemiology was new enough at that time that it was plausible for this to be a part-time job, even at a huge drugmaker.

"Merck has a responsibility to support a study like this," I told Harry, "especially given the questions VIGOR raised. You need to see yourselves as the stewards of the molecules you're offering the public, and that brings some responsibility." He agreed, and we began the lengthy process of negotiating a research contract. I required that we be able to conduct the study as we saw fit, and that we could publish any findings in whatever way seemed best to us. It was the academic equivalent of a film director requiring control over the final cut of the movie. He agreed.

Things got off to a promising start, but as the work progressed Harry was diagnosed with rapidly progressive lung cancer and had to hand over responsibility for the study to others at the company. Our relationship with Merck began to change. I had already learned about the problems that could come up in working with pharmaceutical companies to study the side effects of their products, and thought I knew how to redline proposed contracts to remove any troublesome language. The easiest phrases to delete were those that industry sponsors often tried to insert giving the company the right to approve the final results of the research before we could publish them; I'd cut those out on the first read-through. More subtle were requirements that the final payment would be delivered upon "satisfactory completion of the research," with "satisfactory" potentially meaning that the results were to the company's liking. Those phrases had to go also. Sometimes, there would be a two-part requirement that our unit would not divulge any confidential corporate information provided by the company during the research; that seemed plausible enough. But the other shoe might drop a few pages later in language declaring that all the results of our research were deemed to be confidential information.

The hospital lawyers often didn't catch these issues in those days, and I thought I had learned to deal with all the problematic phrases. But as our Vioxx–heart attack study progressed I realized that I had missed a key one. The basic case-control analysis we planned to use had been signed off on by Merck at the outset. We also agreed that we'd simply inform the company about details of our methods as the study progressed, which would trigger the next installment of payments. Proceeding in good faith on our end in retrospect appears to have been a naive mistake. No one ever told me we couldn't take a planned analytic step, but at several points along the way we were told that the study plan looked good, but that corporate sign-off, while expected, was taking longer than anticipated to work its way through the large bureaucracy. Sure, big company, I get it, I thought.

Slow-Walking the Study

Then came the request that we add an additional component to the research to make sure that the heart attack diagnoses sent to Medicare by the hospitals were valid. That would require working with each hospital to audit a sample of the actual (anonymized) medical records of the heart attack patients, to be certain that they really had had heart attacks. Claims-based pharmacoepidemiology was still a relatively young field, and it would be important to make sure that we got this pivotal study outcome right. We all wanted our methodology to be bulletproof, right? Merck would be pleased to provide more funding to support this additional step, because it was so important. Dan Solomon and I deputized Dr. Kiyota to oversee this painstaking work, which required getting photocopies of thick hospital records for some of the several thousand heart attack patients. We did the extra validation required, and were pleased to find that the data the hospitals had provided to Medicare on heart attacks was indeed reliable.

At the time, I thought of the delays as the inevitable product of dealing with a large corporation, and of a shared desire to do what was needed to get the most rigorous result using a relatively new analytic approach. It was only later that I found out that Merck already had internal data from its own clinical trials showing that Vioxx did indeed increase the risk of heart attack by threefold, which it was keeping secret. I had also failed to grasp some simple arithmetic in thinking about our relationship with the company. By 2003, Vioxx sales had reached about $2.5 billion annually. Divide that by 250 working days per year; if the study came up with findings that were unfavorable for the drug, any delay in reporting those results would protect $10 million of sales per day.

Under Solomon's leadership, despite these hurdles our study progressed well. The team came to include Carolyn Cannuscio, a bright young doctor who was finishing her doctoral work in epidemiology at Harvard and had applied for a job at Merck. Our colleagues at the company proposed her involvement as a link between our group and the drugmaker. She was a sharp researcher who was superbly trained, and it seemed like the plan would work out well for everyone.

As the months passed and the data came in, a clear picture emerged. We were finding a significantly higher rate of Vioxx use in patients who had heart attacks, compared to similar controls taking similar medications. More people were beginning to question the glib "naproxen is protective" explanation for the VIGOR findings, and other observational studies of large numbers of patients in routine care were also suggesting that the risk was real. By early 2003 we had enough information for Dan to write a paper to present that fall at the annual meeting of the American College of Rheumatology, the main professional society of doctors who deal with arthritis and related diseases. As provided in the contract, we informed Merck of this plan, and sent them a copy of the abstract to comment on, but not to change.

Disinformation and Deception

Merck hated the abstract; our new contacts there derided the findings and sent corporate emissaries to Boston to warn us that their internal data proved we were wrong and that we would become a laughingstock if we stood by our research. They told us that since our results couldn't be right, they shouldn't be reported. How could they be so sure? In the heyday of early Cox-2 ebullience, a theory arose that since Alzheimer's disease might be caused by an inflammatory response in the brain, inhibiting inflammation might also prevent the progression of that disease. (It didn't.) "We have data on thousands of patients from our Alzheimer's disease trials that show that this heart attack risk is simply not there," the Merck officials told Dan—an assertion that would become crucial as the drug's story unfolded.

We stuck to our guns. Dan presented our findings at the large national rheumatology meeting in the fall of 2003, and we wrote up the paper for submission to *Circulation*, the premier journal in cardiology. Internal memos within the company later revealed that in September 2003, just before Dan was to present our research, the company sent a note to its sales staff. The all-caps warning stated,

> DO NOT INITIATE DISCUSSIONS ON ANY OF THE UPCOMING ABSTRACTS ON VIOXX THAT WILL BE PRESENTED AT THIS YEAR'S AMERICAN COLLEGE OF RHEUMATOLOGY MEETING.

If a doctor did ask a Merck rep about our work or similar studies, a company guide on "obstacle response" instructed them to reply, "As stated here in the label, the significance of the cardiovascular findings . . . is unknown."

Our concern was shared by many thoughtful medical researchers around the country. Dr. Gurkirpal Singh, a junior faculty gastroenterologist at Stanford, was also worried about the cardiac risk of Vioxx and asked Merck to reveal more of what it knew about that. This displeased the company; he was told that "there would be serious consequences" if he persisted in his inquiries. In later Senate testimony, Singh said that Dr. Lou Sherwood (the Merck senior vice president who made the dismissive "naproxen prevents heart attacks" comment to me) called Singh's superiors at the medical school to complain about his inquiries. The younger doctor later testified that Sherwood had bragged about his "extensive contacts within academia" and said he "could make life very difficult for me at Stanford, and outside" if Singh persisted in expressing concern about the drug. Memos obtained during litigation later showed that Sherwood, a former medical school senior faculty member, bragged to colleagues at the company how thoroughly he had gone after Vioxx critics within academia to silence their concerns.

For me as an academic researcher, it was chilling to read these memos once they became public in the subsequent Vioxx litigation. In one internal note dated just before the publication of the VIGOR trial, Sherwood described a conversation with one of Singh's senior colleagues: "Fries and I discussed getting Singh to stop making the outrageous comments he has made in the past few months. . . . I will keep the pressure on and get others at Stanford to help." His candor was unnerving; he wrote to a Merck marketing executive, "Tell Singh that we've told his boss about his Merck-bashing . . . should it continue, further actions will be necessary (don't define it)." Sherwood then went on to tell his Merck associates how valuable he was to the company on this front:

> Without trying to appear immodest, I believe I am the most respected physician in the pharmaceutical industry among academic chairs and deans. . . . Therefore, when I call them on a matter of urgent concern, they generally take it seriously. . . . This has been a source of strength . . . as I have been able to exert balanced leverage in some difficult situations.

Our team wasn't aware at the time of Merck's concerted efforts to silence researchers who raised concerns about their product. *Circulation* put our study through its usual fastidious peer-review process and accepted the paper. We let Merck know of the result, as required by the contract. The company responded by demanding that we keep some of the most incriminating data out of the paper's abstract, knowing that this section is sometimes all that many busy physicians read. We refused. They quibbled about the wording we used to depict the Vioxx–heart attack risk, and we remained firm. Finally, the company told us we had to remove Dr. Cannuscio's name from the paper, because they didn't want a Merck employee associated with the publication.

"The Case of the Vanishing Author"

We objected that Carolyn had been an active member of the study team, had contributed meaningfully to the project, and by any definition merited authorship. I also couldn't see denying a young researcher the chance to be a coauthor on an important paper in such a prominent journal. Carolyn was on maternity leave at the time, and they didn't make her available to participate in the debate. "It's up to Dr. Cannuscio to talk with us about her authorship," we said, "not the company." The paper moved inexorably through the publication process, going from submitted manuscript through editing and revision to the galley stage, and ultimately to page proofs.

As the paper was about to be published, Carolyn called Dan and requested that we take her name off the paper. It was clear this wasn't her preference, but she wanted to keep her job at Merck. Reluctantly, we deleted her name from the list of authors at the last possible moment. As a poor substitute for coauthorship, in the acknowledgments section of the paper we credited an unnamed epidemiologist who had contributed importantly to the research. Somehow, we didn't omit her name from the "affiliations" section at the bottom of the paper's first page, which stated mysteriously, "Dr. Cannuscio is an employee of Merck." Most readers wouldn't have noticed this odd identification of a person whose name didn't appear on the list of authors. But as with the intimidation of my colleague at Stanford, it seemed important to get the word out about these *ad hominem* shenanigans. Tom Burton, a reporter at the *Wall Street Journal*, had called me on several occasions about medication-related stories he was working on, and I thought he might want to know about this development; such pressure tactics needed to see the light of day. That resulted in an article on the front page of the paper's business section that ran under the headline "Merck Takes Author's Name off Vioxx Study":

> In the sedate world of medical journals, this could be called The Case of the Vanishing Author. Stepping into thorny ethical territory, drug titan Merck & Co. ordered the name of one of its epidemiologists purged from the list of authors on a research paper—after the study produced an unflattering portrait of a blockbuster drug Merck happens to make. . . .
>
> Throughout, Merck was consistent in disclosing that it had sponsored the study. But the effort to otherwise distance itself from the negative findings about its painkiller Vioxx strikes some medical-journal editors as ethically questionable. "It's an

enormous disservice to the reader," says Drummond Rennie, deputy editor of the *Journal of the American Medical Association.* "If the people up there in the list of authors aren't responsible for everything in the article, something's wrong. It's completely unethical. . . ."

JAMA editor Catherine DeAngelis is disappointed that Merck didn't see this as a chance to show that sponsors of research can willingly publish findings that run contrary to their own interests. "They missed a wonderful opportunity to get some good publicity for the pharmaceutical industry," she says. "Aren't they seeking truth?"

Our paper attracted considerable attention. Although Merck had funded the study when we proposed it and signed off on the original design and every step of the protocol, the company immediately denounced it as terrible science that couldn't be trusted. It also continued to maintain that no additional risk of heart attack or stroke had ever been shown in any study in which Vioxx was compared to placebo, rather than to another drug like naproxen that was "cardioprotective."

Sales of the drug continued briskly. State Medicaid programs spent a billion dollars on the drug that year—a big hit taken by perpetually strapped programs tasked with covering the health-care needs of the nation's most vulnerable patients. As the controversy was building, I finished the manuscript of *Powerful Medicines* in mid-2003 and sent it in to the publisher, while Vioxx continued to top the charts of widely prescribed new drugs. In it, I wrote:

> Research led by Dr. Dan Solomon in my division, as well as studies from Vanderbilt University and even Merck's own clinical trial data indicate that Vioxx can increase the risk of heart attacks as well as cause high blood pressure. Nonetheless, extravagant marketing aimed at patients and doctors have made these among the most profitable drugs ever sold. Those of us who work at universities may not be very good at turning ordinary things into gold, but others clearly are.

Powerful Medicines came out in August 2004. A month later, the drug was pulled from the market.

The Fatal Polyp Study

The "naproxen protects the heart" excuse crashed and burned dramatically on September 30 of that year, when the data and safety monitoring board of a totally separate clinical trial sent an emergency message to Merck. That study was known as APPROVe, another neat acronym, for Adenomatous Polyp Prevention on Vioxx. Because Cox-2 selectivity offered the theoretical prospect of protection against all kinds of conditions that might possibly have an inflammatory cause, Merck had launched a large clinical trial of nearly 2,600 patients with recurrent colon polyps, a benign but potentially precancerous lesion. Its goal was to see whether giving them daily Vioxx for years might reduce the progression of their polyps to malignancies. Participants were randomly assigned to take Vioxx or placebo. Enrollment in APPROVe began in early 2000; the ante was raised with the publication of VIGOR later the same year, which put the world on notice that Vioxx might harm the heart. Merck's APPROVe study forged ahead.

At its regularly scheduled meeting on September 30, 2004, the APPROVe data and safety monitoring board reviewed unblinded data showing a striking increase in cardiac events in the patients who had been randomized to Vioxx: they were having heart attacks and strokes at a much higher rate than those assigned to placebo. The difference had begun to appear earlier, at the eighteen-month point of the trial, but a decision had been made to wait nearly until the end of the planned three-year study to halt it, when the ever-more-striking difference in risk became statistically significant. The trial monitors then concluded that it would be unethical to continue. The findings put an end to Merck's claim that the increase in cardiac events in VIGOR had been seen because naproxen prevented heart disease, since the comparison here was with an inert placebo. When Merck officials were shown the results, they understood that they had to take the drug off the market immediately. The company's stock plummeted.

The conclusions of our *Circulation* paper were vindicated, along with similar assessments made in other "unreliable" observational studies of huge numbers of real-world patients taking Vioxx. The globally eminent Cleveland Clinic cardiologists and researchers Eric Topol and Steven Nissen made the case compellingly also. Well, that's that, I thought. End of an era. Done and dusted. But some of the most dramatic developments in my involvement with the story were about to begin.

The Start of the Investigations

Soon after the withdrawal—and this sounds weird in retrospect—I thought I saw a black van with heavily tinted windows parked near my house several times each week when I went to work. Worse, it seemed to be following me. I took to making unexpected turns to see if it remained on my tail, and it appeared to do so. You've been working way too hard, I said to myself, this can't be real. My wife concurred. But the black van with the dark windows kept turning up. Briefly, I wondered whether it might have been sent by Merck to trace my movements—or whether I was just losing it.

It turned out that the van was real, and was indeed tracking me, but not for the reasons I had thought. One morning, my doorbell rang at seven o'clock; I opened it in my robe and slippers to see a woman and a man, both much more clean-cut than the people I usually hang out with. They said they were from the FBI and were there to talk to me about my research on Vioxx and its side effects. I, of course, refused to let them in, and asked why they had turned up at my house so early to ask me about my research instead of just contacting me at my office. "We weren't sure how to find you at your office," they said, which seemed strange, "and we've learned that we get better answers if we talk to people unexpectedly, so they don't have time to check with others or prepare their responses." I demanded to see some identification, and the woman produced a business card with an embossed government seal, stating that she was with the Boston office of the FBI—either that, or someone had a big budget for making authentic-looking phony cards. I told them this was no way to conduct an investigation, and that if they wanted to talk to me, they could call my office and make an appointment like anyone else, in which case I'd be happy to meet with them. It seemed safer to have that talk with lots of people around, in case they weren't really with the FBI—or even if they were. They left, I assume in the black van with the tinted windows. I didn't look; I just ran back inside the house.

Shaken, I immediately phoned Dan Solomon at home and said, "You aren't going to believe what just happened to me." Before I could go on, he said, "The same thing just happened to me. I had people at my house at six thirty this morning claiming to be from the FBI and wanting to talk about our Vioxx research. I didn't let them in." When I got to the office I checked the number on the woman's card, and it matched the listing for the Boston office of the FBI. I called and set up an appointment for Dan and me to talk to them in our division's conference room. In the interview, they said they were conducting a criminal inquiry about Vioxx, but refused to give any more details. Our talk covered unremarkable ground about how I had persuaded Merck to fund our study, our interactions with the company over the ensuing years, the fallout from our abstract and paper in *Circulation*, and other details of the research. After a lengthy conversation, they left; I never heard back from them. But I did wonder how many of my tax dollars had been spent paying for people to sit outside my house in a black van and follow me to work, and then confront me early in the morning for their investigation. Having come of age in the 1960s, I can't say I was shocked, but I was appalled.

From Observation to Litigation

Months later, I got a call from one of the lawyers suing Merck on behalf of clients who had heart attacks or strokes while taking Vioxx.

I'm not drawn to legal dramas about adverse drug effects, even though for some doctors it represents an attractive source of income, with rates for credible experts ranging up to a thousand dollars or more per hour. But since I don't accept payment for any of that work, this appeal was absent. And the rules of engagement in courtroom battles aren't my style. I don't mind the gently adversarial give-and-take that comes with competing for federal research grants or submitting a paper to a medical journal: the worst it usually gets is comments like "This is a poorly chosen analytic approach," or "The conclusions are not fully justified by the data presented." In litigation, lawyers repeat these concerns in a minor key. ("Who's really paying you to say this?" "You don't really like drug companies, do you?")

So why would a mild-mannered, conflict-averse academic allow himself to get drawn into such cases, especially for free? Three reasons. One is a sense of justice: patients ought to be made whole if they suffer preventable damage from a drug sold by a company that should have known better. If a manufacturer was suppressing worrisome reports of damage done by its product and did nothing to warn doctors or patients about it, that's a wrong worth trying to right.

A second reason might be described as pharmaceutical industry quality control: the fact or risk of litigation by harmed patients and their attorneys can be a compelling deterrent of future bad deeds, especially if the FDA is not paying close attention. Sometimes other branches of government will swing into action to penalize bad deeds. A few years after the Vioxx litigation ended, the Department of Justice forced GlaxoSmithKline to admit to hiding safety problems and committing other transgressions and to forfeit $3 billion, at the time the largest health-care-fraud settlement ever; the government's victory over opioid manufacturer Purdue Pharma more recently is another example (see chapter 20). But such federal actions are uncommon, making the role of citizen litigation necessary as well to remind some corporate golem-executives that they can't always act with impunity if they sacrifice patient safety to the demands of spreadsheets.

A third reason I've very occasionally helped out the plaintiff (patient) side in such cases was summarized in a *JAMA* paper I wrote with Aaron Kesselheim early in our years of work together, which we titled "The Role of Litigation in Defining Drug Risks." At a time when even more secrecy surrounded the ownership of information on patient outcomes in industry-funded research, we argued that lawsuits were sometimes necessary to uncover the extent and severity of the side effects occurring in those studies. As occurred with the original CLASS and VIGOR papers, even the peer-review process and the moral authority of prestigious medical journals were not always enough to ensure thorough revelation of all the trial data. In the case of Vioxx, internal Merck documents later revealed the company's ongoing efforts to obscure the risks of its blockbuster, including instructing its sales force how to deflect questions about heart risk that doctors might ask during their promotional visits; it even created a gamified tool to train them how to do this, which it named "Dodge Ball" (*oops*). Without the litigation that followed, no one would have known about those efforts.

Hiding the Truth from Patients

On a larger scale, the distortion and secrecy of trial findings also violates the trust of the tens of thousands of subjects who volunteer to participate in clinical trials each year. A company asks patients to take a new chemical whose effects on people are not well understood—or they might get a dummy pill that will not do them any good. Subjects agree to come in for extra medical visits and extra tests; in the case of the APPROVe study, that included colonoscopies. And they're expected to do it all for free.

The whole infrastructure of new drug development rests on the generosity of these study subjects, their willingness to give their time and take on extra risk to move our knowledge of prescription drugs forward, often with only a fifty-fifty chance of benefiting, and an unknown chance of being harmed. As I received more and more requests to help with the growing number of Vioxx lawsuits, I also thought of those trial volunteers; assisting with the litigation seemed like the least I could offer. Someone has to step forward to help out, as so many clinical trial subjects do each year. And for me, no colonoscopies would be required.

Still, I didn't want to be dragged into a bottomless pit of depositions, trial appearances, and hassles. I was still building the Division of Pharmacoepidemiology and serving as a supervising physician at the Brigham, so I had to protect time for that work. I offered the lawyers a practical solution: I would review all the evidence I could find, write up an expert report for the record, and then sit for a single deposition in Boston, at which the lawyers representing Vioxx patients (or their survivors) and a team of lawyers representing Merck could have their way with me, with the proceedings transcribed and videotaped. That single statement could then be used for free at any of the hundreds of trials that would unfold in the coming months and years. But things didn't work out that way.

CHAPTER 7

Texas Hold'em

> The good thing about science is that it's true whether or not you believe in it.
>
> —Neil deGrasse Tyson

Mike Humeston's attorney was one of those who called and asked me to consult on the Vioxx–heart attack connection. Humeston had been chosen to be one of the lead plaintiffs, and his case would become pivotal as thousands of lawsuits made their way through the courts. I again explained that I couldn't comment on whether any given person's heart attack was caused by Vioxx, and didn't want to be paid for my work, but would walk him through the relevant pharmacology, our epidemiologic research, and what the company seemed to have known and when it knew it.

Attorneys all over the country were signing up potential plaintiffs; many of them were aggregated into a multi-district litigation (MDL) to be reviewed together by a single judge, with the goal of arriving at a settlement applicable to most of the thousands of litigants. Whenever any new lawyers would call, I'd refer them to my written report and my taped deposition. That worked well enough, enabling me to devote most of my efforts to my day job at Harvard and the hospital—until I got a call from the very persuasive Mark Lanier.

I didn't know it at the time, but the silver-tongued Mark, who spoke with an engaging, informal Texas drawl, was one of the most successful plaintiffs' litigators in the country. In 2005, not long after Vioxx was taken off the market, he had won one of the first big cases: a $253 million judgment against Merck on behalf of a woman whose apparently healthy fifty-nine-year-old marathon-running husband died suddenly of heart disease after taking Vioxx; Texas law later reduced that amount by about 90 percent. Some additional important Vioxx cases were coming up, he told me, that he needed my help with. Okay, I responded, feel free to use my report and taped deposition however you like, no charge. "But I need you to be there in person for just this one trial," he implored. One of the two plaintiffs was a guy from Idaho who had originally sued Merck in 2005, the year after Vioxx was taken off the market, and lost. But striking new developments had been uncovered since then, including the company's concealing of some heart attacks in the VIGOR study, as described in the *New England Journal* editors' "Expressions of Concern." Those transgressions led a New Jersey judge to grant him a new trial.

Mark explained that Humeston's case was chosen by the presiding judge to serve as a bellwether, to inform how the thousands of other Vioxx cases could be handled in the years to come. He was working on these cases in tandem with other plaintiffs' attorneys including Chris Seeger, and Mark promised to make the engagement as painless as possible. The appearance in court would be scheduled at my convenience, kept to the shortest possible time, and he'd get me to the courtroom and back as conveniently as feasible. Where was the courtroom? In Atlantic City, New Jersey, since that was the state in which Merck was based. I said that getting there seemed like a real schlep, since it wasn't convenient to any major airport. Don't worry, Mark said, I'll fly you there.

That was my first taste of the persuasive power that enabled Lanier to win hundreds of millions of dollars of settlements for his clients over the years. So it came to be that in January 2007, I found myself in the private aviation terminal at a Boston airport with a few overnight things thrown into a little carry-on and my briefcase in the other hand, stuffed with research work I assumed I'd get done on the plane trip and during my spare time in New Jersey—an expectation that turned out to be ludicrous. At the time scheduled for takeoff, a lanky young guy in a natty leather jacket came up and offered to carry my stuff out to the plane. I figured he was a cabin attendant (did private jets even have cabin attendants?) or the copilot, or Mark's assistant. It was Mark. He filled the short ride on his plane from Boston to an airport outside Atlantic City with strategy discussions about the case Merck was making.

When we landed we drove to the plush forty-story Borgata Hotel and Casino in Atlantic City, with its 2,800 rooms and 161,000 square feet of casinos. It seemed ironic that this high-stakes case, which could help shape the course of billions of dollars in settlement funds and potentially the future of drug-side-effect liability and policy—or not—was being tried in a city best known for its gambling palaces. We bypassed the roulette wheels and slot machines, passed through an astonishing collection of colorful translucent columns, multistory chandeliers, flowers, fronds, and other sculptures by the glass artist Dale Chihuly, and made our way to a big suite Mark was using as his war room. It was a hive of activity, with young lawyers and legal assistants busily preparing for the next day's testimony. I hadn't eaten much that day, so room service brought me a lobster burger, a food I didn't even know existed.

What Did They Warn and When Did They Warn It?

At the trial, Lanier revealed the courtroom dexterity that had gained him such fame. His performances before a jury were a mixture of revival meeting (he was a part-time pastor at his megachurch in Texas), legal exegesis, and compelling rhetoric. He knew that to win he had to pull together a broad range of complicated ideas in pharmacology, drug evaluation, clinical trial design, communication, FDA policy, and legal liability—a man after my own heart. In his opening statement he had shown the jury an animated cartoon he had commissioned featuring a huge truck labeled "Vioxx" driving toward an intersection; a much smaller minivan approaches the intersection from a cross street. Initially, the big truck faces a green light as it moves forward, but then the light turns yellow. As it approaches the other vehicle the light turns red, but the truck just keeps on going and smashes into the minivan. The changing traffic lights, Mark told the jurors, represented the growing evidence of risk that kept accumulating about the drug, even as the 18-wheeler just kept barreling ahead, stopping only after it crashed into what we assume was an innocent and quickly killed family. "Someone has run a red light," he declared.

He then took on the issue of selective Cox-2 inhibition. Mark likes to use props to make complicated ideas accessible to jury members who may not have finished high school; the things he chose this time were a scale and a bag of little green and orange plastic toys. "You can tell I have kids," he drawled with a smile. The plastic tchotchkes represented the two kinds of prostaglandins that the Cox enzymes produced. The orange ones were thromboxane, which helps blood to clot. The green ones were prostacyclin, which keeps the arteries healthy and open and makes it harder for clots to form. With equal amounts, Mark said as he piled them into the pans of the scale, everything balances. He then removed some of the green toys and explained that if you take away the "good" prostacyclin without also reducing the clot-forming thromboxane, the scale tips out of balance and clots can form, causing heart attacks and strokes. That, he declared, is what Vioxx did.

I've been teaching in pharmacology courses at Harvard and MIT for years, and for a moment wished I could have brought Mark and his tchotchkes in to help with that explanation. He kept the scale in the courtroom for much of the trial.

Protecting the Drug or the Patients?

In my testimony, I tried to focus on what Merck knew about the risks of Vioxx, and when they knew it. In October 1996, three years before the drug was marketed, the company had conducted a trial that lasted only six weeks, but nonetheless raised a red flag summarized by a Merck researcher: "Adverse events of most concern were in the cardiovascular system (e.g., MI, unstable angina . . . increase in blood pressure)." As the company was designing the VIGOR study around that time, Tom Musliner, a Merck scientist, wrote:

> There is a substantial chance that significantly higher rates [of] MI, angina, strokes, transient ischemic attacks, etc. will be ob-

> served in the selective Cox-2 inhibitor [Vioxx] group compared to the standard NSAID group.

Some in the company suggested that one way to proceed would be to put study subjects on low-dose aspirin to prevent that risk, but others were concerned that this might dilute or eliminate the new drug's advantage in preventing gastrointestinal bleeding. Musliner stated the design option starkly:

> Prohibit use of low dose aspirin and accept the risk of observing significant differences in [cardiovascular] rates. . . . One could attempt to minimize between-group differences [in heart attacks and strokes] by excluding patients at higher risk.

Of course, this would make the trial population quite different from the higher-risk and older people to whom the company would market the drug. But the purpose of the study wasn't to create generalizable knowledge about patient care; it was to prove the new drug reduced GI bleeds, while minimizing any countervailing problems that might be expected. That is, it was about reducing the risks for Merck, not for patients. So much for the idea of saving the government money by having drug companies design and run the pivotal clinical studies of their products.

In reviewing the internal company memos that had been pried loose by the litigation, I learned that while the company was designing the VIGOR trial, another one of its scientists, Dr. Briggs Morrison, made a point similar to Musliner's: unless you let subjects take low-dose aspirin to protect them against heart attacks during the study, "you will get more thrombotic events and kill the drug." His colleague, Dr. Alise Reicin, responded the same day:

> Low-dose aspirin—I HEAR YOU! This is a no-win situation! The possibility of [cardiovascular] events is a great concern—(I just can't wait to be the one to present those results to senior management!). What about the idea of excluding high-risk CV

> patients. . . . This may decrease the CV event rate so that a difference between the two groups would not be evident.

Here again, Merck seemed more concerned about what might kill the drug than about what might kill the patients.

At a break in my Atlantic City testimony, a member of Mark's team remarked how well I was doing, adding, "The jurors love you!" "How can you possibly know that?" I asked, assuming that the lawyers for either side weren't supposed to talk to the jurors during the trial. But the team had hired a consultant to recruit shadow jurors—people whose demographics and backgrounds resembled those of the actual jury members. That way, the lawyers could learn in real time which arguments were going over well or poorly, to help guide midcourse corrections as the trial proceeded. The shadow jurors were "blinded"—they weren't told which side the consultant was working for, to get a more accurate reading of their impressions. In that respect the methodology used was more sophisticated than one sees in some drug studies.

"They particularly like the fact that you aren't getting paid anything to do this," a member of our team told me, adding that jurors can become pretty jaded about experts-for-hire who inevitably say whatever the side that hired them expects them to say. The fact that I was on the medical faculty at Harvard didn't seem to hurt, either.

It's Not for Patients, and It's Not Inserted in the Package

Determining what side effects a drug can cause, and how often they occur, is a central element of rational medication use. We can learn that from clinical trials and often even better from large-scale observational studies of the kind we were doing in DoPE, our Division of Pharmacoepidemiology. But as that evidence is projected into the health-care delivery system, the depiction itself can take on a reality of its own. In the end, the Humeston case and thousands like it didn't really depend on whether Vioxx caused heart attacks—the APPROVe randomized trial and ample additional data proved that it did. But since all drugs can do bad things as well as good ones, the legal wrangling centered on how adequately and promptly Merck had described that risk in its official labeling.

It seemed weird that the legal fates of all those plaintiffs relied so heavily on the tiny print of a cluttered painful-to-read document often known as the Patient Package Insert (PPI) that hardly any physicians or patients ever looked at. This is an odd name, since it is clearly not written for patients, and is usually not inserted into a prescription's packaging when a patient picks up the drug at a pharmacy. (The PPI is different from the printed information that drug stores include with a filled prescription, which have their own origins and limitations; see chapter 22.) The official PPI is a lengthy, densely packed, many-thousand-word compendium of reams of information about a drug, from its biochemistry to its pharmacology to its approved uses to its risks, depicted in sometimes excruciating detail. And although its information is directed at the prescriber, it isn't something we doctors usually refer to when making a prescribing decision. It acts more as a legal document, in which a drug company states these properties as it sees them, subject to the approval of the FDA. Oddly, risks and benefits are often not provided in any useful comparative way that the physician (or some imaginary patient with a degree in pharmacology) could make the most use of. These problems were well known. In a 2006 *NEJM* article published seven months before the Atlantic City trial, a colleague and I referred to the "linguistic toxicity" of companies' official FDA-approved drug labels, and described them as "notoriously user-hostile." We went on,

> The FDA has now admitted what most clinicians have known for decades: the current labeling is poorly organized; it is stuffed with often irrelevant information; it may include an important fact about safety in any of a number of places (categorized as a "warning," a "precaution," or an "adverse effect"); and it often fails to distinguish between a drug's side effects and problems

> that may not even be causally related to its use. . . . Data on risks included in the official label often lag behind the available evidence by as much as several years—a reflection of the FDA's problems with post-marketing surveillance and of manufacturers' reluctance to accelerate the inclusion of new data about rates of side effects.

But life-and-death decisions, not to mention billions of dollars in litigation claims, still rested on these arcane documents. When I first learned that their contents were ultimately the responsibility of the drug manufacturer, I wondered at the length and detail of the sections on a drug's potential problems. Wouldn't that discourage doctors from using the drug? "No, the companies love it like that," an industry executive once explained to me. "Everyone knows nobody reads these things. These sections are written with heavy input from the company's lawyers. That way, when a patient gets a side effect they can say, 'It's not our fault; don't say we didn't warn you.' It's really a CYA document. The ads and other promotional materials are what doctors and patients really pay attention to." As the first of many Vioxx cases came to trial, this proved to be a wise assessment: the PPI served its CYA function well, covering Merck's ass very effectively in several of the pivotal cases. Our Vioxx research had focused on *defining* the drug's risk; it turned out that the *depiction* of that risk would also be enormously important.

As the evidence of the drug's cardiovascular problems became clearer once Vioxx was in widespread use, the company's internal memos that were pried loose in the litigation showed how hard they worked on figuring out the least risky way to describe it. The marketing department had produced spreadsheets depicting the reductions in sales that might be expected if those risks were explained in different ways. The analysis concluded, Mark told the jurors, that Merck would lose hundreds of millions of dollars if the most clear-cut alert was used, so it chose not to go that route. The company then spent about two years fighting the FDA to block the proposed labeling changes that warned about the heart risk most clearly.

Buckets of Risk

Lanier's explanation of this during Mike Humeston's trial was masterful. To convey how Merck described the risks of Vioxx in its official FDA-approved label, he brought out three big plastic buckets. The red one was marked "WARNING," the section in the label depicting the highest level of concern. Then he brought out another plastic bucket labeled "PRECAUTIONS," used for other bad outcomes a doctor should be aware of. Everything else, told the jurors, gets dumped into a miscellaneous category further down, called "ADVERSE REACTIONS," for which he brought out a third bucket. That's a "catchall" category, he explained, for things like sore throat or constipation or hemorrhoids. He threw handfuls of OTC remedies for these conditions into that bin. Then he pulled out a plastic model of the heart and asked the jury, Where did Merck put the heart attack side effect? He held it for a moment over the red WARNING bucket. Not here, he said, where the serious problems belonged, and moved on to dangle it over the PRECAUTIONS bucket. Not there, either. Then he walked to the "trivial"-side-effects container. This is where they tossed the heart attack problem, Mark exclaimed, along with all that other miscellaneous stuff, in the least important bucket! With a flourish, he dropped the plastic heart into that bin. His approach might have seemed hokey, but it was a faithful and understandable representation of how the company had low-balled the drug's cardiac risk for doctors and patients.

The jury agreed with our side of the case, and in March 2007 determined that Merck's actions represented "an extreme deviation from reasonable standards of conduct" and "malicious, oppressive, or outrageous" behavior. Mike Humeston was awarded over $40 million, an amount that would be put at risk of being decreased substantially later on. But his co-plaintiff in the Atlantic City case, the survivors of a forty-four-year-old Vioxx user who died of a massive heart attack, fared much worse. Lanier and the family were crushed when the jury decided that since the other patient had his heart attack in September 2002, a year after Humeston's, and Merck had finally changed its label description of cardiac harms the preceding April, in the eyes of the law the company had thus provided "adequate warning" about the risk and was therefore not culpable.

On average, typical Vioxx plaintiffs didn't do as well as Humeston. After years of such test cases, the company and the patients' lawyers came together to craft a settlement to be offered to the thousands of people enrolled in the multi-district litigation. Most accepted; Merck ended up paying out nearly $5 billion, at the time one of the largest settlements in pharmaceutical history. But at a per-person level, the amounts were much more modest: Vioxx users who had a heart attack were awarded just $150,000 to $200,000 each, about a third of which they had to hand over to their lawyers. It's sobering to think of the scale of the settlement in relation to the far more billions of dollars that Merck made from Vioxx while it was still on the market. In terms of changing drug company behavior in the future, some critics worried that huge as it looked, in the end the settlement might amount to little more than "a speeding ticket"—just the cost of doing business.

In Texas Hold'em poker, as in other versions of the game, a player has to decide whether the hand he's been dealt is strong enough to play or whether it's better to fold. I don't know whether Mike Humeston was a poker player or if he ever discussed the game with his Houston-based lawyer, Lanier. But its theme was central to the resolution of his case. Because of the much larger award Humeston had gotten before the multiparty settlement, he initially chose not to sign on to the plaintiffs' group award. But by staying outside the collective arrangement, he risked having Merck appeal his case, which it had vowed to do; if the company won on appeal, he could lose everything. This was unfolding just as another side-effect case was making its way toward the Supreme Court. Its unusual history is described in the next chapter; that issue also depended not on whether a drug caused the problem—in this case, gangrene requiring amputation. Everyone agreed that it did, but again the question came down to whether the manufacturer had adequately warned about the problem. Many expected the high court to rule in favor of the drug manufacturer, which had argued that the risk was well described in its official labeling, freeing it of culpability. If that happened, it could favor Merck's appeal and create a risk that Humeston could end up with far less to show for his Atlantic City courtroom win. Fearing that likely set of events, Mike and his wife decided to head off a potentially devastating appeal by Merck and consider a settlement. The amount that would be involved was undisclosed, as often occurs in such cases. I hope it was generous, because the Supreme Court soon afterward issued a surprise decision that astonished most observers. Had he been able to predict this unexpected decision, Mike Humeston might have decided not even to consider the idea of settling with Merck.

Using the Legal System to Pry Out the Facts

As the Vioxx litigation was winding down, my colleagues and I were granted access to some astonishing new information that emerged through the discovery process the lawsuits had unleashed. To address the question "What did Merck know and when did it know it?" the patients' lawyers had demanded access to the raw clinical trial results that Merck collected in its other research. Prominent among these were their supposedly negative Alzheimer's disease studies. Our team was led by David Madigan; he was chair of the Statistics Department at Columbia and later became the dean of its Faculty of Arts and Sciences; he's now provost of Northeastern University. The litigation enabled us to review some previously hidden files. Those trial results showed clearly that the drug did not prevent memory loss; in fact, patients randomized to take Vioxx seemed to be *more* likely to develop evidence of cognitive deterioration. But more alarming, we found that patients given Vioxx in those Merck studies were *more than three and a half times likelier to die of heart disease* than those who were randomized to get placebo. Worse, all three Alzheimer's studies had been completed by April 2003, over five months before the drug was taken off the market following the APPROVe study's "surprising" findings. I was amazed to learn that Madigan's analysis of the data showed the combined Alzheimer's study findings had actually reached the conventional level of 95 percent certainty of an increase in cardiac risk by *June 2001*, three months before Mike Humeston's heart attack.

So these Vioxx-causes-cardiac death data were already in place within the company even as Merck scientists were warning our team in DoPE that their Alzheimer's disease studies proved that Vioxx had no cardiac risk, and its lawyers were fighting the FDA to keep a clear warning of that off the drug's official label. We published our paper, "Under-Reporting of Cardiovascular Events in the Rofecoxib [Vioxx] Alzheimer's Disease Studies," in the *American Heart Journal*. I figured these appalling new findings might influence the litigation somehow, but no. The settlements had been reached and signed off on, the cases were closed, and the lawyers had moved on to other contests.

So Much of This Could Have Been Avoided

One of the ironies of the Cox-2 saga is that in late 1999, just as Vioxx and Celebrex were increasing in sales so dramatically, doctors at the Prince of Wales Hospital in Hong Kong—not an internationally known mecca of clinical research—wondered whether simply giving a patient a drug to prevent ulcers along with one of the older NSAIDs might achieve the same degree of "gastroprotection" as the costlier new selective Cox-2 inhibitors like Vioxx and Celebrex. The ulcer drug was omeprazole, heavily marketed as Prilosec and commonly known as "the purple pill." Its patent was expected to expire in April 2001, potentially making its use with an existing NSAID very affordable if it could be shown to provide adequate stomach protection. Running a trial of an older off-patent NSAID along with a soon-to-be-off-patent ulcer medicine wasn't commercially appealing for the drugmakers that fund most clinical studies, and certainly not for the makers of Vioxx or Celebrex, so the Hong Kong study was supported by research grants from the Chinese University of Hong Kong and the Health Services Research Committee of Hong Kong. The researchers randomly allocated patients with a history of GI bleeding to take either Celebrex or an older, generic NSAID along with Prilosec. They showed that combining the two older drugs provided the same rate of gastroprotection as the expensive new one—with no increase in cardiac risk.

Those results were reported in the *New England Journal of Medicine* in December 2002. In a sense, the trial represented a different kind of natural experiment, making it possible to compare not only two drug regimens but also two ways of disseminating trial findings. The results were reported in the world's most prominent medical journal, but since one drug was generic and the other was going generic soon, the combination offered no prospect of a financial windfall for any drugmaker. As a result, disseminating that discovery wasn't backed by the kind of hundred-million-dollars-a-year promotion that was being put into the enormously lucrative Vioxx and Celebrex franchises at the same time. The "selective Cox-2 inhibition" drum continued to beat loudly well into 2004, driving sales of the newer drugs higher and higher, while the less-hyped findings about the older-drug combination received far less notice.

Informing the Patient

It's an accident of history that we don't have to request informed consent from patients before we prescribe most prescription drugs to them. For a small skin biopsy, an endoscopy, or a tooth extraction—no less cardiac surgery—the doctor must detail all the expected benefits and the possible risks, and make sure they are understood and accepted by the patient. As a thought experiment, I sometimes wonder what would happen if this were also required when we write prescriptions. Given all we know now about Vioxx, I sometimes think about the conversation I might have had with a patient in mid-2004 while the drug was still being used:

> "Mrs. Smith, there's a medication I could prescribe to treat your arthritis that won't provide any better pain relief than similar

drugs that are out there, but it will be somewhat gentler on your stomach and might reduce the chance of bleeding in your GI tract. You could also achieve about the same stomach protection by adding an over-the-counter drug like Prilosec to the old Advil you're currently taking. The new arthritis drug is pretty expensive and will cost about $80 a month, compared to about $15 for generic Advil or Motrin, which you can get over the counter without a prescription. Oh, did I mention that this new drug probably doubles or triples your risk of having a heart attack or a stroke? Well, it does. Do you want me to write you a prescription for it?"

Conversations like that could have saved thousands of lives, tens of thousands of hospital days for the care of drug-induced cardiovascular events, and billions of dollars that were spent on a drug whose hope turned out to contain so much hype. Before it left the market Vioxx is estimated to have caused thousands of drug-induced heart attacks and strokes, the largest epidemic of medicine-induced cardiovascular disease in history.

But the good news is that this realization led the way to some major reforms in how the U.S. health-care system identifies and deals with drug side effects. By creating one of the worst drug crises in the history of American medicine, Vioxx soon took its place next to opium syrups, sulfanilamide elixir, and thalidomide as a trigger for needed policy changes. Its crashing end breathed new life into long-ignored proposals for improving the way we study drug side effects, and set the stage for a public reassessment of how the nation approaches medication risks. In the end Mike Humeston, his fellow plaintiffs, their lawyers, and a small group of researchers opened the way for vital new programs that have enabled us to better understand and manage the inevitable downsides of prescription drugs. These reforms are discussed in chapter 9. But first, a detour into the land of arcane tiny print.

CHAPTER 8

The Label as Protective Talisman

Where should the ultimate responsibility lie for defining a drug's safety and appropriate use? The Vioxx litigation highlighted the outsize role played by a medication's labeling in defining its "official" side effects. Viewed from the perspective of the courts, however risky a product might be, listing its possible adverse effects on the label can confer protection on a manufacturer the moment they are printed. By this logic, the label enables the physician (and even more fancifully, the patient) to read its thousands of words and make an informed decision about whether to take on a particular risk in light of a drug's benefit. It's almost as if those tiny letters on an enormous folded piece of paper confer some kind of supernatural protection for the company, like the words inscribed on the prayer wheels that observant Buddhists spin in a temple, or a blessing tucked inside an amulet dedicated to a saint and worn around the neck of a devout Catholic, or the sacred scroll hidden in a mezuzah on the doorpost of a Jewish family.

So are the courts to be the ultimate arbiter of drug safety?

Other Label Battles Reach the Courts: Who Gets to Define Risk?

The Vioxx case is just one example of this linguistic magic that can be more powerful—at least in the eyes of the law—than the evidence we see through the lenses of pharmacology, epidemiology, and clinical practice. This was just one of several times the courts have been asked to make the final decision about the safety of a medication; another key case also dates back to the Vioxx era. In April 2000, Diana Levine, a Vermont musician, went to a local clinic for treatment of a particularly bad migraine headache. She was given a drug called Phenergan (not a great choice) that was administered by a physician's assistant intravenously (also a bad idea) via an IV "push" in which it was forcefully injected into the vein, rather than dripped in slowly as the manufacturer recommended (a terrible plan). But instead of remaining in the vein, the drug apparently ended up in an artery in her arm (a disaster). Phenergan is toxic to the lining of blood vessels: in a vein it can lead to dangerous blood clots; in an artery, it can cut off blood flow to the body part it supplies, with even worse consequences. The damage Phenergan did to the main artery in Ms. Levine's arm first led to excruciating pain, then to gangrene, and ultimately required an amputation. Wyeth, the company that made Phenergan, had stated on its official label that the drug should never be injected into an artery, and that if given intravenously it should be administered slowly through a well-running drip. The language on the label, like that for Vioxx, was the subject of protracted negotiations between the company and the FDA; in the case of Phenergan, the back-and-forth went on for over a decade, mostly because of very long delays on the FDA side. Levine sued Wyeth on the grounds that although its warning about avoiding arterial injection was made on the official label, it was not made strongly enough.

A state court in Vermont agreed with Ms. Levine, and ordered Wyeth to pay her $6.7 million in damages. The company appealed on the grounds that it had indeed warned against injecting its drug into an artery, and did suggest the preferred method of slow intravenous-drip use. Further, it had to wait years before the snail-like FDA review process was completed on revisions to its label instructions. Moreover—and this is an aspect of the case that received the most legal attention—the company argued that state juries or judges should not be allowed to second-guess the FDA about the adequacy of language about safety in a federally approved drug description.

It's hard enough to negotiate the language of a label once with the FDA—and now that we know what happened between Merck and the FDA over the Vioxx label warnings, we have a better understanding of what this can involve. Once that contentious process is completed, Wyeth argued, does it make sense for every state to decide for itself whether a given warning is adequate or not? Shouldn't a federal decision preempt the states from reevaluating its adequacy? The preemption issue touched on a long-standing third rail in regulatory jurisprudence: settled law seemed to dictate that if a given right is reserved to the federal government, that should rule out allowing individual states or other litigants to prefer their own policies. (That principle began to unravel in 2024; see below.) From my perspective, it seemed okay that Wyeth had warned that its intravenous product should not be injected into an artery. What more was needed—a neon sign? Is such litigation really the best way to ensure that doctors and patients get the information they need about the risks of the medications they use?

The preemption issue also came up later in a case in my own state, when Massachusetts decided to ban use of a new extra-strength narcotic painkiller called Zohydro. It was extremely potent, and we were in the midst of the opioid epidemic. Who needed a new drug in this class that had no clear advantage over any of the other available drugs like it, but did confer more risk of overdose as well as abuse? Its potential for harm would likely have outweighed any incremental benefit it could claim, since doctors could just increase the dose of an older drug and get the same pain-relief result. Let's just make it illegal here, said the Commonwealth of Massachusetts. No you can't, said the courts. The FDA had approved it, so no one state, even one as smart as ours, could preempt that decision.

Back in Vermont, many were surprised that the Supreme Court even agreed to hear the *Wyeth v. Levine* case, since the preemption doctrine seemed so clear. Everyone assumed that once the FDA had approved Wyeth's official label for Phenergan, no lower-level court could challenge that. But the high court didn't see it that way, and in March 2009 voted 6–3 to uphold Levine's claim against Wyeth on two grounds: the company could have made its warning stronger, and state courts indeed could second-guess the FDA if they objected to a statement in a company's product information. (Most of the harm done to Ms. Levine seemed to be the fault of the people who took care of her, but there's usually a cap on how much clinicians and medical institutions can be sued for, and pharmaceutical companies have much deeper pockets.)

On hearing of the Supreme Court's *Wyeth v. Levine* decision I wondered how much blame a manufacturer should incur if its drug is used incorrectly by clinicians. Granted, Wyeth was certainly not a model drugmaker in this regard; in 2008, it was sued multiple times by women who developed breast cancer after taking its widely sold estrogen product Premarin—another blockbuster medication whose risks were not clearly defined or adequately communicated to doctors or patients, and which Wyeth had promoted with enormous zeal. But for Wyeth to have to pay $6.7 million to Diana Levine because someone injected Phenergan into her artery when the drug was clearly intended for oral or intravenous use? If a doctor had injected it into someone's eye and they had gone blind, would that have been Wyeth's fault, too? Is this the best way we can make sure that drug companies warn about the risks of their drugs adequately, and doctors use them appropriately? Apparently, it is.

Diana Levine's case became more vivid for me when I found myself sitting next to her sometime later at a small witness table for a Capitol Hill briefing to update House and Senate staffers about pending legislation on drug regulation. I had never gotten that close to someone with their own eponymous Supreme Court case, especially on a topic so central to my own work. (A third witness was Gregg Gonsalves of Yale, the former AIDS activist we met in chapter 1.) My presentation focused on the need for the FDA to strike a better balance as it evaluated drug efficacy and safety. Ms. Levine was to talk about the problem of adverse drug effects from the patient's point of view.

As she spoke, I wondered if I was confusing the woman sitting next to me with the patient at the center of the famous Wyeth case. She gestured normally with both hands; both forearms, wrists, and fingers looked completely normal, right down to what appeared from just a foot or two away to be symmetrically shaped limbs with their light hairs and small age spots. I figured I was sitting next to a different Levine, although her account of the Wyeth case sounded like a first-person story. Her presentation was compelling in the way that only a patient's own story can be. As she talked about her awful clinical course, the congressional staffers seemed visibly moved. At the climax of her appeal for better warnings about adverse events she declared, "*This* is what a drug side effect looks like!" Firmly grabbing her right hand with her left, she yanked off a remarkably convincing prosthesis and waved the stump of her arm in the air as she appealed to the staffers to make drugmakers more accountable for the risks their products can cause. Several people gasped, including me. I'm sure her presentation left much more of an impression than mine did.

Can a Judge in One State Decide a Drug Is Too Unsafe for Anyone to Use?

In 2023 and 2024, an even stranger legal battle on drug safety called on the courts to decide whether a different FDA-approved drug was safe enough for patients to use. A group of anti-abortion doctors constituted themselves in Texas as "the Alliance for Hippocratic Medicine" and sued the FDA on the grounds that its twenty-year-old decision to approve the abortion-inducing drug mifepristone was unsound because the drug was not really safe. Following the Supreme Court's *Dobbs* decision of 2022 that ended federal protection of a woman's right to terminate her pregnancy, the use of medications to induce an abortion had become more common than surgical abortions, and mifepristone was a key component of that treatment.

The doctors who brought the new case demanded that the court revoke the FDA's approval of the drug because it wasn't safe, and immediately ban its use—not just in Texas, but throughout the whole country. This argument flew in the face of several obvious facts: First, in the twenty years since its approval, mifepristone had developed a very impressive record of safety. Second, it would make no sense for a state-level judge to second-guess the FDA and be able to withdraw a drug from the market not just in their own jurisdiction, but in the nation as a whole. Third, the argument of the doctors bringing the action was based on their own concerns about having to care for women who might in the future take mifepristone and come to them to complete the termination of a pregnancy. But that was a hypothetical problem: no such case had yet occurred, and federal law protects doctors from having to participate in terminating a pregnancy if that violates their religious principles.

The case was implausible on several fronts, but the doctors had chosen their venue well: a Texas federal judge ruled in their favor and declared mifepristone unsafe to use. Worse, he ruled that his decision would be binding throughout the entire nation. Another federal judge in Washington State quickly made a competing ruling to protect the drug's availability, and the Texas decision was also appealed by the Department of Justice acting on behalf of the FDA—guaranteeing that the case would be taken up by the U.S. Supreme Court. Many of us wondered why the high court wouldn't simply dismiss the claims of the anti-abortion doctors and the Texas judge based on the utter implausibility of their arguments. But in a worrisome move the court accepted the case, raising concerns that they were eager to get involved in the medication abortion debate.

In the end, the high court did reject the anti-abortion doctors' case, but primarily on the technical basis that the plaintiffs formally lacked standing to bring the action because they had not been harmed by anyone's use of the medication. The decision was a relief to people across the country who worried that access to mifepristone could be terminated, but the logic of the decision left open the possibility that the court might still be willing to rule on a future case in which the issue of standing is not a limiting factor. On the positive side, in his ruling Justice Kavanaugh did mention in passing that "federal courts are the wrong forum for addressing the plaintiffs' concerns about FDA's actions." But on the negative side, he persistently referred to opposing abortion as being "pro-life."

If a future case demanding local preemption of an FDA safety decision returns to the highest court in the land and has a less weird argument to make, it might come from a neighboring state. Just before the Texas mifepristone decision, a Louisiana case began to make its way through the courts in May 2024, once the state had made nearly all abortions illegal after the overturning of *Roe v. Wade*. That legislation was also motivated by the bogus argument that mifepristone was unsafe, and added two additional features. It made the same charge against another drug often used in medication abortions, misoprostol—a drug that, like mifepristone, also has important medical uses other than electively inducing abortion. The Louisiana Republican state legislature and Republican governor went on to reclassify both drugs as "dangerous controlled substances," potentially subjecting women who possessed them to fines or prison time.

Might we be entering a world in which a judge in one state can legally second-guess an FDA decision about a drug's safety or effectiveness, sometimes for political reasons? That outcome would be welcomed by many on the extreme right who oppose all manifestations of what they call the administrative state, even in matters of science. A few days later, Louisiana also made it illegal for doctors to prescribe FDA-approved medications to transgender patients under eighteen for gender-affirming care, including estrogens or testosterone. Cases like these are often reviewed by the notoriously conservative federal Fifth Circuit Court of Appeals, based in New Orleans, a jurisdiction that some observers describe as "Where the law goes to die." This was the court whose ruling in the Dobbs case paved the way for the Supreme Court to undo *Roe v. Wade*; it is housed in a building named after a judge named John Minor Wisdom, which seems appropriate. Nationally, it is worrisome that the notorious Comstock Act of 1873 is still on the books, and could be used by a future administration to outlaw the contraception as well as medications for abortion.

Not Deferring to Deference

The threat to centralized, evidence-based determinations of drug safety and effectiveness took another big hit around the same time at the end of the Supreme Court's 2023–2024 session, when it dealt a major blow to the authority of government agencies in general by reversing a forty-year-old principle known as the "Chevron deference." The high court had ruled in 1984 that in disputes over the implementation of federal law, the courts were expected to respect decisions made by the relevant federal entity (in that case, a ruling by the Environmental Protection Agency concerning the oil company Chevron) on how to interpret the legislation, rather than opening up every wrinkle of each regulation to potential litigation. The old precedent had rested on the idea that Congress could never pass laws complex enough to anticipate every possible detail of how to put them into practice. By contrast, staff at the federal agencies charged with implementing those laws (such as the EPA, the Department of Agriculture, and the FDA, among many others) had the broad and deep expertise to do so. But protecting the power of federal agencies was anathema to the regulated industries as well as to the conservative movement seeking to dismantle "the administrative state." They much preferred the right to sue the government over restrictions they didn't like. That ruling could have important implications for the power of all federal bodies, including those in charge of making decisions on drug safety and effectiveness such as the FDA, as well as those responsible for paying for them, like the Centers for Medicare and Medicaid Services.

Over decades of ferally clever (or cleverly feral) activity, anti-regulation advocates had been bringing cases designed to erode that governmental authority to implement congressionally mandated programs. With the Supreme Court stacked with ultraconservative jurors, this goal was finally accomplished in June 2024 through two cases involving herring, of all things. The high court had made clear it was accepting these cases specifically to revisit and possibly overturn the Chevron deference issue. The herring industry, pusuing its economic agenda at the expense of the common good (see golems, above), had been overfishing the ocean's stock and driving the numbers of those fish to unsustainably low levels. To address that, beginning in 2020 the National Oceanic and Atmospheric Administration (NOAA) required these boats to carry observers to ensure that each catch stayed within legal limits. Herring (see chapter 18) are hard-working little fish far from the top of the food chain that play a major role as bait for larger, fancier creatures. These characteristics were shared by the fishermen that a conservative activist group enlisted to serve as the plaintiffs in a case aimed at helping the Supreme Court undercut the authority of federal regulators. With the activists' guidance and ample funding, two separate groups of New England herringmen sued the government to overturn a requirement that they had to pay these monitors for their time. What better scenario for an anti-regulatory test case—not one but two sets of earnest fishermen forced to fund a government program out of their own hard-won, modest incomes? Put that way, who would want these guys to lose?

Lower courts had said that the Chevron deference precedent should mean that once Congress had passed a law to prevent overfishing of herring, the agency responsible for implementing it (NOAA) had the final say over how to run and pay for it. But swimming upstream against forty years of precedent, the 2024 court put its own finger on the scales of justice and gutted that concept, creating a sea change in regulatory policy. In a 6–3 decision along ideological lines, it ruled in favor of the fishermen and declared that they didn't have to obey that part of the regulation, whatever NOAA said.

Some observers said this was not as big a change as it seemed, since the increasingly conservative Supreme Court hadn't been enthusiastic about the Chevron deference for years. But others worried that this new ruling could trigger a flood of anti-regulatory lawsuits, drowning the powers of government agencies in litigation that could now be brought by anyone who objected to the rules—a risk that increased dramatically following the November 2024 elections. It could have implications for federal agency decisions from finance to farming to health care, with the latter of greatest interest to us here. Undercutting the clout of federal agencies and opening more drug-related policies to litigation by powerful and deep-pocketed interests could create many problems, especially in a newly conservative governmental environment:

- limiting the FDA's authority to make final decisions about the safety of prescription drugs and their effectiveness for new uses;
- reducing the FDA's control over promotional information for doctors and patients depicting drugs' benefits and risks;
- blocking the authority of the Medicare program to negotiate prices on the medications it pays for;

- modifying a host of existing and future rules concerning Medicaid eligibility and the rights of patients with private health insurance.

The herring case was decided at the same time that the public learned of an ambitious plan that was coming to widespread attention. Known as *Project 2025: Presidential Transition Project*, it had been prepared by conservatives, many close to the former Trump administration, and laid out a bold plan for sharply cutting back on the role of government once Republicans came to power. The changes would include blows to many of the federal agencies we have been considering here, from the FDA to Medicaid to Medicare, among many others—limitations that were now legally facilitated by the Supreme Court's herring decision.

In overturning *Roe* and ending federal protection for abortion access, as well as cutting back on federal protection of voting rights, the high court had ruled that such rules were not really settled law at all. Now it had undercut the idea that the government had unquestionable authority over medication-related issues as well. We also learned how political, ideological, and religious positions could be enforced by presenting them as drug risk issues. So is the way we address the question "Is it safe?" to be based on pharmacologic evidence, or clinical trial findings, or epidemiological observations, or a shared doctor-patient decision, or a legal determination, or politics?

Yes.

CHAPTER 9

A New Era of Reform

The 2004 withdrawal of Vioxx from the market had not been a one-off event. It followed several other medication problems that came to light over the previous few years; the early 2000s had seen the accumulation of the timber that Vioxx would ignite into a conflagration. Earlier in 2004, Pfizer had agreed to pay $430 million to settle a case brought by all fifty state attorneys general over its promotion of the epilepsy drug Neurontin for unapproved uses. In July of that year, Eliot Spitzer, then New York attorney general, sued GlaxoSmithKline over its suppression of results it didn't like from clinical trials of its antidepressant Paxil, including findings that the drug seemed to increase suicide risk in young people. (See Erick Turner's *NEJM* analysis of antidepressant trials in chapter 1.) An internal Glaxo memo had described the company's plan to "manage the dissemination of data in order to minimize any potential negative commercial impact"—that is, to bury research results that would be bad for sales. The company settled quickly in August of that year, just a month before the unanticipated Vioxx withdrawal. Industry observers were surprised that Glaxo got off lightly in settling for a fine of only $2.5 million, much less than many had expected, and much less than its $3 billion settlement for fraud years later. But the 2004 deal turned out to be awesome in another way: Spitzer extracted something much more valuable by getting the company to agree to make public the results of all its clinical trials online, an unprecedented requirement. In an era of "We paid for it, we can hide it," no drugmaker had been obliged to do this; Spitzer's innovative plan presaged a much more ambitious vision for clinical trials data that would be put into place as one of the most important post-Vioxx reforms.

The same years also saw the growth of nationwide concern over the underreported negative outcomes of another drug class, the heavily promoted estrogen products widely used by women to treat the symptoms of menopause—drugs like Premarin and Prempro (both made by Wyeth, of the *Wyeth v. Levine* amputation case). Such products had been on the market since the 1940s, when the FDA approved them on the basis of very scanty evidence without requiring information on their long-term benefits or safety. The manufacturer then failed to look into their risks during their many decades of lucrative sales, because no one made them do so. In 2002 *JAMA* published the results of a landmark NIH-funded randomized trial that further documented that estrogen use caused breast cancer. The report unleashed a wave of litigation against Wyeth by women who had developed malignancies after taking the drugs, and the number of cases ballooned in the next years. In one judgment, a Nevada jury initially ordered Wyeth to pay three women $134.5 million for their estrogen-induced breast cancers. (Wyeth was later bought by Pfizer, which settled such suits by over ten thousand women for about $770 million.)

These examples helped convince the public and lawmakers that neither doctors, patients, nor the FDA really had a good grip on side effects, even for some of the most widely used products. Against this yearslong background, within seven weeks of the Vioxx withdrawal the Senate Finance Committee held hearings about that debacle, warranted by its jurisdiction over the Medicare and Medicaid programs. The session was titled "FDA, Merck, and Vioxx: Putting Patient Safety First?" and the chair, Republican Chuck Grassley of Iowa, began with pointed questions for both the government agency and the manufacturer. In a comment that still rings true over two decades later, he declared, "One of my concerns is that the FDA has a relationship with drug companies that is far too cozy. That is exactly the opposite of what it should be. The health and safety of the public must be FDA's first and only concern.... Consumers should not have to second-guess the safety of what is in their medicine cabinet."

Signaling the pivotal nature of the crisis, Montana Democrat Max Baucus said the hearing "goes beyond Merck. It goes beyond Vioxx. We must think critically about the way we test and evaluate drugs generally to ensure their safety. . . . Why did the FDA not detect the risks associated with Vioxx during the initial approval process, or even in the 5 years since approval?" he asked, posing a question that Congress had never considered before. "Should we be doing more to monitor drug safety after a drug has been approved?" Raising a then-radical concept, he observed, "Clinical trials focused on drug safety should not stop when the FDA approves a drug. Rather, we need to continue testing drugs to thoroughly evaluate the potential risks, not just the benefits." From his Finance Committee perspective, he decried the fact that in the five years that Vioxx was on the market, the government had spent over a billion dollars paying for it, primarily through Medicaid.

Baucus then put forward a radical concept that had long been resisted by drugmakers: "I also support greater use of studies that test the comparative effectiveness and safety of drugs in similar therapeutic classes." A totally sensible expectation, but after it surfaced briefly in the Vioxx hearings, the idea would then be pushed aside for fifteen more years, not returning to the center of congressional deliberations until a 2019 debate over the Affordable Care Act (Obamacare). Then, under continuing industry pressure, it was once again marginalized immediately afterward; this commonsense idea still faces strong opposition at both the federal and state levels (see chapter 13).

One early witness in the Senate's 2004 Vioxx hearings was Dr. David Graham, a physician-epidemiologist in the FDA's Office of Drug Safety. A wiry guy and avid runner, he'd connect with me each year at the annual meeting of the nascent International Society for Pharmacoepidemiology, where we'd commiserate about our anomalous outsider roles in our home institutions. As our group had been doing, David was also studying the Vioxx–heart attack risk in a different large database of patients in routine care, and he was finding results similar to those we had published in *Circulation*. His work was not received well by his agency supervisors. "I was pressured to change my conclusions and recommendations," David testified at the Senate hearings. Because Vioxx was at the time still on the market, "One Drug Safety manager recommended that I should be barred from presenting [my findings at an academic] meeting, and also noted that Merck needed to know our study results. So, I guess Merck needed to know the results, but the public did not. An e-mail from the director for the entire Office of New Drugs was revealing," David went on. "He suggested that since the FDA was not contemplating a warning against the use of high-dose Vioxx, my conclusions should be changed." A clear problem of cart-before-horse.

As of the date of the hearing, the FDA had still not allowed Graham to publish his research findings, even though his paper had been accepted by *JAMA* after rigorous peer review. The drug's trajectory demonstrated "a profound regulatory failure," Graham told the senators. "I would argue that the FDA, as currently configured, is incapable of protecting America against another Vioxx. We are virtually defenseless. . . . FDA and [its] Center for Drug Evaluation and Research are broken." He described a built-in conflict-of-interest problem in his workplace: the division that approves new drugs had most of the power at the agency, often opposing the findings of FDA safety researchers if the results suggested that a green-lighted drug had unexpected side-effect problems. Graham charged that the agency "views the pharmaceutical industry that it is supposed to regulate as its client. It over-values the benefits of the drugs that it approves, and it seriously undervalues, disregards, and disrespects drug safety." Tough language indeed, coming from the inside.

The Vioxx withdrawal had given David a sense of vindication in light of his own research findings, but it worsened his situation at the FDA. A few days after the blockbuster was pulled from pharmacy shelves, proving he was right about its dangers, he wrote to a colleague: "Believe it or not, I'm being treated as if I was Benedict Arnold—with antagonism, hostility, and a strong dose of ostracism." As a civil servant he couldn't be fired, but he later told me that after his Senate testimony and his continuing outspoken comments, "They reassigned me to a remote office and took away a lot of my support staff."

Government agencies and corporations, unlike universities on a good day, have to march to the beat of a common organizational drum. For companies, everything needs to move in the same direction to increase the bottom line. For government agencies, it's seen as vital to present the public with a homogeneous view aligned with the perspective of its leadership: don't reveal cracks in describing the government's position on anything, since consistency is seen as vital to the agency's authority.

Taking the Next Steps

The Senate hearings were followed by other probing investigations into the Vioxx disaster by the Government Accountability Office as well as the Institute of Medicine, a prestigious body representing some of the nation's best physicians and medical scientists. Both groups created informed, thoughtful, lengthy reports that tried to answer the central issue implicit in the senators' questioning that day: How the hell could this have happened? The U.S. health-care system had approved, used, and paid for five years' worth of a very widely prescribed medication that turned out to almost double the risk of heart attack and stroke, and we didn't seem to understand what had gone wrong.

One answer that was appropriately given short shrift was that the Vioxx problem was isolated, created by a small number of "bad apple" people in just one company. Yes, Merck was the mainspring that drove the problem for this one drug, but its problematic corporate behavior was systemic. It wasn't limited to a few rogue actors or overzealous regional sales managers, as some at the company claimed. Once the ensuing litigation pried loose thousands of pages of secret internal memos, it became clear that the whole chain of events—including self-serving and risky clinical trial designs, distortion of the evidence, pressuring the FDA to let the company understate the cardiac risk, and deceptive promotional practices—was all a coordinated process directed from the very highest levels of the company. And as the recent embarrassments of Glaxo, Wyeth, and Pfizer had made clear, the problem wasn't limited to one drugmaker.

But Vioxx and drug-safety problems like it weren't just the result of bad actions by drugmakers or the FDA: other participants in the prescription drug ecosystem also played crucial, if smaller roles.

We clinicians, who, of course, wrote every single one of those prescriptions, were far too willing to accept the too-good-to-be-true story that selective inhibition of cyclooxygenase (Cox) would bring only benefit and no harm. And patients were too easily swayed by the glitzy $100-million-a-year program of direct-to-consumer ads suggesting that the drug's innovative chemistry somehow guaranteed far more effectiveness and far less risk than it really did. Insurers as well, in both the commercial and public sectors, complained about the drug's high price, but bought uncritically into the idea that selective cyclooxygenase (Cox-2) inhibition was safe and worth paying billions of dollars a year for, and found it hard to resist the considerable demand from both patients and prescribers. Manufacturers, the FDA, physicians, consumers, payers—Vioxx and Cox had made us all into suckers.

Some Sensible Changes

Reports from the Senate, the Government Accountability Office, and the Institute of Medicine each proposed specific ways to move forward, opening the next chapter in the country's tradition of fitfully reforming its drug policies in response to tragedy. We've seen that one good attribute of the original Prescription Drug User Fee Act of 1992 was its built-in sunset clause, requiring that it be reauthorized every five years. In the wake of Vioxx, the renewal due in 2007 offered a chance to launch several programs to address the newly notorious but long-ignored problems the crisis had brought into the spotlight.

The user-fee law's new incarnation would be called the FDA Amendments Act of 2007, or FDAAA (generally pronounced as *fa-DAH*, rhymes with "*ta-DAH!*"). It introduced several important new initiatives, even if their goals still haven't been fully realized today. Nonetheless, the reforms put in place then continue to affect tens of millions of prescriptions written by health-care professionals and taken by patients today, primarily for the better.

A New Tool for Monitoring Side Effects

After the 2004 Vioxx withdrawal, the FDA reacted by issuing more and more cautionary statements, mimicking the industry strategy of "Don't say we didn't tell you!" The agency put out sixty-eight major warnings about prescription drugs in 2007, up from fifty-eight in the prior year, compared to just twenty-one in 2003. But self-protective performative caution statements weren't what we needed; the problem required a more fundamental data-driven solution.

After the Vioxx withdrawal, I was asked to write an editorial in *Circulation* about what was needed to fix the problems that had led to the debacle. I argued that the FDA didn't have the clout it needed to force manufacturers to perform needed follow-up studies once a product was on the market, since such requests were so often ignored. I also called for deploying more modern methods to identify drug side effects by using data from large populations to study medications in widespread use—like the research we had been doing for years in my group.

Several of us in academia had been writing about this need for years, with little government or industry reaction. I recall attending a lecture by Dr. David Kessler, the very capable FDA commissioner who served between 1990 and 1997. His talk offered what seemed like a visionary statement to some—that he could imagine a day at some point in the future when researchers would be able to harvest the vast amounts of health-care-claims data already available on health system computers, and somehow use it to study which drugs caused which problems. I could barely contain myself, and wanted to leap to my feet and yell, "Yo, dude! My pals and I are doing exactly that right now in Boston! We've been doing it for years! You should come and look!" But it was a big auditorium, and there was little chance for questions or comments. After Kessler left his post early in 1997, no permanent commissioner was named for another two years.

Over a decade after my non-outburst, such recommendations were codified in the FDAAA. Congress instructed the FDA to build a nationwide system of adverse-effect monitoring that could make use of the ongoing fire-hose stream of computerized data on the prescription drug use and health outcomes of millions of Americans—information already being routinely collected by Medicare, Medicaid, the Veterans Health Administration, and private health insurance companies all over the country. It would be vital to anonymize the data to mask patients' identities, but that was doable. The new government-mandated program would be called Sentinel. Thanks to the FDAAA, the full-grown system is now up and running, routinely sucking in all medication use and health-care episodes of over a hundred million Americans, creating one of the largest repositories of drug use and medical care in the world that can be used to spot early signs of unanticipated medication risks. Researchers from around the country, particularly my colleagues at DoPE, are learning how to harvest even more rich data from patients' anonymized electronic health records to make that information even more accurate.

As with older commonsense reforms at the FDA (like labeling opium products, banning poisons, requiring drugs to work), it took a disaster to bring about an obvious solution. The Sentinel database continues to grow, accruing terabytes of data every day from routinely collected health-care transactions and working with collaborators (including several faculty in DoPE) to develop innovative approaches to this valuable data. But more needs to be done: this publicly funded resource ought to be readily available to research groups around the country, but the FDA limits access to it, with most drug-safety studies that use it conducted by the agency itself and its direct collaborators. Access by other independent research groups outside the FDA is theoretically available through a private foundation, but is rarely granted. When it is, it is usually to pharmaceutical companies; such use is costly, and approval times lengthy. The foundation's website currently describes just seven such studies performed over several years, all with drug manufacturers, and only one lists a completed paper in the medical literature. It's not clear why this is the case; perhaps it's over concern by government or the drug industry that wider access to the dataset, even if limited to established outside researchers, might turn up problems that may not be real, or that neither the FDA nor the drugmaker wants to be responsible for. Whatever the reason, a precious resource that has taken millions of dollars of public money to create and maintain is being used at only a small fraction of its potential.

Preventing Companies from Hiding Trial Results

Until Vioxx, most people (including most doctors) didn't understand that companies could conduct a clinical trial of their product, but weren't required to make its findings public. But as news emerged about the distortion of trial results and the hiding of negative data about Paxil, Celebrex, and other widely used medications, the public and Congress were moved to action. The practice of submerging problematic clinical trial data was an open secret in the pharmaceutical industry, and well known to many of us in the field, but such behavior created a furor when it became widely documented. The FDAAA offered a chance to provide a legislative remedy for that as well.

A new and astonishing example of the problem came to light just as Congress was writing that legislation. In May 2007, I received an urgent phone call from an editor at the *New England Journal of Medicine* asking me to evaluate a just-submitted paper; he gave me only a few days' turnaround time. Normally, such review requests came in writing, the manuscript would be delivered in those days by mail or courier (their offices are just across the street from ours), and the review would be due in a few weeks. What was the rush this time? The paper contained a potential bombshell, but the editors had to be sure it was correct. Dr. Steve Nissen was the respected Cleveland Clinic cardiologist who back in 2001 had coauthored a review of Cox-2 inhibitor trials and concluded that Vioxx did indeed increase the risk of cardiovascular disease. Now he was at it again; with a colleague, he had reanalyzed all the available clinical trial data on a different drug—Avandia, the best-selling diabetes drug in the country. He feared that it, too, increased the risk of heart attack, and thought the clinical trial data proved it, even though this was not highlighted in its official labeling. If true, this would be a major problem for patients with diabetes, who were already at increased risk of cardiovascular disease. We prescribed Avandia and drugs like it in order to reduce that danger, not to increase it.

The FDA's review of the drug was of no comfort on this front. The agency required only that a diabetes medication had to lower blood sugar, but it didn't require that the drug had to reduce the incidence of any of the end-organ diseases (heart, kidney, retina, etc.) that we really care about. (This is one of the oldest examples of the agency's overreliance on industry-friendly surrogate measures that make it possible to approve a drug based on a change in a lab test with no requirement to show patient benefit beyond that, as discussed in chapter 3.) I reviewed Nissen's new Avandia–heart attack analysis for *NEJM*, and found it to be a solid and scary piece of work; the journal rushed it into publication a few weeks later. Just as Congress was turning its attention to FDA reform, the world learned that one of the most widely used drugs for diabetes actually increased cardiac disease; small comfort that it lowered blood sugar.

The FDA had been sitting on all the trial data Nissen analyzed, even though it wasn't readily available to the public, but the agency hadn't noticed the problem. In talking with Nissen later, I asked him how he was able to get hold of all the Avandia study results that hadn't been seen by anybody else beyond the manufacturer and the FDA. He gave me a two-word answer: "Eliot Spitzer." As we've seen, back in 2004 as New York's attorney general, he had let drugmaker Glaxo get away with only a relatively small fine of $2.5 million for hiding the negative findings about its antidepressant Paxil. But as part of that settlement Spitzer also required the company to post all its current and future clinical trial results on the internet—an unprecedented demand. Three years later, Nissen and his colleague used that database to analyze the frequency of heart attacks in trials Glaxo had conducted of Avandia. "It took a lot of clicks to find it, and they didn't make it easy, but in the end we were able to get the data we needed," he told me.

As long as companies controlled the results of the clinical trials they funded, would future studies of drug side effects need to rely on one-off legal settlements before researchers and the public could get to see those results? The Vioxx-*NEJM* hidden-data scandal, Steve Nissen's Avandia paper, and other high-profile examples made it clear a better solution was needed.

Since this problem of data suppression was long known in the research community, a federal registry site had been established years earlier: ClinicalTrials.gov, known as CTG. The idea was that all studies involving humans should be registered there before they began, specifying the study design, numbers of patients, hypotheses to be tested, outcomes to be measured, and so on. It was a great idea, but enrolling a study was voluntary, and compliance spotty. Some top-tier medical journals tried to address the problem by announcing that they would not publish any study that hadn't been prospectively registered with CTG before it enrolled its first patient. This helped, but companies could still launch secret studies that they knew would never make it into these first-rate journals anyway. They could continue the same bad habits of publishing and promoting the results of trials that they liked, and burying the others.

The FDAAA changed that. Part of the new legislation empowered the government to require that all studies involving human beings had to be registered with CTG before they could start, with legal and financial penalties if that wasn't done. The number of trials registered in CTG rose substantially, and the practice is now nearly universal. Eliot Spitzer's innovative settlement was transformed into nationwide policy for all drug studies. Anyone with an internet connection can now learn the details of what studies are being conducted, by whom, the number of people involved, and the trials' design. The new legislation was a milestone in the open and complete disclosure of clinical research and has set a standard internationally.

But as with other FDAAA reforms, more work still needs to be done, and important issues still need to be fixed. Some study sponsors in the drug industry list numerous "primary study outcomes" for a given trial, even though each study should ideally have just one. That leaves a lot of wiggle room over which "primary outcome" a company might choose to feature in a publication if they don't all come out as desired. More crucially, the original vision for CTG was that companies would also eventually be required to include the actual results of those trials in the same publicly available database, not just information on a study's existence and design. That requirement is making some headway, but years after the passage of the FDAAA, compliance with that crucial part of the ClinicalTrials.gov requirement is still very incomplete.

Some follow-ups:

- After Nissen's Avandia paper was published in *NEJM*, Glaxo and the FDA disputed its conclusions, even though both already had in their possession nearly all the data Nissen reviewed.
- Three years later, the FDA acknowledged that Avandia did indeed increase the risk of heart attack and restricted its use to near zero; it is now hardly ever prescribed.
- In the wake of Avandia's demise, the FDA required manufacturers of new drugs for diabetes to test whether they increased the risk of heart disease—not whether they decreased that risk, which is still optional. It's a little like the government requiring that the manufacturer of a car has to ensure that it doesn't explode when you turn it on—not whether it is safe to drive.
- Glaxo's misadventures came to public attention again in July 2012, when it settled with the U.S. Department of Justice for an unprecedented $3 billion for its offenses related to Paxil, Avandia, and other products. One of these was its failure to provide full evidence of its clinical trial findings to the FDA.

Making Companies Complete Follow-Up Studies Once a Drug Is Approved

The Vioxx autopsy had revealed how early the signals of cardiovascular risk were known both before the drug was approved and afterward, as well as the barriers that trial monitors faced in trying to get the company to address those concerns as they grew. Follow-up studies that the FDA expects drug companies to complete after a drug's approval are known as post-marketing requirements (or commitments). But several of us in the field knew that often such requirements weren't really requirements, and the so-called commitments were often not honored completely, promptly, or sometimes at all. Once a drug was approved, the FDA just didn't have much clout to force companies to pursue these questions. The problem became so obvious that the agency was forced to report annually in the Federal Register how many such post-marketing studies it had requested, how many were in progress, how many were completed, and how many had not yet begun. Each year, the figures were (or should have been) very embarrassing, particularly the "Not Yet Begun" column, years after a study was to have been launched or even completed. The problem illustrated the puniness of the idea that simply disclosing a problem publicly will somehow lead to its correction. Even worse, the FDA itself could set very loose expectations for completion, giving companies so many years to do the requested studies that a company could be not-late even if it produced no findings for many years after approval. Research from our team led by Kesselheim and from the group at Yale led by Joseph Ross continues to reveal the embarrassing under-completion of such vital studies, even years after the FDAAA was put into place. In one study from our group, about three-quarters of such studies of approved drugs had not been submitted on time.

These concerns raise a related issue: What should the FDA do if follow-up research reveals that a drug doesn't offer any meaningful benefit or has unanticipated side effects? Even when new studies prove that, the agency has trouble limiting access to the product. As passage of the FDAAA law showed, these shortcomings could be addressed if the nation had the legislative and regulatory will to overcome industry opposition and give the FDA the power it needs. The 2022 FDORA regulations could help address that, if the agency chooses to use the authority it's been given. But the anti-science bias of President Trump and those he put forward for key health-care leadership positions does not bode well for this.

Despite the illness, death, and wasted resources that marked the rise and fall of Vioxx, its demise awakened public and legislative concern over how a disaster like that could have happened, and what could be done to prevent a recurrence. As with earlier drug-safety debacles, it led to an evolution in public understanding as well as a drive for reform that brought about badly needed change. It would be better if we could put such obvious reforms in place proactively instead of waiting for the next unthinkable disaster to surprise us and move us to action. Still, crisis-driven incremental improvement is better than no improvement at all.

– PART THREE –

What Should It Cost?

CHAPTER 10

The Price of a Wonder Drug

> My prescription plan changed. It now costs me $1,700 a month for the [lupus] auto-injectors. Needless to say, I couldn't afford that. I'm a social worker and bring home about $3,000 a month. The medication co-pay cost more than my rent, electricity, cell phone bill, and car payment combined.
>
> —A.M., Florida

> I have to decide which medicines I can do without and which I can't. I end up rationing my medicine, and that is like playing Russian roulette with my health. Because of this, my conditions have worsened. I lost vision in one eye due to my diabetes. It is getting more and more difficult to remain active. I want to be able to live a happy and healthy lifestyle and not be so negatively affected by high-cost medications.
>
> —K.P., Washington

As I was finalizing this chapter, I found myself standing in line at my local chain drugstore trying to deal with a recurring snafu on one of my prescriptions. A small elderly woman came up behind me, looking distraught.

"Go ahead of me," I said. "Maybe your problem can get resolved quicker." She thanked me and asked the person behind the counter why her prescription would cost $120, since she had health insurance. The staffer explained, "Your insurance company covers a lot of the charge; this is the part you have to pay by yourself—your co-pay." The woman clutched her pocketbook and said quietly, "I can't afford that; don't fill the prescription." She walked away, seeming a bit more hunched over than she had been a few minutes earlier.

I wondered which drug she decided to forego. Was it a treatment for her heart failure that might avoid an emergency hospitalization? Was it one of the injectable biologic drugs that work so well to contain the symptoms of inflammatory conditions like Crohn's disease? Was it an overpriced new antidepressant that was no better than older medications that are much cheaper?

We doctors review patients' pharmacy records far too rarely, but this little episode would probably not have been recorded in any case. If anyone did look at her "fill history," perhaps when she was admitted to the hospital, all that is likely to appear would be this: "Patient was noncompliant with her prescribed regimen."

"Because I Can": The Origins of High Drug Prices

While people in all countries face rising prescription drug costs, nowhere is the problem as out of control as it is in the U.S. The Organization for Economic Cooperation and Development (OECD) tracks the economies of its thirty-eight relatively wealthy member states across a variety of sectors, from agriculture to technology to health; the findings in the last category are particularly sobering. The U.S. spends about 17 percent of its gross domestic product on medical care expenditures, compared to the average for comparable countries of about 11 percent. Likewise, the U.S. spent twice as much per person on medications as people in these other advanced countries, and that doesn't necessarily include costly hospital-administered drugs.

Those rankings might be acceptable if we also had overall better clinical outcomes or patient satisfaction—that is, if we really believed the slogan that the U.S. has the best health-care system in the world. But our health outcomes don't lead the pack globally. The life expectancy of Americans is nearly four years below the average for OECD countries and falling; our opioid death rate is higher (see chapter 20), and our death rate during the Covid pandemic was higher than those of most other developed countries—the worst except for Peru, according to an analysis from Johns Hopkins University. (By contrast, our leadership in inventing effective and safe Covid vaccines was exemplary, even if we performed poorly in rolling them out to our citizenry.) Also concerning are the facts that we rank near the bottom of wealthy countries in the equitability of our health-care delivery, and that our level of patient satisfaction doesn't match our much greater spending. The Kaiser Family Foundation, now known as KFF, reported that between a quarter and a fifth of Americans say they have trouble paying for the prescriptions their doctors write, a shortfall that can clearly impact health substantially. I've cared for such patients, and some readers may have been in this situation themselves. Our drug payment system has been compared to the hospital gown we ask people to change into before a physical exam: flimsy, cheap, and embarrassing in what it leaves uncovered.

We doctors are often clueless about the prices of drugs or the ability of our patients to pay for what we prescribe. Part of the problem is that we're usually unaware of what anything we order costs, from an MRI to a lab test. But it's much worse for drug prices, which depend on what health insurance company a patient is enrolled in, which drugs are on a "preferred list" for that company, and even how far a person has gone in spending down their annual deductible. Often, it isn't until the patient arrives at the pharmacy that they learn they can't afford the prescription we wrote—or even the co-payment share their insurance company requires them to cover, which itself can run into thousands of dollars a year for many drugs. A health insurer or pharmacy benefits management (PBM) middleman may try to disincentivize use of a given costly drug by slapping a large co-pay on it, making it more costly even for patients with coverage. (Sometimes they'll do the opposite, to maximize the rebates they receive; more on that later.) I've had this happen to patients who were too embarrassed to tell me about it. For some, that means that their blood pressure remained elevated or their blood sugars too high despite what I thought I prescribed, defying all apparent pharmacologic logic. That can lead to new medicines being added by the doctor, while the underlying cause of this "poor control" of a chronic disease remains undetected. Having to choose between filling a prescription or paying the rent or putting food on the table isn't a choice anyone should have to face in a wealthy society, but it happens often in the richest nation on earth.

The consequences of our health-care-cost overruns aren't limited to the medical care system: the expense of our drugs and our medical care have an impact on payrolls as well. Health insurance costs are often borne by the employer, and that affects what it pays its workers, since the total cost of hiring and retaining someone must take into account the expense of their benefits as well. As a result, our highest-in-the-world health-care costs make it more expensive to employ a worker in a U.S. car plant, for example, than a similar person in a car plant elsewhere. Finally, medications join the rest of our supersized health-care costs in contributing to higher taxes and the budget-busting spending on government programs snarkily referred to as "entitlements," such as Medicare and Medicaid, which are among the largest drivers of rising government expenditures. Thus, the unrestrained costs of our medications and other health care ripple throughout the economy, to our collective detriment.

As we're about to see, one remarkable drug illustrates what can happen to specific patients when a medication becomes unaffordable. In this chapter we'll consider how prescription drugs in the U.S. became more expensive than anywhere else on earth. The next chapter will detail the steps that got us here; later, we'll consider actionable steps we can take to deal with the problem.

Breathing Room

The Edinburgh Fringe Festival is the world's largest performing arts event. Each August musicians, actors, singers, acrobats, stand-up comics, and other performers from around the world arrive at over two hundred venues throughout the Scottish capital to present over three thousand different shows. While I was there in 2023, a particular event caught my eye: a one-man performance called *Wonder Drug* in which a British comedian with cystic fibrosis used puppets, props, and blow-up dolls to describe what it's like to live with that debilitating condition, and the medication that saved him. How could I miss that?

Cystic fibrosis (CF) is a genetically based chronic illness in which the body can't produce internal secretions properly. About one in thirty people carries the gene that can cause it, even though that usually doesn't result in full-blown disease. In the lungs, the defect can transform the normal fluid lining the airways into a viscous glop that leads to a chronic cough, shortness of breath, and frequent bouts of pneumonia. Effects on secretions in the digestive system lead to problems absorbing nutrients. Until recently, patients with CF suffered progressive difficulty in breathing, frequent hospitalizations, and early death—usually in their thirties or forties. Historically, all that doctors could do was try to prevent the inevitable complications and treat them when they occurred: inhalers to help with the lung secretions, enzymes to ameliorate the digestive problems, antibiotics for the recurring lung infections. When the disease progressed too far, some patients faced the last-resort prospect of a lung transplant.

The star and only performer in *Wonder Drug* was a young British comedian named Charlie Merriman (a great name for that job), who described his own experience living with CF: the constant cough and frequent shortness of breath, the need to use nebulizers several times a day, the gastrointestinal problems, the frequent infections and periodic bouts of pneumonia. Like his internal secretions, the plot thickens when he meets a love interest in Italy at the start of the Covid epidemic, while they are making a film together about the bubonic plague. In the Edinburgh performance Merriman, wearing a hand-painted T-shirt to remind us where his lungs and stomach and pancreas are, used puppets, dancing antibiotics, singing syringes, and politicians in their underpants to vividly illustrate the disease as well as his long wait to access the drug that could tame it. All this to a soundtrack of 1980s pop favorites.

The show was both amusing and heart-wrenching. Its title referred to the new medication Merriman was waiting for that could repair the underlying mechanism of the disease, offering for the first time the prospect of a more normal existence and even the hope of a near-average lifespan. Months passed; his symptoms persisted and his disease progressed. The relationship with his new love interest faltered. He kept up with his daunting daily schedule of treatments and wondered each day whether he would ever get access to the new medicine, with its promise of normal functioning and escape from an early death.

More months passed; his doctor said the new drug wasn't available yet, but she hoped it would be eventually. He waited. The Fringe performance climaxed when he was finally able to get the new pills. They worked quickly and thoroughly, at last enabling him to live a near-normal existence. The show's finale features Merriman doing aerobic exercise effortlessly at a pace that would have left most of us in the audience breathless.

The show didn't explain that his long wait for the new drug was because its American manufacturer, Vertex Pharmaceuticals, put a six-figure annual price tag on it, an amount that the British National Health Service found exorbitant and unjustified, and which it said it couldn't afford to pay. Merriman's monologue didn't get into the fact that health insurance companies and state Medicaid programs all over the U.S. were also struggling to cover the product at its even higher list price here, about $300,000 a year per patient. But it *was* a life-changing medicine, if you could just get access to it.

Where do wonder drugs like this come from? The pharmaceutical industry depicts the process as involving white-coated company scientists working through the night and spending billions of dollars of corporate funds to develop cures for devastating illnesses like CF. Yes, that happens sometimes. But an enormous amount of the research underlying these products is funded by public sources, like the National Institutes of Health. When that happens, who owns the resulting molecule, and how is its price set? For Merriman, how did all these forces come together so that even after this wondrous treatment for his illness was on the market in the U.S., he still had to endure months of continuing shortness of breath, inhalers, wheezing, and lung infections before his doctor could prescribe it for him so long after it had been discovered and proven effective and safe? How did Vertex come to price it at around $300,000 per year here—a daunting price for uninsured patients and for public- and private-sector insurers alike?

Sometimes a breakthrough medicine is created almost wholly within the labs of a drug company, and at their expense. When that happens, especially when the new treatment reaches the market after a drugmaker has invested in dozens or even hundreds of other products that didn't pan out, the innovator company deserves a lot of credit, and a lot of revenue. But that is often the exception rather than the rule.

Where Wonder Drugs Come From

I still remember a vivid 1963 cover story in *Life* magazine that I saw as a tenth grader, describing the discovery of DNA. It depicted a colorfully imagined double helix with the headline "Scientists Close in on THE SECRET OF LIFE." The article explained that the new science of DNA would soon make it possible to decipher a body's genetic code and enable doctors to understand the causes of diseases and—even more exciting to a fifteen-year-old—to invent new medicines that could fix whatever went wrong. We now know that this promise was a bit too broad and the timeline off by several decades, but the core revelation was true, at least for some deadly conditions: the discovery of the genetic code opened up an unprecedented new era in biology and drug development. I don't know whether that article was also seen by little Francis Collins, a boy a bit younger than me who had been homeschooled in Virginia's rural Shenandoah Valley. But eventually he caught on to its message magnificently. After getting a doctorate in biochemistry and a medical degree, Collins focused his career on identifying the genes that caused specific diseases.

In 1989, a bit over a quarter century after that landmark *Life* magazine article, Dr. Collins and Dr. Lap-Chee Tsui of the University of Toronto Hospital for Sick Children (known in Canada simply as SickKids) announced that they had identified and cloned the gene that caused cystic fibrosis—an accomplishment that was then called the greatest applied discovery in human genetics in decades. Tsui's research had been supported by Canada's NIH-like national research agency and by the Cystic Fibrosis Foundation of Canada. Collins's work was funded by the National Institutes of Health and by the Howard Hughes Medical Institute (HHMI), an enormous nonprofit committed to biomedical research. (Hughes, an eccentric aircraft executive, had given HHMI most of his holdings in the enormously successful aviation company Hughes Aircraft, effectively making the profitable defense contractor a tax-exempt charity. But during his lifetime the institute spent relatively little on medical research, leading to charges that it primarily served him as a personal tax dodge. One of the richest men in the world, Hughes died in 1976 without a will; after lengthy court battles, his fortune of over $5 billion was given to HHMI, making it the largest medical philanthropy in the country. It eventually started making research grants in earnest to scientists like Collins and hundreds of others; its assets currently exceed $24 billion.)

After his discovery of the gene for CF and several other diseases, Dr. Collins was appointed in 1993 to run the federal government's Human Genome Project, an ambitious national program designed to map all thirty thousand or so genes in the human body. The hope was that this multibillion-dollar taxpayer-supported project would lead to new treatments to address genetically based diseases like CF. Collins then went on to serve as director of the National Institutes of Health from 2009 to 2021.

Many steps lie between finding a gene that causes a disease and coming up with a treatment for it. Identifying the faulty gene is a huge step forward, but researchers then have to figure out how to undo the damage it causes—and as we saw with muscular dystrophy, this doesn't always work. In the case of CF, the gene mis-coded the instructions for transporting chloride into and out of the cell—the deficit that caused Merriman's lung and digestive secretions to gum up into dysfunctional, sticky goo. That process had to be repaired; a great deal of additional federally supported research went into building that connection. In addition, other large investments were made by the Cystic Fibrosis Foundation, a U.S.-based nonprofit whose support came primarily from family members of CF patients. One donor who stood out was Joe O'Donnell, a very successful Boston businessman whose son was afflicted with the disease. He led the foundation's fundraising efforts and contributed substantially to that effort from his own personal wealth.

The CF Foundation began an innovative program of what it called "venture philanthropy": giving support to researchers and drug companies to entice them to do research that might lead to a cure for CF—a condition rare enough that most drugmakers had little interest in developing products to treat it. In exchange, the foundation would get a share of the royalties from any drugs that resulted from the partnership. In 2000, the foundation gave an initial $40 million to a small Cambridge biotech firm called Aurora Biosciences to induce it to study drugs for CF that could address the damage done by the misbehaving gene that Collins, Tsui, and their many collaborators had identified; that amount eventually increased to $150 million. In 2001 Aurora, its scientists, and its intellectual property were bought for $592 million by another biotech firm, Boston-based Vertex Pharmaceuticals. At the time, Vertex had only one drug on the market and had yet to turn a profit, but its officers liked Aurora's drug development portfolio. On the day of the announcement Aurora's stock went up by 44 percent. "We are going to seize as much of this ground as we can," said Vertex CEO Josh Boger of the acquired research portfolio. Another Vertex official later said the company hadn't been sure it wanted to keep Aurora's CF drug development program, but did so because the CF Foundation's funding covered so much of its cost, offering "a less expensive form of financing."

After buying Aurora and its team of CF scientists and its platform for developing new drugs, Vertex continued the demanding and costly agenda of building on the basic science insights into what goes wrong in the cells of CF patients, and turning that knowledge into drug development, a process heavily "de-risked" by the ample funding from the CF Foundation and other philanthropic and public sources. Vertex's first CF drug, Kalydeco (ivacaftor) was discovered in 2005 and approved in 2012, but it treated only about 4 percent of CF patients. Other new drugs followed, and then a three-drug combination built on these concepts, Trikafta. It worked in the vast majority of CF patients and was approved in 2019. The drugs have been a major commercial success for Vertex, which now makes nearly $10 billion per year on sales of its CF drugs. The discoveries were also a boon for the CF Foundation's venture philanthropy approach; the venture part meant that in exchange for its funding, the foundation acquired a share of the rights to any drugs that resulted from that support. In 2014 the CF Foundation made $3.3 billion by selling its royalty rights to the drugs whose development it had funded. A 2020 deal for its remaining CF drug rights brought in over $575 million more.

Vertex did extremely well with its sales of its CF drugs, and the CF Foundation, whose funding heavily underwrote that development, also got a breathtaking windfall from its share of the royalties. Patients now had a treatment that treated their symptoms remarkably well and held the promise of a normal lifespan for those afflicted with a once-fatal disease. Everyone wins, right?

Not exactly. Those billions of dollars in sales came from somewhere. A number of scientists did very important work building on the insights of Collins, Tsui, and their many collaborators who identified the CF gene, taking on the daunting task of creating molecules to undo the damage the faulty gene caused, including those who did the key original work while employed by Aurora Biosciences. But when all the pieces came together in the end, it was Vertex that would come to own the patents on the miraculous drug molecules, and would therefore be able to charge whatever it wanted for the resulting medicines.

This ability of U.S. drug companies to charge anything they choose for their products is not seen elsewhere in the world. The situation came to widespread attention in 2015 when a small-time hustler named Martin Shkreli set up a company that bought control of Daraprim, a very old drug that had become available generically; it was a key treatment for the parasitic infection toxoplasmosis, that affects vulnerable AIDS patients. Shkreli used a technicality in the patent laws to gain total ownership of the drug, and increased its price by 4,400 percent from $17 per capsule to $750 per capsule. Why? he was asked. "Because I can," was his reply. Crude, but accurate. (He later did prison time for unrelated financial crimes, and a federal judge banned him for life from any future work in the pharmaceutical industry.)

Despite the extensive public funding that led to the discovery of Kalydeco and other CF products, and despite the CF Foundation's pivotal funding for the development of the drugs themselves, Vertex owned the patents, it owned the products, and it was legally entitled to price them as it saw fit, at about $300,000 per patient per year. That created a major hurdle for patients and insurers both private and public; even families with good health insurance could be hit with many thousands of dollars a year in co-payments. A paper in the *Journal of Cystic Fibrosis* surveyed nearly 1,900 people living with CF and found that two-thirds reported facing food insecurity, housing problems, or debt burdens—not solely because of their drug costs, but partially. Nearly half said they had to forgo or delay their CF care because of cost, and 39 percent said they had been contacted by debt collection agencies.

Despite the billions it received in royalties on the drugs whose development it funded, the CF Foundation did not see its role as making those funds available to patients who had trouble paying for the drugs. Instead, it chose to invest its now-substantial endowment in other drug-development opportunities to expand its venture philanthropy program. For CF patients having trouble affording the cost of their treatment, the foundation provides advice on how to get onto Medicaid or seek help from private insurance companies, patient assistance programs offered by drug companies, and food stamps.

A pediatric pulmonologist colleague demanded a meeting with a senior Vertex executive about their drugs' prices. "How dare you charge $300,000 a year for this drug?" he demanded, angrily. "Why not $100,000 a year, or $50,000, or less?" The Vertex executive was unmoved. He could have channeled Shkreli, but he offered a more revelatory answer. "Funny you should say that," he answered, according to the lung doctor. "Just a few days ago I had a shareholder sitting in that very same chair. He asked me, 'How dare you charge only $300,000 a year for our drug? Why not $400,000 a year, or $500,000?'"

Drug companies have to listen to their investors. They don't have to listen anywhere near as much to patients, insurance companies, ethicists, policy analysts, or the government. And in the U.S., alone among industrialized countries, they can in fact charge whatever they want—even for a product that the public helped in part to develop. Like golems, they need be faithful only to their fiduciary responsibilities to investors.

Pharmaceutical manufacturers aren't allowed to do that in most other countries, including Great Britain. That country's National Health Service provides free care to all British residents, including the medications they need. But to be able to do so, it has to set strict limits on what it will pay for goods and services. The NHS operates on a fixed central budget: health-care expenditures for a given year are capped, and if more is spent on *x*, then less is available for *y*, where *x* may be a medication, a costly radiation treatment, or nursing home care, and *y* can be everything else, such as family planning and obstetric services, routine surgeries, care for the disabled, and all other drugs. This zero-sum-game concept isn't an idea we Americans are used to. Here, if something in health care costs more, then you spend more, and the sky's the limit.

The economic constraints of the British National Health Service make our approach look like that of an entitled drunken teenager wielding his parents' credit card in the mall, secure in the knowledge that someone will pay the bill and there won't be any consequences. On the other hand, the Brits spend a lower proportion of their gross domestic product on health care than most other European countries. For a wealthy country, this is probably too low, explaining the queueing, shortages, and other limitations that patients there must often endure. All the same, until recently the British have traditionally had a fondness for their NHS despite fourteen years of underfunding by a succession of Conservative governments, leading to greater stinginess and longer waiting times. More and more each year, many of them are asking whether that extreme stringency yoked to orthodox cost-effectiveness analysis has become a tool for denying needed medicines and services to its citizens; we'll take that problem up in chapter 13.

To pay for its universal coverage of virtually all health-care needs, the NHS evaluates the appropriate price that each drug warrants. To keep its health expenditures affordable, the country established the National Institute for Health and Care Excellence, with the nice acronym of NICE. That group calculates a reasonable price for all new medications based on their benefit to patients, and that's what companies generally agree to be paid. The UK has over ten thousand residents with CF—more than any other country outside the U.S. In Britain, Vertex had priced its earlier CF breakthrough drug, Orkambi, at £105,000 per year ($138,000), well above the costs of most other drugs in the NHS and much greater than the price that NICE and other groups had calculated as fair; Vertex refused to sell it at the price NICE had calculated. When the NHS and the company couldn't come to an agreement, the NHS offered Vertex £500 million over five years (over $650 million) for NHS beneficiaries to access the drug, while guaranteeing the drugmaker a secure source of ongoing profit—the largest financial offer ever made by the NHS. The company refused.

Many patients asked, "How can the company be so heartless as to demand such an exorbitant price?" Vertex executives asked, "How can the NHS be so heartless as to refuse to pay for this life-saving drug?" Remarkably, the standoff went on for several years, during which time that first breakthrough drug wasn't available to British CF patients unless they paid for it out of pocket, which few could do. In 2019, a group of frantic parents of children with CF wrote to the prime minister and the health secretary:

> We cannot explain, let alone expect you to understand, the sheer dread and helplessness it causes us to know that we are likely to outlive our children. The anguish in knowing that a drug exists that can change that—sparing them unnecessary suffering and decline in health—but that they are denied access, is unbearable.

Vertex said it needed the money for its research, but a Canadian researcher found that the company had already made up its investment in the disease many times over and would continue to profit handsomely from the medication for many years even at much lower prices. The impasse between the company and the NHS dragged on as CF patients endured continuing daily symptoms that the drug could have prevented; they also developed recurrent pulmonary infections, with each new episode further reducing their lung function and increasing their risk of developing new infections with antibiotic-resistant bacteria. Some died. In early 2019, Vertex announced that it had thrown away 7,880 packets of Orkambi that had gone unused during its UK price standoff, on the grounds that they had passed their sell-by date. The *Guardian* reported that this would have covered the population of UK cystic fibrosis patients who needed the drug for decades.

In October 2019, the NHS and Vertex finally reached an agreement on a price for Orkambi that both could live with; the amount was not disclosed. But soon thereafter, Vertex brought to market a much better follow-on product, the even more effective three-drug combination Kaftrio, that worked impressively well in a far larger proportion of CF patients (it's sold as Trikafta in the U.S.). The new drug was approved in the U.S. in 2019, where Vertex assigned it a list price of $322,000 per patient per year. Back in Britain, it took until 2020 for the NHS to reach an agreement with the company about its price; that's when Merriman finally got the wonder drug he needed. After years of debilitating chronic illness, it made him feel better almost immediately.

In the U.S., the respected Institute for Clinical and Economic Review estimated that taking into account its remarkable clinical benefits, a fair price for the drug would be between $67,900 and $85,500 a year, including a profit margin for the manufacturer. It invited Vertex to participate in discussions of that recommendation, but the company refused.

Defenders of high drug prices in the U.S. argue that many American patients have health insurance. And, they argue, those without coverage can try to get onto Medicaid, the publicly funded state-based program of health care, which will cover their medications. But many private insurers require patients to pay a fixed percentage of a drug's cost, so a 20 percent charge for Trikafta could come to over $60,000 per year owed by the individual. Some drug companies offer "patient assistance programs" that can help those without insurance or cover a portion of the patient's co-payments, though their level of generosity and very existence are at the will of the manufacturer. Such charity, often provided in the form of coupons given to patients to use for their co-pay costs, can substantially reduce the consumer's share of the bill, while sidelining them as combatants in the debate on prices and preserving the much larger part of the cost charged to insurers—raising premiums for all subscribers.

Facing financial hardship, many families become impoverished—at which point they may be able to qualify for state-supported Medicaid. But that just pushes the problem up a level, as we'll see below. Unaffordable drug charges covered by Medicaid have to be offset by reducing expenditures on other medical care, or by seeking extra taxpayer funding from state legislators. The situation is much worse in other parts of the world. After Trikafta was approved, Vertex did little to make it available affordably in most of the developing world, and blocked attempts by generic manufacturers there to license or produce it.

Our PORTAL research group has been working with several states struggling to deal with the high drug expenditures impacting the budgets of families and of health insurers, including Medicaid. Led by Dr. Ben Rome, we've been trying to help several states decide which drugs to focus on and what fairer payments would be: amounts that would reward pharmaceutical innovation and compensate for all the blind alleys companies have to go down before they come up with a viable new product, but prices that would also not be unbearable for patients and financing programs.

Colorado was one of the first states to move forward in this direction: in 2022, its legislature authorized the creation of a state-based prescription drug affordability board (PDAB). Its bold mandate was to identify which medications were the most "unaffordable" for the state's residents, and to assign each a more reasonable price—an unprecedented step for any state to take. The first drug it chose to explore was Vertex's Trikafta. Since that company was one of the most aggressive drugmakers when it came to price, and in light of the NHS experience with those very drugs, I worried that this was a risky choice.

Across the Atlantic, things had been more fraught for CF patients like Merriman. The British National Institute for Health and Care Excellence had continued its evaluation of the affordability of drugs for CF. In late November 2023, NICE agreed that "there is a large and robust evidence base for the acute benefits" of Kaftrio and other Vertex CF drugs. However, given the very high price Vertex put on these drugs, NICE ruled that despite the clear benefits, its cost was well above the value-for-money levels that would be affordable without requiring cuts in other parts of the fixed-budget National Health Service. Its report concluded, "Even when considering the condition's severity and [the drugs'] effectiveness on quality and length of life, the most likely cost-effectiveness estimates are above the range that NICE considers an acceptable use of resources. So they are not recommended." (Not recommended means not covered.)

Patients like Merriman who were on the drugs could continue to have the drugs paid for within NHS, as could others already taking them as of the date of NICE's pending final ruling. After that, access for new patients was not certain. The nation had recently allowed its use in children age two to five, so a scramble ensued to get these kids "grandfathered in" and started on the medications before the looming deadline. But in no case would the NHS provide the drugs to children under age two, even though many authorities believed that beginning their protective effects early was the best way to prevent ongoing damage to the lungs and other organs.

This put parents of babies born with CF in an excruciating position. If a baby didn't turn two before the new NICE deadline, the ruling—unless it was modified—would mean that it could never get started on the life-saving drug. The price of Kaftrio in Great Britain was estimated at about $235,000 per year, although the exact amount is kept secret. Pharmaceutical scientists estimate that the cost to manufacture the drug is about $5,700 for a year's supply.

When the NICE edict was issued, an English television station interviewed the mother of a nine-month-old girl in Norwich who was born with CF.

> "We were reassured she would have a healthy long life, she would outlive us," the distressed mom said. "And now that chance is

> being robbed and it is a possibility if [the drugs] are pulled we are going to be planning our daughter's funeral and burying her one day. No parent should have to bury her child, and a price should never be put on a child's head."

Separately, in a submission to the U.S. Securities and Exchange Commission, Vertex forecast that 2023 revenues from its cystic fibrosis drugs would amount to nearly $10 billion, and announced a stock buyback program of up to $3 billion. In early 2023, the company also said it would slash its patient assistance programs from a maximum of about $100,000 per patient annually to a ceiling of $20,000. The announcement caused chaos in the U.S. CF community, as many patients depended on that program to be able to afford their medicine, even if they had health insurance.

> "We felt pretty helpless," a Utah nurse told the STAT news service about the prospect of affording the medicine for his two-year-old daughter with CF. "We talked about what we could do financially, like if we needed to sell our house . . . but that would only help for so long."

How did we end up here, and what should these drugs really cost? We will rethink these issues in the following chapters.

CHAPTER 11

Giving It All Away

> Capitalism without competition isn't capitalism; it's exploitation. Without healthy competition, big players can charge whatever they want and treat you however they want. And for too many Americans, that means accepting a bad deal.

That statement was made by the noted socialist extremist Joe Biden in a 2021 White House ceremony marking his signing of an Executive Order on Promoting Competition in the American Economy. He recognized many of the ways our free enterprise system has become distorted to favor the "prize" part over the "free" part, especially in the area of pharmaceuticals.

We Have Created Our Own Affordability Crisis

How did we end up here, with wonderfully effective drugs that people can't afford, or that place unbearable financial burdens on healthcare systems and family budgets? The missteps are pretty clear, and each could be undone if we had the understanding and political will to do so. It was you and me and our forebears who made medicines so expensive, by yielding to pharmaceutical companies the right to charge whatever they want for their products. Each step of our collective march into this national quagmire was the product of years of lobbying and bad legislative decisions. But because of that, the good news is that each is fixable.

Of course, drugmakers often make very important contributions to the development of new medicines, and they deserve to be paid fairly—even very handsomely—for that role. Drug discovery is a daunting task, even if much of it is "de-risked" by taxpayers, as we'll see below; manufacturers ought to be compensated for all their false starts and failures as well. Unfortunately, fair to handsome compensation hasn't been enough to satisfy most companies. Instead, they have argued that *any* limits on prices or their revenues will cripple the irreplaceable innovation that they alone provide, and will strangle the pipeline of new cures. Too often, that's where the discussion begins and ends, even though studies from our group and other researchers demonstrate that the presumption is patently untrue.

The largest engine driving the nation's prodigious ability to bring new drugs to market is the hundreds of billions of taxpayer-generated dollars we have invested in the National Institutes of Health and other public and philanthropic funders of biomedical discovery. We've seen the key role played by the federally funded Human Genome Project in discovering the genes that cause cystic fibrosis, and the follow-on NIH and foundation support that led the nation to the doorstep of very effective treatments. Because of the pervasiveness of the myth that extremely high prices are needed to get new medications, and the powerful effect this misconception has had on shaping legislation and public beliefs, my colleague Kesselheim has made it one focus of his PORTAL research program in our division. In an early paper, we traced the public-funding contribution of twenty-five of the most influential drug discoveries in the preceding decades, and showed how each of them had vital origins in federal support. Our team has gone on to dissect the beginnings of other enormously important drugs, tracing their original patents and the NIH grants that preceded them, and found the same thing. A few compelling examples are presented below.

As lifesaving drugs have fascinating origin tales, so do the policies that make them unaffordable. Just a few pivotal moments shaped the evolution of our price-it-anywhere rules; important milestones occurred in 1789, 1980, 2003, and 2008. The first date is the creation of our innovative patent policy around the time of the nation's birth; 1980 saw the passage of key legislation that made it possible to privatize publicly discovered knowledge. In 2003, an industry-influenced

Congress passed a law forbidding the nation's largest public health insurer, Medicare, from negotiating any of the prices it pays for drugs, later requiring it to cover most of the costliest medications on the market. Finally, the period during and after the 2008 elections marked a quantum leap in the rhetoric against the idea of measuring the actual worth of health-care interventions, when vice presidential candidate Sarah Palin warned that if Barack Obama were elected he would institute "death panels" to ration care, inevitably leading to withholding medical goods and services from the elderly and disabled. We can rethink each of these watershed moments to understand how each policy went wrong and what we can do now to repair each misstep.

Yes, the Government *Is* the Problem, in Part

We doctors often hear patients exclaim, "The government should do something about high drug prices!" Sure; but with great irony, we can recall Ronald Reagan's infamous statement that the government is actually the *cause* of most of the nation's difficulties. In general that's a terrible rule of thumb to guide policymaking, but in this case the dirty little secret is that there is some truth here, but not at all in the way Reagan intended: the federal government is one of the key reasons U.S. drug prices are the highest in the world. The nation accomplished this feat through several different mechanisms, beginning in the first years of its existence.

The Founding Fathers were prescient in placing enormous value on innovation to drive the newborn country forward. So they created a system of patents—socially useful government-backed monopolies designed to foster and protect inventors and their inventions. That value was so central to the Founders that it was enshrined in Article I of the Constitution, which states, "The Congress shall have Power . . . To promote the Progress of Science and useful Arts, by securing for limited Times to Authors and Inventors the exclusive Right to their respective Writings and Discoveries." The novel but very sensible logic was that innovators should be able to own all the rights to their inventions for a reasonable period of time in order to reward their creativity. But the other side of the patent coin is the second and equally important part of that social contract: after the end of that reasonable period, those monopoly rights come to an end. That will enable others to produce the once-protected product, driving down its price and making it more widely available. And if innovators want to have a continuing source of revenue, they'd have to invent something new.

A patent that would last forever would not only make the product unaffordable by permanently prohibiting competition, it would also provide no incentive for the original creator to keep creating. At first, the awarding and expiration of patents was one of the major success stories in the prescription drug market. Inexpensive generic versions of once-patent-protected drugs are now produced by multiple competitors and make up 90 percent of all prescriptions written in the U.S., but they've become so cheap that they account for only 20 percent of our national drug expenditure. That's the good news. The less good news is that while still-patented drugs make up only about 10 percent of all prescriptions written, they account for the other 80 percent of our drug expenditures. That's because their manufacturers can set any price they want for them, and the price is usually very high. Companies can then manipulate the patent system to block competition well beyond what the framers of the patent idea intended.

So despite the good news on generics, in which the system works as it should, for non-generic drugs the federal government too often gets this wrong on both the coming and going sides—how patents are issued, and how they expire. On the coming side: The U.S. Patent and Trademark Office (USPTO) is supposed to issue a patent for a new product if it is "non-obvious, novel, and useful." Yet when it comes to medications, the government has slid into issuing patents for products that lack some or all of these key characteristics. An editorial in the *New York Times* charged that the USPTO is "a backwater office that large corporations game, politicians ignore and average citizens are wholly excluded from. As a result, not only is legal trickery rewarded and the public's interest overlooked, but also innovation—the very thing that patents were meant to foster—is undermined." In the notorious case of Theranos, the billion-dollar company that made phony clinical lab test devices, the Patent Office granted numerous patents to machines that didn't work and in some cases didn't even exist.

One well-known drug example is in the medicine cabinets of most Americans: AstraZeneca's Nexium, the "purple pill" so widely used to treat a variety of stomach complaints. Its first incarnation was as omeprazole, first marketed as Prilosec. The drug very effectively shuts off acid production in the stomach, giving impressive relief to millions of people with peptic ulcers or gastroesophageal reflux. It was also widely overused, but we can't blame the Patent Office for that.

What we can blame them for is their decision several years later to grant a brand-new patent to omeprazole's virtually identical twin, esomeprazole. The "es" prefix refers to *S* for *sinistre*, Latin for "left." It contrasts with the *D* prefix for right-handedness, from the Latin root that gave us words like "dexterity." These initials are also used in medical jargon to refer to the sidedness of any paired organ, like eyes and ears. As a left-handed person I used to take offense at their semantic origins, but I'm getting over it.

Why name a medication "left"? Many molecules exist as a mixture of mirror-image versions of the same substance, slightly different geometrically from each other in the same way that pairs of shoes or gloves are. Concerned that its lucrative patent on Prilosec was expiring (as the Founding Fathers meant for it to do), AstraZeneca engaged in some chemistry sleight of hand to create a product consisting solely of the "sinister" version of the molecule, slapped an *S* (actually an "es") on its generic name, and called it esomeprazole. The company gave it the brand name of Nexium—the "next" purple pill—and marketed it as a new medical breakthrough.

Sometimes this asymmetry can have pharmacological implications about a drug's effects, but often not. AstraZeneca didn't demonstrate any convincing evidence that the *S* version of the drug had clinically meaningful properties different from the original right-plus-left product. Instead, the company just engaged in what might be called hand-waving in its patent application, and the new drug was granted a patent of its own, renewing the clock on one of the most lucrative franchises in medication history. The company then handily converted the older right-left mixed product to over-the-counter status ("OTC Prilosec") and handed its marketing to a different part of the company, through which it continues to generate enormous profits. The newer left-side-only drug remained the only medicine of its kind on the prescription drug market for several years. Heavy promotion implied that the newer, "next" purple pill was somehow preferable to the existing product. Many doctors and patients seem to prefer widely advertised prescribed medications more than OTC drugs, and many drug insurance plans will cover the former but not the latter. The underhanded scam produced a brand-new government-granted monopoly for the "new" drug that cost the nation billions of dollars of clinically unjustified additional costs, and handed the manufacturer fistfuls of dollars in unwarranted additional profit.

How did that happen? Patent Office examiners guard the gates of these lucrative federally granted monopolies and thus govern hundreds of billions of dollars a year in sales of all kinds of products. They tend to be earnest, underpaid, and overworked. One analysis reported the average amount of time allotted to a federal examiner to evaluate a product for a new patent as just nineteen hours. That's the average for all kinds of patents; a Patent Office publication broke it down a bit more, explaining that an examiner gets 16.6 hours to review a fishing lure application, and 25.9 hours for an immunotherapy drug application, even if billions of dollars may ride on the second decision. The examiners often find themselves in over their heads, facing off against an army of extremely well-trained and exorbitantly paid patent attorneys working for a drug's manufacturer. And once a patent is granted with the full authority of the federal government behind it, given all the other imperfections of the prescription drug market, it can become a license to print money.

A more recent example is the antidepressant nasal spray Spravato (esketamine), the left-handed version of the anesthetic agent and recreational drug ketamine. For several years, patients and clinicians had noticed the remarkable (some said "miraculous") effect that occurred when depressed people were given ketamine as an anesthetic for a surgical procedure. Some patients who had been suffering from intractable long-standing mood disorders awakened from their operations and proclaimed that for the first time in years they no longer felt depressed. This finding also cast an entirely new light on our primitive understanding of the neurochemistry of depression, since existing medications took weeks to have any effect; for ketamine, the result when it occurred was virtually immediate. The ketamine anesthetic had long been generic, first approved in 1970, but the marketplace was ripe for a new product that could be separately patented and therefore ownable. Drugmaker Janssen created a left-handed version of the molecule, added the "es" to the previous drug's generic name, compounded it into a nasal spray, and gave it the trade name of Spravato. (A colleague speculated that the name conjured up a spray that could give you bravado.)

The new product was reviewed on the FDA's "breakthrough" and "fast track" pathways and evaluated in three randomized trials against placebo. The studies were said to be double-blind, though it's hard to imagine how patients couldn't tell whether they were given a drug that could make you feel drowsy, dizzy, nauseated, or disassociated (a temporary psychotic-like state) versus a saltwater spray. So much for the blinding. In two of the studies the drug failed to show an advantage over placebo, so the FDA and the manufacturer went with the third study, which did. Questions have recently arisen on whether its side effects were fully reported. But now, for any patient with depression who ever said, "Doc, can you give me a treatment that may or may not work better than squirting salt water up my nose?"—Spravato was the drug to choose.

Suicide in a depressed patient is the nightmare outcome that most terrifies prescribers, patients, and families. The old intravenous ketamine isn't officially FDA-approved for depression, no less suicidality; it's been off-patent for so long that no manufacturer was motivated to conduct the costly clinical trials that would be needed to win that approval. In contrast, Spravato's promotional material and official FDA-approved description note that it is approved for "major depressive disorder with acute suicidal ideation or behavior," which seems encouraging. But there actually wasn't much convincing evidence that the drug really did reduce the risk of suicide; one line later, under "Limitations for Use," the official product label says, "The effectiveness of SPRAVATO® in preventing suicide or in reducing suicidal ideation or behavior has not been demonstrated."

A *JAMA* study from Yale evaluated a series of several other such patented left-versus-right one-handed drugs; it found that the new products were rarely compared with their both-handed or opposite-handed twins to see if they truly had any superior clinical effects; when they were compared, differences were generally not seen. What does that say about the "novel" attribute we expect for a patentable product? But they're pretty busy over at the USPTO, evaluating all those new fishing lures and stuff. Comparisons of drug patents granted in the U.S. versus other countries have found that in our pharma-friendly environment, we issue dubious drug patents far more readily than other nations do. And challenging a dumb patent can be difficult, uncertain, and consume a lot of time and money.

Generic ketamine costs about $187 per IV dose and has many manufacturers; none of them would be motivated to promote it at that price, and such promotion would be illegal anyway, since the older drug has no official FDA authorization for that use. As a result, many insurers won't pay for it. But doctors can prescribe any FDA-approved drug as they see fit, even if it hasn't been granted an official "indication" for a given condition on its label. That has given rise to hundreds of IV ketamine clinics all over the country that offer anesthesia for outpatient surgical procedures as well as treatment for depression as well as psychedelic psychotherapy. Spravato costs about $1,300 a dose; its official FDA blessing enables its manufacturer to promote it heavily for depression. More recent clinical trials have found that the intravenous and intranasal versions of the drug are about equally effective, with some studies finding that the older drug works a bit better. By 2023, Spravato had become the fastest-growing product for Janssen's parent company Johnson & Johnson, expected to bring in over $600 million a year.

Stuck in a Thicket

Handedness is only one small part of the government-granted monopoly problem. Companies can also obtain additional exclusivity rights on trivial aspects of a medication that are unrelated to any clinical benefit: that creates a "thicket" of patents surrounding the drug, each one further extending the original exclusivity in time and further blocking competition. The congressional House Oversight Committee has found that twelve of the medications that account for Medicare's highest expenditures are covered by no less than six hundred separate patents. Researchers in our PORTAL unit have identified a host of such abuses, as has an intrepid nonprofit known as I-MAK (the Initiative for Medicines, Access, and Knowledge), along with the productive group at Yale headed by Dr. Joe Ross. Al Engelberg, the spunky octogenarian lawyer who helped establish the legal basis for the generic drug industry in the 1970s, has written compellingly about these issues, and several professors of law have also been leaders in examining the relationship between patents and medication access—Robin Feldman at the University of California and PORTAL collaborators Michelle Mello of Stanford and Sean Tu at the University of West Virginia, among other scholars. Together, the combined budgets for all of us are a tiny fraction of the salaries of the patent attorneys hired by the drug industry, but we and other public interest researchers are doing our best to bring considerations of equity and reality to this contested area.

AbbVie, maker of the costly and lucrative immune suppressant Humira, one of the best-selling drugs in the world, also surrounded its drug with a thicket of derivative patents to ward off generic competition. Examination of these patents and the drug's sales revealed that such extra patents enabled AbbVie to earn an additional *$114 billion* in revenue after its main patent had expired. As our colleagues at I-MAK discovered, several of those patent applications were shot down by European patent authorities or were revoked there after challenges. As a result, a more affordable biosimilar version of Humira became available in Europe more than four years sooner than in the U.S.

In its striking report titled "Overpatented, Overpriced: Tackling the Root of the Drug Pricing Crisis," I-MAK made several other disturbing observations:

- Pharmaceutical companies filed over 140 patent applications on average for *each* top-selling drug.
- Two thirds of these patent applications were filed after the drug was approved.
- Each of America's ten top-selling drugs is protected by an average of seventy-four patents apiece.
- Four times as many patents are granted on the top ten drugs in the U.S. compared to Europe.
- Lower-cost versions of America's three top-selling drugs became available in Europe an average of nearly eight years earlier than they did in the U.S.
- That delay accounted for an estimated $167 billion more spent by Americans on just three drugs (Enbrel, Humira, Eliquis).

Sometimes the patent thicket is built up with legal protections that aren't based on any medical properties at all. For new drugs that pose major safety concerns, the FDA will sometimes require a company to deploy a risk evaluation and mitigation strategy (REMS), to inform prescribers, patients, and pharmacists about important precautions related to its use. This may involve requiring a negative pregnancy test before dispensing a drug that can cause birth defects. Or a pharmacist will have to check a white blood cell count before dispensing the antipsychotic drug clozapine, since the medication can drive those counts to near zero if that isn't caught in time. So far, so good. Informational and safety provisions like that can't be patented to thicken the thickets of exclusivity claims built around a drug, can they?

You bet they can.

One sinister development (not in the left-handed molecular sense) involved Xyrem, a liquid sleep-inducing medicine; in chapter 16 we'll see how its misleading overpromotion was justified as "free speech" in a notorious case that threatened much of the FDA's regulatory authority. Xyrem returned to the public eye a few years later with another daring gambit. Its manufacturer had changed its corporate name from the poignant sounding "Orphan Drugs" to the perhaps more revealing "Jazz Pharmaceuticals." The medication itself was a simple molecule that had been developed and tested by others in the 1960s, and was even sold over the counter for a while as a "nutritional supplement" before it became clear it had problematic uses, including as a date-rape drug. Through the magic of patent law it was then transformed into a prescription-only medication to treat the rare condition of narcolepsy, and Orphan/Jazz came to own the rights to it; the company then increased its list price dramatically year after year, reaching an annual cost of about $200,000. The FDA was concerned about its potential misuse, and ordered the drugmaker to put in place a system to track who was filling these prescriptions. The company did so, and then patented the tracking system itself. As its underlying monopoly rights over the medication were expiring and a generic drugmaker sought to sell it at a much lower price, Xyrem's manufacturer sued them on the grounds that the newcomer's tracking plan violated the patent on its REMS approach, which it considered a proprietary "method of use" property of the drug.

This was not an outlier strategy. We again meet up with thalidomide, the sedative-antinauseant that in the 1950s and early '60s caused severe birth defects in most countries except for the U.S., where it was kept off the market by an astute FDA medical officer (see chapter 5). Like Xyrem, thalidomide surfaced again in a novel kind of patenting controversy. In the new century it lost its pariah status when the drugmaker Celgene picked through research studies and found some that suggested the notorious product might be useful for treating leprosy, and then as a drug for the blood cancer multiple myeloma. The company obtained a new patent on the drug for these uses—it's legal to patent a novel use of an old drug—and gave it the brand name of Thalomid. It also made some small changes to the molecule to create a separate new product, which it called Revlimid.

Fine; innovation is good, repurposing of old drugs for new purposes can be a worthy undertaking, and should be rewarded. Less fine are attempts to game the patent system to block generic manufacturers from producing a medication at more affordable prices once the original reward-granting patents expire. Celgene did exactly this in several ways. The FDA requires generic manufacturers to test their products against the original drug to make sure they're equivalent, but Celgene refused to make its drug available to its competitor for that purpose, cutting off potential generic manufacturers at the knees and blocking entry of a more affordable version. Less plausibly, the FDA also required prospective generic manufacturers to use the *same* REMS safe-prescribing program—in this case, for the simple purpose of ensuring that a patient not become pregnant. Celgene claimed ownership of its REMS program as well, obtaining fourteen patents on it. Competitors could pay the company dearly to use its pregnancy-prevention surveillance program, or not be allowed by the FDA to market the drug.

It's not unthinkable that as patents expire, the federal government could require a brand-name company to sell a small amount of its drug to a potential competitor to perform the required equivalence studies without undercutting the very structure of the free enterprise system. (In fact, doing so would support it.) Nor is it clear why the FDA couldn't accept a different pregnancy-prevention program that wouldn't violate the patents taken out on a prior one. But such abuses of the patent system enabled Celgene to keep monopoly control for many years over this ancient drug—once sold over the counter outside the U.S. for a pittance—and its slightly modified cousin. And naturally, that right enabled them to keep raising the price they charged. The list price of Revlimid doubled every few years, reaching about $17,000 per month, or $204,000 a year by 2019. The two drugs both remained in use to treat myeloma, generating the lion's share of the company's revenues. That year, the company's aggressive pricing posture and combative use of the patent system paid off. It was bought by Bristol Myers Squibb for $95 billion, then one of the largest pharmaceutical acquisition deals ever.

In the words of one patient:

> I have a blood cancer, multiple myeloma. It's incurable, but treatable with very expensive drugs. The four-drug combination I am

> on now carries a list price of $875,000 a year. I am completely dependent on innovation to survive. But innovation and new drugs should not come at prices that bankrupt people. . . . Drugs don't work if people can't afford them.

The patient is David Mitchell, then seventy-four. In 2016, reeling from his own drug-cost burden, he founded Patients for Affordable Drugs, which has become a formidable presence nationally working for lower medication prices. It is unusual among patient advocacy groups because he refuses to accept support from any companies in the pharmaceutical supply chain.

An Allergy to Competition

The website of Mitchell's organization also contains this account from another patient:

> I am a retired Tucson police department detective and middle school science teacher. . . . I am supposed to carry an EpiPen with me at all times to avoid hospitalization for my severe allergies. I am 66 years old and recently switched to Medicare. I can't believe how expensive my EpiPens are on Medicare. Because of the price, I have a difficult time refilling my prescription. There have been times where I could not afford to carry an EpiPen and ended up hospitalized with anaphylactic shock after being exposed to latex. It is unfair that seniors like myself should have to worry as much as I do to afford our prescriptions. I shouldn't have to spend my retirement praying that my small business sales go well so that I can finally purchase my EpiPen. It isn't right.
>
> —Brenda, Arizona

Some of the most egregious monopoly-lengthening strategies are so-called tertiary patents, which prolong the period of government-granted exclusivity by patenting the *device* used to administer a drug. One familiar example is EpiPen—the syringe used by patients with dangerous allergies in order to self-inject epinephrine, also known as adrenaline—a naturally occurring hormone first synthesized in the lab in the 1950s. Its use can prevent a potentially fatal reaction and be lifesaving. The patent on epinephrine expired decades ago, but the EpiPen manufacturer, Mylan Labs, obtained monopoly rights over the simple injector device as well, blocking generic manufacturers from entering the market for years. That kept the cost of the product at around $600 per prescription. This was a source of terror for patients susceptible to these severe allergic reactions, since having the vital antidote on hand was often unaffordable. Rising public ire led to congressional hearings that hauled in Mylan's CEO Heather Brescher to testify, but she withstood their rage, pointing out that there was nothing illegal about what the company had done. (It may not have hurt that her father was former senator Joe Manchin.) Finally, after years of indefensible unaffordability, generic versions of this age-old medicine have started to become available.

Similar patent scams have long been used with the inhalers needed by patients with asthma and other lung diseases, to enable them to breathe. As with the EpiPen, many of the medications themselves have been around since the last century, and long off-patent. But for decades, these inhalers have been protected by patents on the devices, blocking generic versions from entering the market. The industry got an additional lucrative reboot on its monopolies when the FDA announced in 2005 that to comply with international treaties, it would ban the use of chlorofluorocarbons (CFCs) as a propellant in inhalers, since they are potent greenhouse gases. Switching to new propellants restarted all the monopoly clocks. The companies did deserve some additional patent protection to make that change, as well as for inventing nifty inhalers that get the medicines effectively into the lungs. But it's hard to see how these considerations could justify keeping generic inhalers off the market for so many years.

Dr. Will Feldman, a pulmonary specialist in our group who cares for many such patients, has seen firsthand how difficulty affording their inhalers has impacted them. He set out to study how these old medicines were packaged into delivery systems that made them so expensive. Sometimes it was a patent on the counter dial that measures how many doses have been administered, sometimes on another minor mechanism of the inhaler. In an op-ed written with Kesselheim in the *Washington Post*, Feldman noted that inhalers have contained virtually no new drugs to address novel cellular targets since 1986, but abuse of the patent system and the FDA's conservative rules on approving generics meant that only branded products were available for most of that time. They calculated that of the $178 billion that drug companies were paid for inhalers from 2000 to 2021, fully $111 billion was paid *after* the main patents on their active ingredients had already expired, because of the thickets of secondary and tertiary patents. This part of the industry is so lucrative that in 2022 tobacco company Philip Morris bought an inhaler manufacturer for over $1 billion, to reap additional profit from treating a disease it helped cause, as well as to expand its nicotine-vaping business.

Our colleagues in Europe are more savvy about such matters: the inhalers sold there can be one-tenth or one-twentieth the prices that the same companies charge here for the same products. In 2024, based on Will's work and that of others, Senator Bernie Sanders announced legislation to speed the breakup of the monopolies that made these products so hard to afford for millions of patients suffering from asthma and other chronic lung diseases.

Drug patent abuses don't just maintain artificially high prices and keep medicines out of the hands of the patients who need them. As we've seen, they also undermine actual innovation: investing in legal patent battles can become a more profitable and far less risky way for a company to prosper, compared to the more important but less certain route of developing truly creative new products. Many have faulted the American pharmaceutical industry for losing its edge in innovation. I disagree: drugmakers' capacity to innovate in the field of patent law is exquisite and impressive, even if many companies have lost their mojo when it comes to discovering new medicines for patients.

Pay for Delay

Once a drug's patents do eventually expire, what if no other manufacturer comes forward to make a generic version of it? The price would stay high. But why would that happen, if the market works as it is supposed to? For decades, this commercial magic was facilitated by the strategy of "Pay for Delay." A drug company owning an expiring patent on a costly product would collude with a potential generic competitor and simply pay them not to make a low-cost version of the drug. Basic calculations would clarify how much the innovator drug company would lose with generic competition, and how much the new generic entrant could expect to make by manufacturing its own cheaper version of the medication. Somewhere in between these two numbers would be the size of the corporate bribe needed to make sure everyone comes out financially ahead—except for patients, taxpayers, and insurers.

For years, the Pay for Delay practice slowed generic competition for many lucrative drug products. Then the Federal Trade Commission stepped in and declared it anticompetitive, ending the most flagrant versions of the practice. But lower-profile versions of the process persist, in the form of payments to settle litigation around patent challenges and other workarounds. These patent-based shenanigans continue to tarnish, if not totally defeat, the Founders' original great idea. Further action by the FTC, as well as reforms at the Patent Office, were seen as far less likely in the second Trump presidency.

The Nasty Dance of Product Hops

Descriptions of patent abuse in the pharmaceutical industry are laced with adorable euphemisms that mask the nasty nature of these strategies to keep drugs expensive. Adding layer upon layer of extraneous patents to extend a government-granted monopoly is called "evergreening"; doing so helps create a patent "thicket," conjuring images of Br'er Rabbit stuck in the bushes rather than a perversely impenetrable intellectual property scam. Keeping monopoly control long after it should have ended is known as "product life-cycle management." And a strategy to keep drugs away from patients who need them has been dubbed "product hopping," which brings to mind a benign image of bunnies romping in a meadow, or maybe a children's board game. Actually, it's a mean-spirited strategy to snatch away drugs whose patents are expiring, forcing doctors and patients to switch to a different but similar product made by the same manufacturer that remains under patent and therefore expensive.

One strange example was "Aricept 23," a new dose of a minimally effective drug for Alzheimer's disease known generically as donepezil. Aricept was originally sold in 10 mg and 5 mg doses by Eisai (the same company that brought us Leqembi and Aduhelm for that condition). It barely worked, and doctors questioned whether a higher dose might help patients more. That study was not done for years, until Eisai's patent on the 10 mg pill was expiring—it accounted for the lion's share of the company's total sales. At that point, Eisai ran a trial comparing the old 10 mg dose with its soon-to-be-marketed 23 mg dose, and concluded that the higher dose worked somewhat better. FDA scientists and outside experts disputed this conclusion, but noted that the new dose clearly led to a higher incidence of side effects, particularly nausea and vomiting.

Despite the drug's failure to meet its prespecified outcome criteria, the FDA approved the 23 mg dose as a new form of treatment for Alzheimer's just as Eisai's patent expired on the older pill sizes. That gave the company, now partnering on marketing the drug with Pfizer, an additional three years of exclusivity to promote the "new" medication, enabling the company to sell it as an important development in the care of patients with Alzheimer's disease; the new dose size cost ten times more than the older pill. A trivial clinical development, nearly all of us in the field concluded, especially for a drug that barely worked in the first place. Doctors who really wanted a double-ish dose could easily prescribe two generic 10 mg pills, or two tens and a five, and get essentially the same dose. Who would fall for that? Heavy promotion ensued. Sales soared.

A Sinister HIV Hop?

More troubling accusations of product-hop manipulation have dogged Gilead Sciences (the maker of the hepatitis cure Sovaldi—see chapter 12) over its marketing of essential drugs for the prevention and treatment of HIV infection, such as Truvada. In November 2023, a California federal court approved a $246 million settlement for plaintiffs who argued that Gilead paid a generic manufacturer to keep a less expensive version of Truvada off the market so it could maintain the high price of its own product. But more disturbing was a separate court judgment in January 2024 allowing plaintiffs to proceed with litigation over what looked like an even more cruel gambit. The central ingredient in many HIV medications is tenofovir, first synthesized by a Czech scientist in the 1980s. Gilead bought the rights to the compound and incorporated it into its products to treat or prevent HIV. In the early 2000s, Gilead scientists developed an improved version of tenofovir that would cause less damage to the kidneys and bones—important problems for some patients. The new litigation revealed internal company documents showing that its executives worried that the improved drug could "cannibalize" sales of its existing medication, and seemed to urge delaying its development until the patents on the current product expired. That appears to be what happened; the new, improved drug was released in 2015 as Descovy, just as the patents on the older drug expired. As expected, generic competitors came in and the price of the older drug went from about $22,000 a year to under $400; Gilead gave its new drug a list price of about $26,000 and has actively promoted it as a more effective and safer alternative, especially in preventing kidney and bone side effects. The company is now being sued by patients who suffered bone and kidney side effects for years from the older drug while Gilead appeared to be slow-walking release of its newer product that had less toxicity.

Selling Off the Public's Property: The Bayh-Dole Act of 1980

Patent manipulation is just one piece of our drug affordability puzzle. Another, separate issue has to do with giving away the farm.

By 1980, the nation had been pumping more and more public funding into the growing biomedical revolution, particularly in universities and academic medical centers. What was happening to all those discoveries? According to a narrative embraced by conservatives and corporations, many of those findings were withering on the vine because no one had enough economic incentive to commercialize them. Ostensibly, cures for dread diseases were being kept from the public because the results of all those federally funded studies were lying inertly in dusty file cabinets in medical schools all across America. To accept this, you'd have to assume that researchers who had committed their lives to combating specific illnesses had used NIH funding to uncover their causes and ways to address them, made important discoveries, and then somehow wrote their final reports to the feds and lost interest, letting the matter drop. Really?

According to the withering-on-the-vine narrative, companies (in the biomedical space, that usually meant drugmakers) would have been happy to help get these neglected advances to the citizens who need them, but as long as publicly funded discoveries were owned by the university or teaching hospital that made them, there was no economic incentive to get involved. This vision sharply contrasts with the actual history of some of the most important drug discoveries ever made. In the early 1920s, a physician-scientist named Frederick Banting at the University of Toronto was working with a medical student, Charles Best, to isolate insulin to treat the then-untreatable condition of diabetes. They succeeded in purifying and refining it so it could be administered to patients, an insight that forever transformed the treatment of this potentially fatal disease. In January 1923, along with a chemist colleague, they were awarded the U.S. patent for insulin, and promptly handed it over to the university for one dollar each. "Insulin does not belong to me, it belongs to the world," said

Dr. Banting. It was only when subsequent patents on new forms of insulin were filed by drugmakers that this lifesaving product became one of the most unaffordable medicines anywhere, forcing many patients to stretch out their doses in a clinically risky way to pay for it—until reforms enacted by President Biden made it affordable again, at least to Americans over sixty-five.

That form of diabetes was lethal but uncommon; but for children growing up in mid-century America, as I did, we were all terrified of catching polio; the fact that its grown-up name was "infantile paralysis" just made it seem scarier. The mode of contagion was poorly understood by laypeople, but the idea that it might have something to do with swimming (which it did, through fecal-oral transmission of the virus) left many summer days tinged with terror. Previously healthy children (and even adults, in the case of FDR) would become wheelchair-bound or even confined to metal contraptions that replaced their paralyzed breathing muscles—"iron lungs." Jerry Lewis had his muscular dystrophy telethons, and polio had its equally compelling March of Dimes campaign. No cure was found: you either recovered or you died, or you'd have some degree of paralysis for the rest of your life. Then, in 1955, the world learned that an obscure New York–bred doctor named Jonas Salk had developed a vaccine that could protect people from the disease. Barely ten years after the end of the Holocaust, this mild-mannered working-class descendant of Eastern European Jewish immigrants would save the world from one of its most dread diseases. I lined up with all the other children in my elementary school grade to get the shot that would protect us from this terrifying illness.

Asked by journalist Edward R. Murrow to explain who owned the patent on the vaccine, Salk famously replied, "Well, the people, I would say. There is no patent. Could you patent the sun?"

Getting Tough about Ownership

Fast-forward to 1980, and the old-fashioned sensibilities of Banting, Best, and Salk had become hopelessly out of date. With generous help from drug industry lobbyists, Congress accepted the idea that publicly funded university-based medical discoveries were indeed withering on the vine, and looked for ways to rescue the fruits of the research of all those distractible professors and turn them into something commercially useful. In 1980 Birch Bayh, a liberal Democrat from Indiana (home of pharma giant Eli Lilly), teamed up with Robert Dole, the conservative Republican from Kansas, to write legislation that would create a new pathway for private companies to obtain rights to the publicly funded discoveries flowing from university labs across the country. The resulting Bayh-Dole Act was passed in 1980. It allowed universities and other nonprofit institutions performing publicly supported research to license the rights to those discoveries to corporations, who could then create products to sell to the public. The companies would collect the revenues from those sales, and depending on the deal that was made, a share would go to the university or academic medical center where the discovery was made, and a slice to the researchers themselves. There was no provision for any of those dollars to go back to the original public entity that paid for the research, or to the public that underwrote those costs. Universities and academic medical centers are not widely known for the aggressiveness or acumen of their intellectual property offices, and the outcome of many of these deals reads like a pharmaceutical version of "Jack and the Beanstalk." Companies were also focused on the fact that their *raison d'être* is income maximization, with hundreds of millions or even billions of dollars potentially riding on a given deal. By contrast, many of us in academia are often happy to make a useful discovery, write some high-impact papers, and maybe one day get promoted to professor. Not exactly a level playing field, businesswise.

At first, the new Bayh-Dole law seemed to have some sensible protections built into it. As part of this new social contract, the companies selling drugs based on publicly funded research would make them available to the public "on reasonable terms," to reflect that high-risk early-stage investment by taxpayers. Bayh and Dole were also clever enough to anticipate the foreseeable problem that an important new medication might be discovered through federal funding and licensed to a drug company to commercialize it, only to have the public left in the cold if a company failed to do so appropriately. To address that potential problem, the legislators included so-called march-in rights that would allow the government to reassert its control over a federally generated product if a manufacturer didn't get it out to those who needed it.

Neither safety valve has worked. The pharmaceutical industry successfully adopted a policy of "It belongs to us now, so shut up" for products it licenses from universities. The "on reasonable terms" part of the social contract was deemed to have nothing to do with pricing. In fact, President Trump issued an executive order explicitly saying so during his last year in office. As for march-in rights, Kesselheim and I examined several instances in which public advocates called on the NIH to exert those rights for drugs that were either inaccessible or unaffordable. In each instance, NIH director Francis Collins refused to do so, unwilling to infringe on what was now the property of the drugmakers.

The rights many of us see in the Bayh-Dole language have a lot in common with the well-known eminent domain authority that federal, state, and local governments have invoked for centuries. The logic is similar, and convincing: sometimes a public need, such as building a railway or a new road, is so compelling that it justifies overriding the traditionally sacred right of private property. If land titles were as sacrosanct as drug patents, we wouldn't have any interstate highway system or intercity railroads. But farmers, city dwellers, and other landowners haven't had the same clout as the pharmaceutical industry in enforcing their rights at the expense of the public good.

While the government has backed away from using its power to enforce march-in rights over NIH-funded drugs, it has been willing to use a similar authority in other situations. Eminent domain is normally invoked in the public's vital interest, but a notable exception was made in 2001. Pharmaceutical giant Pfizer wanted to expand its facilities in New London, Connecticut, on land in a nearby low-income neighborhood; the state obligingly declared the zone a "blighted area," condemned it, and gave the land over to Pfizer and other developers along with an 80 percent reduction in the drugmaker's tax bill that would last for a decade. Dozens of homes were razed and their residents forced to move, and Pfizer got to build its complex, though much of the rest of the area was never developed. Several townspeople sued the city in a landmark land-use case that made it all the way to the Supreme Court, which ruled against the residents and supported the unusual seizure of their homes for a commercial purpose. But eight years later, Pfizer's business needs changed and it closed most of the expanded facility, eliminating 1,400 jobs. It's not clear what happened to the people who used to live there.

Some property rights are more sacrosanct than others.

CHAPTER 12

A License to Print Money

We've seen how after taxpayers function as early-stage investors in drug development, paying for the most risky, likely-to-fail, and expensive stages of drug development research, Bayh-Dole makes it possible for universities to license the resulting product to a drug company or a biotech start-up to sell at any price it chooses. Of course, there is often more to the story than this. Sometimes a pharma company will expend large sums to develop a new product mainly in-house, even if it builds on years of external basic science research. Or a company may take the very important and costly final steps to modify a publicly discovered molecule to improve its effectiveness or safety. Further, the drugmaker pays for the costly clinical trials necessary to prove that it works and win FDA approval (though sometimes the public helps fund those studies as well), and navigates a new medicine through the regulatory maze. These steps can be pivotal, difficult, and expensive. When they are, a drugmaker richly deserves to be compensated for the important work it did—as well as for all the blind alleys it had to go down to develop several failed drugs for each one that succeeds. But sometimes the company that ends up owning a medication has had little to do with its creation. One of the most striking examples is a breakthrough drug that changed the way we deal with hepatitis C infection. While a clinical godsend, it nearly wrecked the budgets of patients, state Medicaid programs, and private health insurers in the process.

Buying a Lucrative Asset

Hepatitis C is caused by a virus usually spread by exposure to the blood of an infected person; it's most commonly seen today in intravenous drug users. While many people who carry the virus don't have any symptoms, if untreated it can silently home in on the liver to cause cirrhosis, cancer, hepatic failure, and death. During most of my career, the drugs we had available to treat it required injections over several months, worked only about half the time, and caused major side effects such as nausea, depression, anemia, fatigue, and a host of other symptoms so severe that many patients never finished their prolonged treatments. As a result, we didn't routinely screen for the disease in patients who felt well. Then came Sovaldi, the first in a new class of medications that could be taken by mouth, were remarkably effective and easy to tolerate, and eradicated the virus in just two weeks. (Its generic name is the less pronounceable sofosbuvir.) The drug utterly transformed treatment of this condition: it now made sense to screen large numbers of people for the virus, since we had an excellent way to treat it; widespread use of the new drug could prevent hundreds of thousands of cases of cirrhosis, liver failure, and death.

The problem was that the manufacturer that controlled the patent on the drug priced it at $1,000 per pill, or $84,000 for a two-week course of therapy. Because so many hepatitis C patients were enrolled in their states' Medicaid program or were in prison, where their medical costs were likely to be covered by a separate corrections department health-care budget, the sudden appearance of a new drug with a cost of $84,000 per patient wreaked havoc with these strapped programs' finances. Unlike the federal government, states can't print new money and are generally not allowed to exceed their annual budgets. Some found that to pay for the new drug they had to cut back on other expenditures for schools, roads, or prisons, or other state-level expenditures. The impressive evidence on the effectiveness and safety of Sovaldi meant that from a clinical and public health perspective it should be offered to every patient infected with the virus. Our group performed a cost-effectiveness analysis showing that despite its astronomical cost, its capacity to prevent future cirrhosis, liver cancer, organ transplants, and early deaths meant that over a patient's lifetime it would actually be cost-effective, even at its sky-high price. But state Medicaid programs hadn't budgeted for the appearance of a new drug that would cost them tens of millions of dollars *now,* and they couldn't draw on the money that would be saved many years in the future. Besides, many of those preventable problems would occur when patients were over sixty-five and on Medicare, so most future savings would benefit that federal program, not the state programs that had to come up with the money to pay the enormous drug bills now—another odd consequence of our fragmented health-care system.

As a result, most states were forced to limit use of the drug. Most of that rationing wasn't so rational, rooted as it was in economic desperation rather than clinical considerations. Some programs would pay for it only in patients who already had liver damage, rather than trying to prevent that damage in those who didn't yet have it. By contrast, some decided that it should be reserved for patients who did *not* yet have severe liver disease. Others ruled that the drug could only be prescribed by a specialist, even though it's so easy to use that any health-care professional can prescribe it. Some required evidence that a patient had stopped substance abuse before it could be given. Still other programs went back to their state legislatures to beg for emergency funding to meet the millions of dollars of unexpected new costs that hadn't been budgeted for. We were in the familiar territory of having a remarkably effective drug to treat a serious medical condition whose manufacturer priced it so high that it was out of reach for thousands of patients who needed it. A 2023 analysis by the Centers for Disease Control found that in the U.S., only about a third of people infected with the hepatitis C virus were being adequately treated. All those British patients with cystic fibrosis would have understood.

Where did that $1,000-a-pill, $84,000-per-patient price come from? What enormous research expense was incurred by Gilead to warrant such a huge price tag? Hardly any.

A key innovation that made the drug possible was the discovery by researchers at Rockefeller University and the University of Heidelberg of a method to replicate the RNA of the hepatitis C virus in the lab; that made it possible to test thousands of compounds to see which ones might inhibit its growth. To look more deeply into the trail of public funding that led to Sovaldi, Kesselheim deployed Rachel Barenie, a postdoctoral trainee in our group who was a lawyer with a doctorate in pharmacy—skills that enabled her to move seamlessly across the realms of patents, patients, and potions. Rachel and her colleagues ferreted out all the patents associated with Sovaldi, all the research papers in the medical literature about it and its precursors, and all the NIH grants linked to each. We knew that a key role had been played by Dr. Raymond Schinazi, a full-time faculty member at Emory University and its affiliated Veterans Administration hospital. Rachel's team connected the dots and traced the web of funding from numerous taxpayer-supported NIH grants to Schinazi and his research collaborators. NIH had extensively supported basic research on the hepatitis C virus and ways to combat it, tissue culture methods that made it possible to grow the virus in the lab, studies of how it could be neutralized, and even many of the vital clinical trials that ultimately proved the effectiveness of drugs like Sovaldi. All such NIH grants and contracts are a matter of public record, listed online in a federal website in considerable detail. Strikingly, however, the grand total for one of these grants was officially listed at just one dollar, an implausible number. Rachel and the team made a Freedom of Information Act request to the federal Department of Health and Human Services to find out the right number; after months of delay, it turned out to be hundreds of thousands of dollars.

Taking It Private

Besides his brilliance as a medical researcher, Emory's Dr. Schinazi also had a remarkable talent for doing drug-development research using federal support and then overseeing the transfer of its ownership to private companies. For Sovaldi, the company that came to own its immediate precursor made very important modifications to the molecule, completed the clinical trials necessary to gain federal approval (NIH support is often used here as well in such scenarios), moved the product through the necessary regulatory hurdles, and brought it to market—vital and costly tasks in their own right. But then through a kind of legal alchemy, by the time the product was ready to be prescribed to patients, it was owned by a company that had done little of this work.

As the drug that would become Sovaldi was nearing its final evolution, Schinazi and Emory University transferred their ownership to a start-up company they helped establish called Pharmasset. "I coined that name," Schinazi proudly said later. "It's actually 'pharmaceutical assets' and the idea was to create assets that would be sold to companies. That was the initial business plan." The firm was at first incorporated in Barbados. Key modifications to the molecule were performed at Pharmasset by Michael Sofia, to whom the generic name of the drug, sofosbuvir, is attributed. But it wasn't always supposed to be so expensive.

After Sovaldi eventually hit the market with its thousand-dollar-a-pill price tag that wreaked such havoc on health-care budgets, Congress held hearings in 2014 to discover where that price came from. Testimony revealed that Pharmasset initially planned on selling Sovaldi for just $36,000 for a course of treatment—still a lot for a drug based so heavily on publicly funded research, but less than half the price it ended up selling for. The hike occurred when pharmaceutical giant Gilead Sciences bought the rights to the drug for $11 billion shortly before the drug went on sale. Gilead's executives reassessed its financial potential and decided to charge much more for the product they hadn't invented, because they could, choosing a price of $84,000 for a two-week regimen.

The congressional hearings disgorged reams of confidential documents from Gilead's files. One interesting internal company chart depicted its assessment of what the health-care system might tolerate as the drug's launch price. In vivid red (for a likely threat) through yellow (intermediate) to green (an unlikely threat), the company listed the factors it would consider in deciding what to charge.

The columns running from left to right were different possible price points, from $60,000 to $125,000 for a course of treatment. Ranged against that, horizontal rows listed possible threats from a variety of sectors. These included physicians' professional organizations and other advocacy groups "reacting negatively to price, and affecting public opinion": this problem was listed as "very likely" for nearly all the listed price points. For "Likelihood of losing some key opinion leader endorsement/support as priced too high," the rankings started out as "very unlikely" for the lower prices, but became an angry red "very likely" for the higher prices modeled.

Gilead's analysts covered all the bases. One row described the "Likelihood of public outcry if [the drug's] revenue exceeds $2B as government trying to contain healthcare cost": this was modeled as going from "possible" to "very likely" as the price increased. Perhaps most telling was the company's estimation of the "Likelihood of a Congressional hearing if [the drug's] revenue exceeds $2B." Such government oversight was ranked as "unlikely" for all price points except the very highest one, where it was ranked as merely "possible." As things turned out, the drug's revenue far exceeded that annual figure; it's concerning that the company expected such a low probability of political scrutiny. And it's amusing that the only way we know about this chart was because of a congressional hearing.

In its first year on the market, Sovaldi generated $11 billion in sales for Gilead, coincidentally and totally recouping in one year the entire amount it had paid to buy Pharmasset. While the price of the drug has come down in the years since, nearly every dollar spent on Sovaldi after its first year of sales represented pure profit for Gilead—a company that simply purchased rights to the product from another company, which itself made small but vital alterations to a molecule that was built on a therapeutic approach largely paid for by public sources.

Xtandi—the Long Road to a Cancer Cure

On April 21, 1980, Rosie Ruiz was declared the winner of the Boston Marathon, the oldest and most prestigious long-distance running competition in the world. The twenty-six-year-old marked a time of just under two hours and thirty-two minutes for the twenty-six-mile distance—the fastest ever recorded for a woman in the Boston race, and the third fastest female time in any marathon. Born in Havana, Rosie had emigrated to the U.S. in 1962 when she was just eight. She qualified for the Boston race by finishing its New York counterpart the preceding year in under three hours, coming in eleventh among all female competitors there. (Her application to compete in New York had arrived after the cutoff date, but officials exempted her from the deadline when she revealed she was suffering from a brain tumor.) Ruiz's Boston time was an impressive twenty-five minutes faster than the time she had achieved in the New York race six months earlier.

At the finish line in Boston's Back Bay, near the iconic Trinity Church and the nation's first public library, Rosie was wrapped in a Mylar cloak and escorted to the winner's podium; the traditional leafy garland was placed on her head. The running world was excited to see the honor bestowed on a fresh new female talent who escaped Castro's Cuba and had now reached the pinnacle of American long-distance running.

The old saw about prostate cancer is that many older men die *with* it, but far fewer die *of* it. Malignant cells are frequently discovered at autopsy in the prostates of men over seventy as an incidental finding. That is why routine blood tests to measure PSA (prostate-specific antigen) are no longer recommended in men over that age because they so often come back modestly positive—leading to workups, anxiety, and surgery that are often unnecessary. The metaphorical bestiary of cancer screening tests describes turtles, rabbits, and birds. It's an oversimplification, but conveys some useful concepts. Turtles represent diseases that move so slowly that there's no need to catch them; they're not going to get far. Birds are much scarier—cancers that are elusive because they've often gotten out of control before they're even detected. Rabbits represent the "best" kinds of cancer to screen for: they're on the move, but you can still catch them.

In that old simplistic typology, most prostate cancers are turtles. Discovering them with a screening test in an older man usually produces more terror than healing. But once a prostate cancer had spread—become a bird—little could be done to catch it. The tumor has a predilection to metastasize to bone, where it causes excruciating pain. Historically, there was little hope of effectively treating the disease once it took off like this. Male hormones seem to encourage growth of the tumor, so castration—both surgical and chemical—have been used, along with a variety of chemotherapies, but the success rate was poor. As one of my professors once said, "This is the kind of disease that gives cancer a bad name." Then along came Xtandi. It was developed by scientists at UCLA in the early 2000s almost totally on the basis of U.S. public funding; their work built on years of additional research that generated a more nuanced understanding of how those male hormones interact with prostate cancers at several points within the cell, and how to block those interactions in multiple ways. Following that research, randomized clinical trials of patients with advanced prostate cancer showed an impressive reduction in disease progression, far fewer side effects than the older chemotherapy treatments, and an increase in overall survival.

In our division, Kesselheim's Program On Regulation, Therapeutics, And Law (PORTAL) sought to trace the origins of Xtandi, employing an approach similar to what we had used in our Sovaldi research and led by oncologist Bishal Gyawali. The trail was simpler here: the lion's share of its development occurred in the labs of the small group of UCLA researchers, virtually totally funded by federal grants. As before, we traced the relevant grants, patents, and research reports, building on extensive work done by Knowledge Ecology International (KEI), a Washington-based nonprofit dedicated to affordable access to medications. We identified about $75 million in public support provided by NIH and the Army to fund the work of Drs. Michael Jung and Charles Sawyers, the UCLA researchers who developed the drug, and their colleagues. Additional grants had come from several other philanthropic sources: the Howard Hughes

Medical Institute (funder of some of the original cystic fibrosis drug research); the Prostate Cancer Foundation (established by the fallen junk bond billionaire Michael Milken in 1993 when he was released from prison and diagnosed with the disease); and the Doris Duke Charitable Foundation (founded by the late heiress to a tobacco fortune; the group now supports public-interest work).

Soon after Rosie Ruiz was crowned winner of the 1980 Boston Marathon, questions about her victory began to come up. At the finish line, observers were surprised she didn't appear more exhausted or sweaty. Front-runners didn't recall seeing her pass them. Other questions arose: her limited familiarity with running terms, her less-than-spartan physique, and her resting heart rate didn't seem to fit those of a record-breaking marathoner. Over the next few days, people in New York recalled seeing her riding the subway to the finish line during that marathon half a year earlier.

"We knew that she had jumped in," said Bill Rodgers, who won the men's race that day. "We, who knew what the marathon was, we got it." Eight days later, Ruiz's victory was nullified.

"Doing a Rosie" has become a slang term among runners for taking a shortcut on a race and claiming credit for an accomplishment they didn't deserve. Later in life, Rosie Ruiz was arrested for embezzling, grand larceny, forgery, and cocaine dealing. She eventually found a job with a health-care company in Florida. Throughout most of her life, Ruiz maintained that she had won the Boston marathon fairly, and never gave back her medal.

Since about the tenth century, pilgrims have come from all over the world to walk the Camino de Santiago, a trek culminating in northwestern Spain at the cathedral where the remains of

St. James are thought to be buried. Those who make the journey on foot are awarded the *compostela*, a certificate confirming that a person has completed the trip. Although in past eras people would spend months hiking hundreds of miles, in modern times the Church's Pilgrim's Office requires that a person has to complete only the last portion on foot to get credit. Documentation of having done so is variable.

Following the procedures made possible by the Bayh-Dole Act, UCLA and its scientists obtained three main patents on Xtandi, each of which credited the government funding for its discovery. Then UCLA set out to find a company to work with; in 2005 it licensed its intellectual property rights to the drug to a company called Medivation "in order to bring the innovation to the public," in the words of the university president. His statement continued:

> UC's primary goal in licensing its inventions is not to generate revenue but to serve the greater public. Licensing agreements are routinely necessary to convert University inventions into medications that benefit the public. The costs of drug development are prohibitive to UC, and granting patent rights incentivizes companies to transform innovations into products. Universities, like UC, generally are not in a position to commercialize their own medical innovations and therefore rely upon industry partners do so [*sic*].

Pfizer bought Medivation in 2016. The same year, UCLA sold its royalty interests in the Xtandi patents to Royalty Pharma, whose name, like that of Pharmasset, says the quiet part out loud. Royalty's business model is to work the Bayh-Dole Act by buying up lucrative discoveries coming out of universities and then selling them to interested pharmaceutical companies. The company paid UCLA $1.14 billion for the rights to Xtandi, to be shared by the university and the researchers who developed the drug. As is usually the case, the agreement had no provisions for a payback to the federal government, or to ensure that the drug that was developed with taxpayer money could actually be affordable by taxpayers. Nor was there any consideration about what it might cost in poor countries.

True to its name, Royalty Pharma sold the rights to the drug to the Japanese company Astellas, which now markets the drug along with Pfizer. The companies presently sell it for about $160,000 a year in the U.S., five times the price they charge for the drug in countries like Japan and Canada. As a result, Xtandi has ranked among the top ten most expensive drugs for Medicare annually, which spends about $2 billion a year to pay for it. Worldwide, Xtandi now brings in about $6 billion annually to the Astellas-Pfizer partnership. UCLA and its scientists, having received their windfalls, are not getting new royalty dollars on the drug commercially, but continue to reap the investment dividends of their original $1.4 billion payment from Royalty, amounting to tens of millions of dollars each year.

In India, where prostate cancer is the second most common cancer in men, the daily cost of Xtandi is about forty times the daily income of an average Indian. Ironically, India is also the largest supplier of affordable generic drugs to the rest of the world, and the drug was becoming available there generically at a price that would get even lower as more generic manufacturers entered the market. But Astellas and Pfizer could not abide India's refusal to respect their monopoly rights. The Bayh-Dole Act meant that the university is still the ultimate owner of the patent, even though it sold off its economic rights to the drug years ago. That put it in the awkward position of having a contractual obligation to defend Astellas-Pfizer in their attempts to ban more affordable versions of the drug in poor countries like India.

The situation on the ground was summed up in an article in *Los Angeles Magazine*:

> Rajeev Kumar, a urologist at a public hospital in Delhi, says if the patent were approved [blocking generic versions of Xtandi], almost none of his patients could afford the medication. Already, his patients struggle to afford the generic brands. Many of them

> run out of money a couple weeks into the treatment plan and stop taking the pills. Others, aware they'll inevitably exhaust their resources, refuse the prescription from the beginning. With the patent, even his wealthiest patients would be unable to afford the medicine. . . . In India, Kumar estimates less than 20 percent of his patients have insurance. If they do, their insurance policies usually cover a fixed amount of medical expenses for the entire family, which Xtandi would quickly deplete.
>
> "I know if I offered it to [a patient] he would take it and that'll end up destroying his family," he says. "The next generation (will be) in debt for the next 10 years."
>
> Even as an established doctor and professor at the most widely respected hospital in Delhi, one box of Xtandi would cost his entire monthly salary.

Still, the demand for patent enforcement had to be made by UCLA as the ultimate owner of the patent. So even after new dollars had stopped flowing, the university had continuing obligations to its industry partners that required it to turn up for a command performance in an Indian courtroom to defend an unaffordable price for the breakthrough drug its faculty members had invented, and to block the availability of generic versions of it. I read the university president's statement on this carefully, and did not find the term "Faustian bargain"; it appears that the prostate cancer patients weren't the only ones who had been castrated. Or, as my mother used to say, "If you go to bed with dogs, you wake up with fleas."

I am sure the scientists who developed Xtandi never wanted this to happen, nor do I think the senior executives of the companies controlling its sales necessarily felt good about this outcome. The golems just took over.

Marching Around in Circles

American patients' access to Xtandi has been a particularly compelling target for attempts to get the federal government to use its

Bayh-Dole "march-in" rights to enforce control over that publicly funded research, since the legal case here is much clearer than for many other drugs: all the main patents on the drug acknowledge the government funding, and there is not an impenetrable thicket of secondary patents surrounding them. The argument, as Kesselheim and others of us in our PORTAL group wrote in a letter to the secretary of Health and Human Services, is pretty straightforward: those prices meant that the drug was not available "on reasonable terms" to U.S. patients with prostate cancer. Based on the work of Knowledge Ecology International, several members of Congress have also made this case forcefully and repeatedly. In March 2023, the Department of Health and Human Services rejected that argument, but later that year the Biden administration announced a new "framework" for considering when to use its march-in rights for drugs that were developed through federal largesse. However, the plan would allow for such intervention only for prices that were "extreme and unjustifiable," whatever that means. International comparisons were not mentioned, so the up to sixfold difference in what Pfizer-Astellas charged American patients compared to those in Canada and Japan might not qualify as evidence of this.

Xtandi is just one of the most notable examples of a drug company jumping into the marathon of pharmacological research shortly before the finish line and claiming they won the race; but it's not the only one. One common chestnut about federal support for drug development is that the NIH funds very early-stage basic science research, but the heavy lifting of the costly later-stage clinical development work is funded by industry, a rationale for its getting to keep all the marbles even when a product has its origins in earlier publicly supported studies. It turns out that isn't true, either. With a medical student, Kesselheim and I looked into the research support culminating in new products, using the same strategy of chasing down the relevant webs of patents, research papers, and NIH grants. In a paper we published in *BMJ* we demonstrated that public funding was common even in the latest stages of prescription drug development.

The Risks of De-Risking

This process has been called by critics "the socialization of risk and the privatization of gain." It's the opposite of what happens with other kinds of innovative work, in which early-stage venture capital investors are rewarded handsomely for the greater risk they take, generally with a generous ownership share in the new company. But in another example of pharmaceutical exceptionalism, empowered by the structure of our patent laws the drug industry has avoided that requirement, at least when it comes to taxpayer dollars. That was made even more clear in late 2011 when NIH director Francis Collins created a new institute within the NIH, with heavy encouragement from the Obama administration and congresspeople from both parties: the National Center for Advancing Translational Sciences (NCATS). Its stated mission was explicitly to "de-risk" early-stage investment in the discovery of new drugs, so that the public could bear the brunt of such often-unsuccessful expenditures, making it more attractive for a drug company to come in and own a product once it was past its most vulnerable stages of development. A more recent incarnation of the same idea was the establishment in 2023 of a new federal agency, ARPA-H: the Advanced Research Projects Agency for Health. Designed to pay for even earlier de-risking work, its name resonates with DARPA, the Defense Advanced Research Projects Agency, which underwrote the development of the internet. ARPA-H was expected to have an annual budget of $2.5 billion in 2024.

As in Bayh-Dole, ARPA-H doesn't seem to have any mechanism for payback to the public for products developed through this latest example of government generosity, whether through some kind of royalty arrangement for the NIH, or lower prices, or rebates to patients or purchasers—especially to federally supported programs like Medicare, Medicaid, the VA, or the extensive Department of Defense health-care system. But that was never part of the plan for NCATS or ARPA-H: both are designed to be all pain and no gain for the public, and no pain and all gain for the industry that would own and market the resulting products.

Kesselheim and I thought there should be more discussion of these issues as the NCATS program was being rolled out, so we sent an article voicing our concerns to the *New England Journal of Medicine*. It was greeted well by the section editor, then judged very positively by the outside peer reviewers, and scheduled for publication. Close to the planned publication date, as we were expecting final page proofs to review, one of the editors called to say that because our piece might be seen as a bit controversial, the editor in chief wanted to publish it alongside a counterpoint article by NIH's Dr. Collins. This was unusual: if an article elicits a countervailing view, that's often published as a letter to the editor in a subsequent edition. But Dr. Collins had been shown our article before publication and he wanted to rebut it concurrently, so we agreed. Weeks passed. How was Dr. Collins's counterpoint article coming along? we asked our editor. It was taking longer than expected, came the reply. More time passed. Collins remained very busy (hard to fault the NIH director for that) and hadn't gotten to write his rebuttal. Then could he have a colleague write it with him or for him? we asked. No, Collins wanted to be the one to write it, since NCATS was his pet project. Could his article appear in the next issue, after publication of ours? No, it had to be concurrent, and our piece couldn't be published without the accompanying antidote penned by the NIH director.

More weeks passed, and Aaron and I were getting worried that the timeliness of our piece might be fading. Then came the last word from *NEJM*: no counterpoint article would be coming from Dr. Collins, so it would probably be best for us to publish our own piece in another journal. We submitted it to *Nature Medicine*, which enthusiastically accepted and published it with the title "The NIH Translational Research Center Might Trade Public Risk for Private Reward." It was also a respected journal, but without the enormous readership or visibility of *NEJM*. Maybe that was the point.

In September 2023, a Republican-controlled congressional committee held an industry-sympathetic hearing on Medicare's plan to negotiate drug prices the same way that it negotiates the price of all other goods or services it purchases; the power to do so had been created for the first time by Biden's Inflation Reduction Act (IRA) of 2022. Tellingly, they titled the session "At What Cost? Oversight of How the IRA's Price Setting Scheme Means Fewer Cures for Patients." (In Europe, "scheme" is used as a synonym for "proposal" or "structure." In the U.S., especially in politicized debate, it means "plot.") One of the most powerful weapons wielded by the pharmaceutical industry to combat restrictions on pricing (second only to their massive lobbying clout) is pushing out the idea that drug companies are the main wellspring of new drug innovation. Therefore, the industry argues, since the drug companies plow back so much of the revenue they get into innovation to discover new drugs, crimping that revenue will just reduce the number of drugs that they will discover. They redubbed the IRA the "Innovation Reduction Act," and Pharma even bought the URL innovation.org; clicking on that link automatically redirects you to the site for the industry trade group.

That formulation is wrong in many ways. Of the half-trillion dollars in revenue the industry takes in each year in the U.S., far more goes to advertising and marketing and shareholder profits than to research. Extremely high salaries for senior management also consume a decent (or perhaps indecent) fraction. And as we've seen, much of that research budget goes to develop derivative products that may be patentable, but don't necessarily represent clinically important new advances. Even the usually staid Congressional Budget Office was lured into this logical trap in 2020 when it was asked to cost out the consequences of various legislative approaches to limit runaway drug prices. In an analysis of the effects of the IRA on drug development, the CBO calculated that this would have only a tiny effect, potentially resulting in just 1 percent fewer drugs coming to market over the next thirty years. Leaving aside how anyone can possibly know this, it seems safe to assume that if any drugs don't make it to pharmacy shelves, the ones left behind are more likely to be a new me-too eczema treatment rather than a cure for cancer. But this helped industry change the conversation from "Drug prices are so high that patients and health-care systems can't afford medicines" to "How many new lifesaving drugs will we lose if we contain drug prices?" This faulty logic is based on the following suppositions:

- Nearly all new drug discovery comes from innovative research within the pharmaceutical industry.
- That research is expensive, costing $2.6 billion for each new drug, and is funded by drug company revenues.
- This is made possible because the industry plows back a substantial amount of its revenues into the research it conducts.
- If those revenues and the profits it generates are reduced by ham-handed legislative interference, it will crimp the pipeline of new drug creation, innovation will dry up, and new drug discoveries won't be brought to market.

Once the public debate goes down that errant path, it's hard to get the discussion back onto the right track. But reality is quite different. To review:

- The $2.6 billion-per-drug estimate is an erroneous industry-funded number based on suspect methodology applied to secret numbers, ignores the contributions of the public sector, and is grossly exaggerated.
- Drug companies actually plow back only 10 to 15 percent of their revenues into research; the share that is put into truly innovative studies (as opposed to trivial but patentable changes that don't add much patient benefit) is even less.
- Every year, more and more new drug products are being developed, tested, and brought to market outside the for-profit pharmaceutical industry model.

Yes, the industry plays an important role in this high-risk enterprise, and we need to make sure that it receives a fair and even generous return on the work it does perform. But skewing the analysis with exaggerated claims doesn't do the country any service, and leads to a continuation of bad policies.

The Mistake from 2003: Wrecking the Free Market

After the Bayh-Dole Act of 1980, another national step toward legalizing unaffordable prices involved taking the "market" out of "marketplace." By the early 2000s it had become clear that the Medicare program, established in 1966, had succeeded in paying for hospitalization costs and doctors' bills for Americans over sixty-five. Prescription drugs hadn't been included when it was written, since they were so cheap in 1966 that this didn't seem necessary; yet that expense had become unbearable for many. Enthusiasm rose to finally include a drug benefit as part of Medicare, and that addition was enacted in 2003. Surprisingly, its language exempted the drug industry from most of the usual give-and-take of normal commercial transactions, instead requiring the government to pay any price they were charged. This made medications the only product, from computers to uniforms to soybeans, for which the government is legally prohibited from negotiating the cost of what it buys. We can all thank Billy Tauzin for that.

A conservative Louisiana Democrat-turned-Republican, Tauzin by 2001 had become chair of the powerful House Committee on Energy and Commerce, which has jurisdiction over Medicare. As the provision to create a Medicare drug benefit was making its way through his committee in 2003, Tauzin pressed for an unusual industry-promoted law forbidding the government from pushing back on the prices of any of the medicines it would pay for: they would cost whatever their manufacturers wanted them to cost. Fiscally, that represented all gas pedal and no brake. The unusual measure passed in December 2003, and a few days later Tauzin announced he would retire from Congress the following year. The day after his term ended, he started work as head of the Pharmaceutical Research and Manufacturers of America (PhRMA), the drug industry lobbying group, at an estimated annual salary of $2 million. In 2010, the year he retired from that post, the group was reported to have paid him $11.6 million, making him the nation's highest-paid health-care lobbyist.

The Check Is in the Mail

A second part of the one-two punch in the face of the marketplace came in 2006 just as the new Medicare drug benefit was being implemented, when the Department of Health and Human Services defined six "protected classes" of drugs, comprising most of the costliest medicines—treatments for conditions like cancer, mental illness, HIV—and required Medicare to pay for every drug in those classes, also at whatever price their manufacturers charged. A separate regulation forces Medicaid to cover virtually every FDA-approved drug. These measures preempt the prospect of most government buyers doing any comparison shopping among similar products that could be far less costly and equally effective.

By spring 2021, Congress was again debating ways to get on top of runaway drug prices; House Speaker Nancy Pelosi was spearheading that attempt in the massive $3.5 trillion reconciliation bill making its way through the legislative process. It contained a reasonable drug price–containment provision that seemed destined to be included in the final package. But that language was torpedoed when several key Democrats, led by Representative Scott Peters of California, wrote to Pelosi to object to it. They argued that it would harm innovation in the drug industry; their opposition, along with that by nearly all Republicans, killed it.

It's known that the pharmaceutical industry spends heavily to support congresspeople on both sides of the aisle, but the *chutzpah* underlying the largesse in this instance was astonishing. The day after Representative Peters wrote to Pelosi objecting to the drug price–reduction measure, he received a $5,800 personal check from Pfizer CEO Albert Bourla, $5,000 from Eli Lilly CEO David Ricks, $2,900 from Merck CEO Kenneth Frazier, $2,900 from Bristol Myers Squibb CEO Giovanni Caforio, and $1,000 each from two PhRMA officials. Soon afterward he got $5,000 from each of the PACs for Pfizer and Lilly. Many of us have called for greater transparency in government, but this isn't quite what we had in mind.

It should now be clearer why the same medicine made by the same manufacturer in the same factory can cost half as much in Canada or England or Japan as it does here, or even less. The paradox is that in the name of preserving the free enterprise system, these laws have eviscerated it, eliminating the need for companies to compete on the basis of a product's quality or price. But if we could wipe away these dysfunctional policies, what would replace them? What *should* a prescription drug cost, to reflect its clinical value and public investment and also fairly reward its manufacturer for any contributions it made to a product's development? It is possible to figure this out: researchers around the world have gotten reasonably good at doing so, and such methods are in use in most other wealthy countries. But as we will see in the next chapter, using those approaches has been made illegal—yes, illegal—in the U.S.

CHAPTER 13

Old Whines in New Battles

> Price is what you pay; value is what you get.
>
> —Warren Buffett

In November 2008, Barack Obama and his running mate, Joe Biden, defeated John McCain and his running mate, Sarah Palin, in a lopsided victory. But Palin wasn't done with politics; as the new administration tried to shape and pass its landmark Affordable Care Act, soon to be known as Obamacare, Palin returned to the spotlight to disparage the whole idea of the government getting more involved in funding health care. This fit well with a zany but then-popular slogan referring to the most popular federal program that demanded, "Keep the government's hands off my Medicare!" With the encouragement of many companies in the health-care industry, Palin got out in front on this theme the summer after her electoral defeat, posting on social media:

> The Democrats promise that a government health care system will reduce the cost of health care, but . . . government health care will not reduce the cost; it will simply refuse to pay the cost. And who will suffer the most when they ration care? The sick, the elderly, and the disabled, of course. The America I know and love is not one in which my parents or my baby with Down Syndrome will have to stand in front of Obama's "death panel" so his bureaucrats can decide, based on a subjective judgment of their "level of productivity in society," whether they are worthy of health care. Such a system is downright evil.

Her rant extended a growing trend on the right. A few months earlier, a conservative commentator had written that setting up health information technology programs resembled the eugenics programs of the Nazis. Crazy as all this sounds, these positions represent the most extreme versions of a view that still resonates in some circles: that the government should play no role in assessing the appropriateness or the cost of any health-care service or technology, especially medications. Given enough freedom, the marketplace will sort all that out. (See the Albigensian Crusade, chapter 1.) Smacking into this view has been our need to figure out a fair and rational way to determine how much specific medical interventions are worth—again, especially medications—and how we can use those insights to pay for them fairly, but not excessively. At present, the U.S. health-care system operates on the principle that we can afford *everything.* But we can't, and we've seen what happens when we act as if we can.

So how can we estimate more reasonable prices that could move us beyond the current "Because I can" approach? If we could blow away all the irrational legal idiosyncrasies and ill-advised policies, if we could make a fresh start based only on the best evidence, how *would* we ideally decide on what a new drug is worth? There is a rich realm of research on this subject that brings together clinical medicine, economics, ethics, the psychology of choice, and other disciplines to propose appropriate prices for medications. Beginning in the 1970s, economists began trying to put an accurate value on all sorts of expenditures: building a railroad, drilling an oil well, opening a factory. Because I dealt with these issues at some length in *Powerful Medicines,* I won't take on a detailed discussion of them again here. But the way these issues have played out in the years since then has gotten pretty interesting, so we'll focus on some recent developments.

By the 1990s drug prices were rising inexorably, taking up an ever-larger share of the national health budget and the economy overall. Great new medicines were introduced into practice along with others that cost a lot but weren't any better than products we already had. Imagine yourself a state Medicaid director whose job is to work within a fixed budget to cover all the health-care needs of poor patients in your state. You have to figure out how to handle several new treatments:

- A diabetes drug that will prevent the heart and kidney damage caused by that disease several years down the road, but has a list price of about $1,000 a month vs. $20 a month for an older drug that just lowers blood sugar.
- Gene therapy that can replace a defective section of DNA in a patient with sickle cell anemia, a condition that strikes mostly African Americans and causes frequent agonizing pain crises; it eventually leads to disability and death. The new treatments offer the prospect of curing the condition after a single treatment, but costs $2 or $3 million per patient.
- Genetic treatment for spinal muscular atrophy, a degenerative condition that causes paralysis in children; those with the severe form of the disease usually die before age three. Its price is $2.1 million.
- The gene-skipping technology (see chapter 3) that makes tiny changes in muscle protein levels in children with muscular dystrophy, but doesn't result in evident clinical improvement; its price is $300,000 per year.
- A new monoclonal antibody to manage psoriasis; it works about as well as existing older prescriptions, but is about thirteen times more expensive.

If you pay for all of them, you'll have to reduce the budget for other treatments or services. Do you cover them all? If not, which ones? How do you decide?

As consumers, we make decisions on more mundane purchases every day; so do corporations and the government. But in no sphere of life does anyone (except perhaps for some spoiled trust fund offspring) say, "Hey, let's just buy everything, whatever the cost!" In the U.S., we still don't provide adequate health care for everyone, and some employers still oppose offering health coverage to large groups of people because it would cost too much, and about ten red states have refused to expand their Medicaid programs although the federal government would pick up nearly all the tab. Even ignoring such nasty penuriousness, there will always be more on offer in the way of medications and other health care than any system can easily afford. One solution could be to say that expensive medical coverage, goods, and services will simply go to those wealthy enough to afford them, and others would just have to go without. (This approach would be compatible with the view of a conservative economist I once debated about this, who asked me, "Why is this even an issue? The country doesn't provide everyone with National Beer Insurance!") But most of us understand that medications and medical care have a special moral dimension, since access to them is what makes literally everything else possible. (By contrast, some may feel that beer is necessary for survival, but that is not a widely held view. We call those people alcoholics.)

So if we want to move away from a pricing system in which a pharmaceutical company gets to say, "The price of this drug is whatever we say it is," then what can we move *toward*? A good start would be to think about how prices are determined for everything else in the economy—by corporations, by governments at all levels, by households, by regular individuals.

The main idea here is that the price of an item—whether it's a car, a laptop, a potato, or a drug for cancer—ought to reflect its value to the entity that buys it. Right away, we can see some ways that cancer drugs differ from potatoes:

- the purchasing decision for a drug is made by a person (the doctor) who is different from the person using the product (the patient);
- the entity paying for the product (the health insurer or the government) is likely to be different from either of these, and have its own incentives and preferences;
- in a normal marketplace transaction, the vendor and the purchaser are expected to have or be able to access information about the relative attributes of all purchasing choices (e.g., a Kia vs. a Lexus, a fingerling vs. an Idaho spud) that they can understand and assess in considering price differences. Not so with medications.

Those are three major differences, of many. Others worth keeping in mind are:

- I can shop around in choosing a new house or laptop; not so if I'm trying to choose among medications to use while I'm having a heart attack—just as it wouldn't be a good idea to have to negotiate the price of water with the fire department while your house is burning down.
- People have a different view of the value of drugs that can impact their health or even their life, versus everything else that they buy. If you're dying or severely ill, all other purchasing choices, from computers to vegetables, fade into the background.

So how can we assign a fair price to a drug that reflects its benefit to patients and its safety, and also provides a fair profit for its manufacturer? This is not an imaginary academic exercise. Medicare will have to impose such determinations for the first time in 2026, if the lawyers and lobbyists allow them to proceed with that legislative mandate from President Biden's Inflation Reduction Act of 2022.

For the most crude way of determining drug prices (all right, the second most crude way, after "Because I can"), let's imagine a hypothetical new cancer drug whose manufacturer wants to charge $100,000 per year, a common number for such drugs. How can we know if that's a fair price? We could look at what we pay for another drug that treats the same condition and has equivalent clinical outcomes, say one that costs $50,000. If the new drug is no more effective or safe, why would we pay more for it? Or we can look at what its manufacturer sells it for in other wealthy nations, where the company presumably still makes a profit. That simple approach is known as reference pricing, and has been advocated by radical left-wing activists like Donald Trump as a reasonable way to decide what a drug should cost.

But basing a new drug's price on what similar drugs cost has a major drawback. Just because one or more drug companies have been successful in taking the Shkrelian position of setting an arbitrarily high price on a medicine in the U.S. doesn't mean that it's a reasonable number. My skin crawls when I read of a company executive justifying a huge launch price for a new drug by saying something like "The figure is compatible with the economic landscape that's been established for this sort of therapy"—sort of the pharma-bro equivalent of "But, Mom, all the other kids are doing it!"

What if we didn't live in a world where drug prices are dictated by the pharmaceutical industry? Just how much better would a new drug have to be compared to an older one to warrant paying more for it? "Twice as good"? And what would that mean, exactly? Half as many side effects? Enabling the patient to live twice as long? What if that meant four months instead of two months? And would that be the same as four years versus two years?

For conditions like cancer, we can start by asking how many life-years a new drug would add, compared to existing treatments. Then we could calculate the number of dollars the medicine would cost for each life-year it adds. So in our example, a cancer drug that cost $50,000 and adds six more months of survival could be seen as costing $100,000 more per twelve months of life added. Is that too much, or too little? We can do an end run around the imponderability of that question by looking at what the U.S. health-care system is already spending on treatments we've been using for years, like statins to lower high cholesterol levels, or blood pressure medicines to treat hypertension, or kidney dialysis for end-stage renal disease. It turns out that when you calculate the cost of these treatments per life-year added when they first came into widespread use, most came in at a cost of roughly between $50,000 and $100,000 spent per year of life added. That's a big relief, because the way we practice medicine every day suggests that we don't feel that's too much to pay per additional year of life—in fact, we do it all the time. The British use a much lower standard for what they're willing to pay for an additional quality-adjusted life-year (QALY; see below); it's more like £30,000 per QALY, or about $38,000.

This appeal to decades of standard practice in American medicine enables us to escape for now the thorny question of what a year of human life is "worth." These numbers will make much less sense in resource-starved countries that may spend just $30 per person per year on all health-care expenditures, compared to about $5,000 per person on average in the wealthier OECD countries, and an implausible $13,500 per person in the U.S. The Princeton ethicist Peter Singer and adherents of the effective altruism movement would argue at this point that the very best thing to do with $100,000 would be to send it to Africa to support programs that address malnutrition, malaria, and sanitation, where that amount would save many more life-years than a few months of extended longevity for a single American cancer patient. That would be numerically accurate, but our goal at the moment is to consider a much more local, narrow, and actionable problem—how to price drugs in the American health-care system.

Even inside the rarified context of American medicine, surely all life-years aren't the same. What if the six months of life added by that new cancer drug were marked by frequent vomiting, hair loss, weakness, and occasional infections, as often occurs with some cancer treatments? Should that half a year of life be counted in the same way as a treatment that offered the same life extension, but one marked by robust good health? Medications, like diseases, can lead to excellent functioning as well as abject misery; that obvious insight led early on to the idea that we shouldn't consider every year of life as identical. So why not count years of misery and sickness differently from years of vibrant health? This gave rise to the idea of a quality-adjusted life-year. Using that metric could allow us to talk about a drug that cost $300,000 for every QALY added, or perhaps just $30,000 per QALY added. This core idea led to a host of analytic opportunities, as well as pitched ethical and political battles.

Here's a recap of the basics of this approach at it applies to pharmaceutical prices, covering up for now some very substantial warts with a thick layer of over-the-counter makeup. (We'll peel that off, layer by layer, shortly.)

- On the benefit side, we can look at the results of clinical trials and extrapolate them into the future, making it possible to predict whether starting a patient on the new drug will extend life by a certain number of years compared to prescribing the current standard of care. This advantage is described as the *incremental life-years* offered by the new drug.

- Whether or not the new drug extends life, we can try to measure how much it improves the *quality* of that life in a given year, compared to other available treatments. This is particularly relevant for drugs that can help people suffering from disabling rheumatoid arthritis, for example, or the distressing gastrointestinal symptoms of Crohn's disease, or severe eczema or psoriasis, even if the lives of these patients aren't extended much by a new treatment.
  - That can be done by a variety of methods, none of them wholly satisfactory, but you work with what you've got. We can ask people how a year of life with a particular kind of severe arthritis would compare with a year of perfect health. Would a year with the disease be worth only 70 percent of a year of good health? 85 percent? 50 percent? Other methods, equally squishy, are also used.
  - Of course, this determination will vary from person to person and can't be measured with much precision. And this very attempt is loaded with assumptions about values (more on this shortly). But it's a start.
- We can then multiply the number of additional life-years offered by the new treatment, if any, by the quality of those years compared to the quality of life on the standard treatment, or no treatment. That gives us the added *quality-adjusted life-years* the new drug can offer.
- Next, we can measure all the dollar costs associated with the new and old drugs: the price of the medication as well as the costs of treatment for the disease being addressed, both with vs. without the new treatment. The extra expenditures associated with the new drug (assuming they are higher) are its *incremental costs.*
- The next step in this oversimplified overview is to calculate all the extra dollars that come with use of the new drug, let's say in a hypothetical population of a thousand patients, compared to all the expected additional benefit these people would derive—the extra quality-adjusted life-years they would gain. Plug the new drug into the projected care of those thousand people, and we can figure out the number of dollars it would take to buy how many additional quality-adjusted life-years.

- That number can answer the question "In any population of patients with this condition, on average how many dollars would I have to spend for each additional QALY gained with use of the new drug?"

This is the basic idea behind the most common form of cost-effectiveness analysis. It won't tell a health-care system whether to pay for a given drug or not. But it's a good starting point to define the component parts of what a drug may be worth compared to alternative treatments—its effect on symptoms and longevity, its downsides in relation to side effects caused or prevented, how patients on average value those benefits—and thus allow us to take a first crude stab at what it should cost. In doing so, it also clarifies where each of those numbers comes from. If we disagree with any of the component assumptions (such as what it's worth to eliminate a year of cramping and diarrhea in a patient with a chronic GI disease), once these numbers in the analysis are made explicit we can vary them and see how the outputs of the model change.

Some of the best work in the U.S. in this area is being done by the Boston nonprofit Institute for Clinical and Economic Review, referred to above, founded by a Brigham residency alumnus named Steve Pearson. (The group's name is a bit of a pun, since the working metric of QALY analysis described above is the incremental cost-effectiveness ratio, known in the field as the ICER.) In other wealthy countries, this function is fulfilled by their own official health technology assessment organizations, often linked to their health-care systems; NICE in England is one example. But since the U.S. has legally distanced itself from this vital work, the brave souls at ICER do their own analyses of the cost and value of new medications independently, vet them openly for criticism, and offer up the results of their calculations transparently on their website for anyone who is interested. Despite their lack of official standing, ICER's cost-effectiveness benchmarks have become a vital starting point for debate on the prices of new drugs both in the U.S. and internationally.

A nuanced approach to cost-effectiveness analysis looks like the fairest and most sensible way to determine a reasonable price range for a medication, one that would value a major advance and offer a generous profit for its inventor, while cutting down to size a new product that is expensive but offers little or nothing over existing drugs. But sensible as it seems, cost-effectiveness analysis has become a major target for the pharmaceutical industry, since it can clarify how many of its products are terribly overpriced in relation to the good they do, compared to alternative medications. As a result, it has become one of the most politically radioactive topics in medication policy. Some industry advocates have argued that independent of the clinical benefits of a drug, its price should also be based on how much money a company spent to develop it, even if the resulting product wasn't particularly remarkable. (This sounds to me like a student handing in a so-so paper and arguing that it should be awarded an "A" because they really, really worked hard on it, even if it didn't come out so well.) Other attempts to justify a higher price for a drug beyond its clinical worth are built into a formulation known as the "value flower," which has petals for attributes separate from a medicine's effectiveness, as manifested in attributes like "the value of hope," "the value of knowing," and a medication's capacity to reduce fear of contagion and disease.

The Sad History of Medical Technology Assessment in the U.S.

In 2009, as the Obama administration was crafting the legislation that became the Affordable Care Act, its framers took this very reasonable position: if the government is going to take a larger role in funding health-care expenditures for more people, those dollars could go further for everyone if we knew more about which goods and services are worth their cost, and which aren't. This could be a big problem if your company makes a product that isn't worth anywhere near what you are charging for it. But you couldn't object in those terms; better to say that even asking this question is paving the way toward rationing care or disadvantaging the disabled and minorities.

With the final implementation of Obamacare I naively thought that these arguments had been relegated to the dustbin of history, but it didn't take long for the very survival of the Affordable Care Act to be jeopardized by this newly roused monster. Part of the original vision for Obamacare was that we could contain the out-of-control expenditures of U.S. health care by creating an ongoing process of comparative effectiveness research. That would provide us all with continuing assessments of new and old treatments to help us judge which ones work best and which are the most cost-effective. In this way, patients could be getting the most up-to-date therapies, as well as those that provide the most value for money—essential to making the Affordable Care Act affordable.

Who could possibly object to that? As it turned out, a lot of people. Even after Palin began to fade into the sea of failed vice presidential candidates, the bogeyman spirit of the "death panels" that she let loose remained alive, ready to be invoked after any call to measure the value of health-care interventions—especially drug prices. Subtle debates about the best way to measure the benefits and costs of medications got transformed into a misleading but effective message that could be snarkily restated as: "ASKING THESE QUESTIONS WILL HURT DISABLED PEOPLE. THIS APPROACH COULD KILL YOUR GRANDMOTHER." A key component of the original Obamacare legislation was to have been the creation of a new research agency, to be called the Comparative Effectiveness Research Institute. Given the self-serving nature of the way pharmaceutical companies sometimes designed the trials they ran, this new publicly funded group would support systematic research on the clinical value and the expense of common health-care interventions, as Senator Max Baucus had called for in the Vioxx hearings a quarter century earlier. It could help us understand which treatments were worth their cost and which would sap the nation's health-care budget without providing much health in return. For medications, we might finally be able to move beyond the false economy of having drugmakers take the lead role in designing, conducting, and reporting most studies of how well their products worked. People embraced the obvious logic that if the government was paying for the lion's share of medical interventions, including drugs, maybe it could save money and improve quality if it also designed and funded the key studies to evaluate them. It was a heady time: researchers across many medical disciplines put together lists of topics for study: the best way to treat atrial fibrillation, how to optimally manage chronic back pain, and dozens of other pressing unresolved questions. To take advantage of this new opportunity, the prestigious Institute of Medicine convened experts from around the country to assemble such an optimistic wish list in 2009.

It was an exhilarating agenda, but the excitement lasted only a few months. The very approach was seen as a threat by many in the pharmaceutical industry, as well as purveyors of all high-dollar, low-value medical goods and services. Years earlier, the nation had dismantled its federal Office of Technology Assessment because it was seen as a threat to some business interests; the government's National Center for Health Services Research was to have taken up part of that agenda, but also had its wings clipped and was reformulated with a new name and a more timid mission after those objections returned. The diminution of the Comparative Effectiveness Research Institute was performed in several steps. First, the name had to go; the term "comparative effectiveness" was deleted, and the new agency was renamed the Patient-Centered Outcomes Research Institute (PCORI). Next, a new piece of law was written (Section 1182) making it illegal to use standard methods of cost-effectiveness research to measure . . . cost-effectiveness. It stipulated that nothing in the authorization of PCORI could be construed as allowing the Department of Health and Human Services "to deny coverage of items or services under such title solely on the basis of comparative clinical effectiveness research."

When PCORI's initial agenda for its proposed funding portfolio was announced, many of us looked in vain for the Treatment A vs. Treatment B clinical research agenda; it wasn't there. In fact, the new funding agency specifically noted that it would not support research that used cost-effectiveness methods. A high-profile 2010 article in the *New England Journal of Medicine* was titled "Legislating against Use of Cost-Effectiveness Information." While other wealthy nations went ahead building organizations to look critically at the clinical worth and economic reasonableness of specific medications and other health-care interventions, the U.S. did not; we were legally barred from doing so.

The States Go It Alone

In the face of rising medication costs crushing the budgets of state and private insurers, and with minimal action at the federal level, several states began to take matters into their own hands. Several set up their own prescription drug affordability boards, or PDABs. Progressive forces took a lesson from the movements on the right like the American Legislative Exchange Council (ALEC), a conservative consultancy that worked with state governments to promote business-friendly laws and policies, crafting pieces of model legislation and advising states how to get them passed. Belatedly, the left caught on to this approach and began to support similar groups with an opposite perspective. One was the National Academy for State Health Policy (NASHP, a less friendly acronym than the chummy ALEC); it offers guidance to state legislators on laws and regulations designed to produce more equity and affordability in health care at the local level.

The emerging PDABs were set up by bright, committed officials; they knew what they wanted to accomplish, but most had little background in clinical medicine or cost-effectiveness analysis. So several of them asked PORTAL to consult on their efforts, including Colorado, Washington, and Oregon; that work was spearheaded by Kesselheim and Ben Rome, the sharp young internist and health services researcher who joined our group while still in his residency at the Brigham.

Closer to home, Massachusetts announced that it would permit the state's Medicaid program to assess the value of some extremely costly prescription drugs—many of which were unjustifiably overpriced and were putting growing pressure on its mission of caring for a population with a high proportion of minorities and people with disabilities; the state approached PORTAL to help with that work.

Industry-supported opposition to these efforts appeared quickly and adopted a paradoxical strategy. With support from the pharmaceutical industry, a group calling itself PIPC, the Partnership to Improve Patient Care, teamed up with another new entity called the National Minority Quality Forum. They complained that all these cost-effectiveness analyses would hurt patients, especially minorities and the disabled. The groups argued that evaluating how well a given treatment enhanced the duration and quality of life was inherently prejudiced against sick people.

It was an illogical argument, but as a public relations move it was clever. Protecting the elderly, disabled, and minorities was a more convincing rallying cry than protecting the revenue stream of pharmaceutical companies. The PIPC and its allied groups became plausible-seeming front organizations to transmit the views of their industry sponsors.

Ghosts of the Death Panels

In one of its broadsides the PIPC played the race card with a statement titled "Traditional Value Assessment Methods Fail Communities of Color and Exacerbate Health Inequities." The PIPC criticized the state for partnering with us and with ICER, since we "seem unable to innovate beyond traditional methods for assessing value," and argued that our doing so will just "entrench health inequities." The intimidation seems to have worked: over several years, despite its spiraling Medicaid pharmacy budget, Massachusetts has not yet asked us to evaluate the appropriateness of the cost of any drugs. This course of action was likely viewed favorably by the state's influential biotech industry.

Many of the most argued-about value propositions involve very costly new drugs to treat chronic conditions like Crohn's disease, psoriasis, rheumatoid arthritis, eczema. These drugs vary widely in price, and also in how well they manage these diseases. But the irony is that their major impact is on the *symptoms* these diseases cause; they generally have little or no effect on length of life. So stripping out consideration of the *quality* of life—how much your joint pain or skin condition or gastrointestinal disease affects how you feel and function—is the only clinical basis for comparing these medicines. Take that out of the analysis, and there's no sensible basis for comparison.

By 2024, the PIPC was aggressively advocating for a bill in Congress called the "Protecting Health Care for All Patients Act," which sought to impose further restrictions on the legality of using cost-effectiveness analysis to evaluate the prices of treatments. "People with disabilities have long fought for this!" the group tweeted, adding that the nation needed more "protections against the use of QALYs and similar measures to make coverage and reimbursement decisions." In February 2024, with strong Republican backing and support by the drug industry, the House voted along party lines by a three-vote margin to make the use of QALY-based cost-effectiveness analysis illegal in virtually all government health-care programs. Such cost-effectiveness analysis had already been banned in Medicare; the new legislation would seek to extend the ban to drug purchasing decisions by Medicaid, the Veterans Health Administration, Medicare Advantage insurance programs, and other federally supported prescription medication coverage. The Congressional Budget Office calculated that the law would add $1.1 billion more to federal drug expenditures over the coming decade. Its fate is not yet clear, but similar bills are introduced regularly by industry-backed foes of cost-effectiveness analysis. With the rightward thrust of the U.S. government after the 2024 elections, economic analyses of medication costs are likely to be even more vulnerable in a government increasingly sympathetic to the needs of companies.

The Wonder Drug, Revisited

By late 2023, the Colorado State Prescription Drug Affordability Board had chosen Vertex's cystic fibrosis drug Trikafta as its first product to assess for "unaffordability"; its decision would even attract the attention of *Rolling Stone*, the first time anything I was involved in had overlapped with that iconic publication since the 1960s. Colorado's CF drug announcement unleashed a torrent of public concern spearheaded by patient advocacy groups close to the manufacturer. Some of them worried that if the board ruled that the drug's price had to be lowered, Vertex could retaliate by cutting its patient assistance programs, or even refusing to sell its CF drugs in Colorado, as it had done previously in England. A local network affiliate ran a lengthy and gripping segment about an appealing young woman with CF whose life, like Merriman's, was transformed by the "wonder drug." Now, she said, she feared her devastating symptoms would return if the board's actions caused Vertex to refuse to sell the drug in her state, and worried that she might need a costly lung transplant. She decried the fact that the PDAB wasn't considering the enormous quality of life improvements the drug made possible—even though the board's industry-influenced mandate explicitly prohibited considering such matters in its assessments.

In early December 2023, the Colorado PDAB met and announced the nation's first ruling by any state drug affordability board. Local CF patients and advocates had argued forcefully that the drug wasn't really "unaffordable" to Coloradans because people on Medicaid didn't have to pay for it at all, even if the state had to do so at a level of nearly a quarter of a million dollars a year per patient. For those with private insurance, Vertex's patient assistance program helped defray their hefty co-pay share of the cost. Taken together, these strategies co-opted individual patients, while leaving payers like Medicaid and health insurers on the hook for the remainder of the charge. But according to the PDAB's legislative authorization, Trikafta thus wasn't really "unaffordable to Coloradans," even though *someone* was paying around $300,000 per patient per year for it. Whether such drugs were unaffordable to the system as a whole did not get addressed.

Across the Atlantic, at the end of 2023 the *Guardian* assessed the ongoing NHS-NICE battle over Vertex's CF drugs in light of the British fixed-budget approach to funding health care: "If the NHS chose to pay the price for these drugs and had no extra cash, what would it have to cut? How many hip replacements? How much cancer care?" On the other hand, it noted that Vertex "says that it needs billions to invest in research. But what is the point if children are still condemned to suffer and die prematurely because nobody can afford to buy the drugs?"

After months of torturous waiting for patients and their families, in late June 2024 the NHS announced that it would back down, agreeing to cover Vertex's three-drug treatment and related drugs for all CF patients in England, nearly five years after the drug was approved in the U.S. NICE said it had revised its original assessment by adjusting its economic model to somehow take greater account of the severity of the condition and the benefits of the drugs on quality of life and longevity. There may also have been an adjustment to the cost component of the cost-effectiveness analysis following discussions with Vertex about prices, but that part of the calculation remains secret. With similar arrangements expected in Scotland and Wales, these very expensive "wonder drugs" would now finally be available to all CF patients throughout the UK, at the government's expense.

CHAPTER 14

Conflicted Interests

When it comes to medication choices, doctors, like regulators, function as judges: we are expected to weigh the evidence carefully and dispassionately and make decisions solely on that basis—without fear or favor, as the saying goes. Some of us also are tasked with that judging function in making such choices at a systems level, in deciding which drugs will be approved for use at our hospital or health-care system, or teaching our trainees about the medications they will use. Still others are called on to help determine whether a new product will be approved for use nationally. We all understand that in court, it's not okay for the judge to also work for one of the litigants; with medications, what happens if that commonsense principle is ignored? The descriptions that follow come from my own institution, but these practices and attitudes are widespread nationally. Beyond that, the policies and norms at our university help set the tone for approaches elsewhere: what happens at Harvard doesn't stay at Harvard.

Like most other medical schools, the institution allows its faculty to spend up to 20 percent of our time on outside consulting, although we're required to report such work each year. This practice is not just condoned by the medical school and its teaching hospitals, it's often encouraged for a variety of reasons. One eminent department chair had a standard response to faculty recruits who balked at the paltry academic salaries he was offering them: "Just think of it as a base. You can earn much more, maybe double that amount, by consulting for drug companies. Being a member of the Harvard faculty makes that easier." Generic drug companies rarely retain consultants to give lectures to practitioners; that's more likely to be done by the manufacturers of costly brand-name drugs, who have both the wherewithal and motivation to pay doctors generously to teach others about their products. Sometimes that's a useful way to spread new knowledge about innovative treatments. Sometimes, not.

A number of years ago the Brigham took over a local community hospital to join its network, and I was asked to give one of the first grand rounds presentations after the merger. On reaching the podium I was troubled to see the following note left for the incoming chief resident by a predecessor from the previous regime: "To set up Grand Rounds talks each week, reach out to the following people; they will provide the speakers and take care of the honoraria." Then followed a list of local drug company sales reps. I felt like I was in the bathroom of a seedy dive bar that had a scrawl on the wall reading "For a good time, call Teeny," along with a phone number.

The provenance of such funding wasn't as apparent then as it has become. Early in my career, when I didn't know enough to pay attention to such things, I'd be asked by area hospitals to come give a talk on appropriate medication use in the elderly, and was paid a hundred dollars or so for doing it. Among other things, I'd talk about diagnosing and managing memory problems in older patients, and sometimes mentioned the uselessness of a drug called Hydergine that was widely used in those days, but didn't work. At the end of one such talk I was approached by a well-dressed man whom I had seen in the back of the audience at other talks I had given; I should have realized that his natty attire meant he was probably not a local GP. "We aren't going to pay for these talks anymore," he said, citing my comments about Hydergine. "Why should we give you money to bad-mouth our own products?" It turned out he was a sales supervisor for Sandoz, the company that made the useless drug. Although the small honoraria I got were issued by the hospitals that hosted me, the money had actually come from drug companies that underwrote the institutions' "education funds." I've learned that any of us in academia who get paid to give talks need to know about the ultimate source of that money, laundered though it may be.

Drug company researchers are sometimes incorporated more directly into the medical school curriculum, and often they are uniquely qualified to teach in their area of expertise. Many are eminent scientists in their own right, and some hold joint appointments as university faculty—as well as strong opinions about the benefits of academia-industry relationships. Even if they don't state those views overtly, their very presence embodies the concept. Of course, those ties can be very useful to both sides, and it's not their existence that is the problem: students just like to know who's paying the people who teach them. The situation came to a boil in 2008 after an eminent researcher affiliated with the Dana-Farber Cancer Institute made a presentation to the Harvard first-year class on the effectiveness of an excellent new drug to treat a form of blood cancer. He had played a key role in its development, and it was a real breakthrough. But students who attended the talk were concerned that he hadn't mentioned he also worked for the company that sold it, and made their concerns public. Harvard admitted it had no consistently applied rules requiring such disclosures and set about to develop them. The students were given a stern talking-to by the dean's office for complaining about the issue openly; some were sent to meet with me so I could try to set them straight. Instead, I praised their activism. The incident led to new Harvard Medical School guidelines requiring all speakers to reveal any financial ties to drugmakers before giving a lecture. Such disclosures don't mean that the information presented will be problematic in any way; it's just that audiences have a right to know about them.

An Embarrassing Exposé

Much larger corporate relationships came under scrutiny in a 2021 series by the *Boston Globe*, which found that for nearly all the CEOs of the city's large academic medical centers, each of whom were senior faculty at their respective medical schools, their day jobs seemed to leave them with a fair amount of free time, and their hospital salaries of $1.8 to $2.7 million a year for that activity were apparently inadequate. The *Globe* found that nearly all of them supplemented that work with lucrative positions on corporate boards, often of drug companies. That work paid them several hundred thousand dollars a year more, sometimes along with stock options that could range into the millions. The Brigham's president, Dr. Betsy Nabel, had served on the corporate board of the medical device manufacturer Medtronic and was also on the corporate board of Moderna, the Boston biotech start-up that helped develop the Covid vaccine, at a time when an important part of the evaluation of that vaccine was being conducted at the Brigham. (Moderna got into an embarrassing dispute when it shut out its NIH colleagues from the vaccine's patent; that was followed by a fight with the federal government over the windfall profits the company made on $36 billion in sales of its only product.)

Critics wondered why running the Brigham wasn't a big enough job to fill Dr. Nabel's time, and why her $2.4 million hospital salary for doing so wasn't enough to live on. She also had an additional side gig advising the owner-dominated National Football League on sports-induced traumatic brain injury, although she was a cardiologist and not a neurologist. Such outside activity was defended by the board chair of the Mass General Brigham, the corporate entity that controls two of the three primary Harvard teaching hospitals:

> We have long believed that it is incredibly helpful to our organization that our leadership gain valuable experience through board-level exposure to how other significant organizations are structured, organized, and managed.

By contrast, when I established DoPE as a division in the Brigham Department of Medicine I decided that none of us would accept any personal consulting payments from pharmaceutical companies. I put in place an identical rule when we established our educational nonprofit, Alosa Health, to provide non-commercial information to doctors about prescribing choices (see chapter 17). Such prohibitions are uncommon in our environment. I didn't do so because I think such activity is immoral, since I don't. It was simply because so much of our work in both settings is about making judgment calls and recommendations about medication decisions that it just seemed more straightforward that way. I'm constantly surprised at how strange these policies sound to many colleagues.

The *Globe* series caused major embarrassment and was followed by an unusual transformation: three years later, the paper did a 2024 follow-up analysis and found that most of those problematic outside entanglements weren't present anymore. Following a petition signed by faculty and students demanding higher ethical standards, most of the academic executives were no longer in those jobs, and nearly all their successors now avoided such outside corporate positions. So, progress. But not universally. The only holdout was Dr. Laurie Glimcher, CEO of the renowned Harvard-affiliated Dana-Farber Cancer Institute, who retained an outside corporate board position that came with compensation of over $300,000 a year, beyond her nearly $4 million salary for running the cancer center. In September 2023, Dr. Glimcher had surprised the medical world by announcing that Dana-Farber would end its decades-long affiliation with the Brigham, located next door, to build its own free-standing cancer hospital in a deal with rival Beth Israel Hospital several blocks away, disrupting hundreds of clinical and institutional relationships that had worked well for years. If patients in the new facility needed attention for other medical problems, they would be transported by a system of bridges and tunnels to the Beth Israel. The corporate entity that controls the Brigham and Mass General Hospitals didn't make a compelling counter-offer, preferring to go it alone in the very lucrative cancer space. Others objected to what some called Dr. Glimcher's edifice complex. They argued that this realignment of institutional relationships belonged more in the corporate world than in the setting of clinical medicine, and worried that the bridge-and-tunnel patients might get worse care if they became acutely ill.

In January 2024, an outside whistleblower called attention to data integrity problems in numerous cancer research papers that had been published by Dr. Glimcher and her colleagues. Several of these had to be retracted or corrected; scientific misconduct investigations ensued at Dana-Farber and Harvard. Later that year Dr. Glimcher unexpectedly announced that she would be resigning her position leading the Dana-Farber in a month, leaving it to her sudden successor to oversee the ambitious program she had spearheaded to overhaul the cancer center's future.

Dr. Glimcher was not the only leader to have a dramatic job

change at Harvard that year. With the abrupt resignation of the university's president Claudine Gay at the start of 2024, Alan Garber, Harvard's longtime provost and a doctor, became interim president; it was later announced that he would continue to serve as president through the 2027 academic year. In recent years, if the provost was a physician, as was the case for Alan and his predecessor, the university's president would look to the provost to help guide decisions related to the schools of medicine, public health, and dentistry. Alan and I had spoken for only a few seconds during all his years as provost, when we found ourselves at the same conference. (That itself was interesting, as he was a noted health economist–physician, and I ran the university's largest program on the cost of medications. But somehow our paths never crossed.) "I'm a markets guy," he said, disagreeing with something I had said about drug prices. Apparently he was indeed. When Garber took on the president role, the *Globe* reported that in addition to his $946,000 salary from Harvard for his job as provost in the most recent academic year, he had been paid a larger amount—$963,000—for his part-time service on the corporate boards of two drug companies; one was Vertex Pharmaceuticals.

Such arrangements are common, and have important implications for the values and culture of our teaching institutions. Earlier in my career, the chairman of the Department of Medicine at Massachusetts General Hospital, Dennis Ausiello, was receiving several hundred thousand dollars a year to serve on Pfizer's corporate board of directors. Also at MGH, Dr. Sam Thier was the founding president and then the CEO of Partners HealthCare, the entity that owned both MGH and the Brigham, making him my boss's boss's boss. Sam had served on Merck's corporate board of directors since 1994, the same year he took on the teaching hospitals' presidency. In the wake of the drugmaker's institutional chaos following the Vioxx debacle, he became half of a two-person executive committee that according to the SEC "functioned collectively in the role typically played by a chairman of the board." To be clear: neither was a science-advising or senior physician consulting position; they were corporate boards of directors, conferring on each member a fiduciary responsibility to further the economic well-being of a given drug company. Besides raising questions about conflicts of interest, these outside entanglements invite questions about what the university calls "conflicts of commitment." That is, how can you run a major teaching hospital or an enormous clinical department and still find time to play a central role helping to run a large multinational corporation?

On Being a Skunk

The relationships I worried about went far beyond Harvard's huge teaching hospitals; they were abundant in the medical school's basic science departments as well. Leonard Valentinovich Blavatnik has been a remarkably generous donor who has given Harvard more than a quarter of a billion dollars over the past decade. According to Wikipedia, he "made his initial fortune after the collapse of the Soviet Union in the privatization of state-owned aluminum and oil assets." His worth was estimated by *Forbes* at $31 billion, and he has donated hundreds of millions of dollars to universities and causes all over the world, as well as to political candidates of all stripes, including many on the right. One result of his philanthropy at Harvard was the creation of the Blavatnik Biomedical Accelerator, a program that funds research "to develop preliminary observations into robust intellectual property positions. Its primary goal is to advance technologies to the point where an industry partnership can commence." The Accelerator supports much cutting-edge research that will undoubtedly lead to important new cures that will help patients. It also is a source of key information about the latest university-based biological research that could be transformed into valuable new drug products. If I had a multibillion-dollar holding corporation that owned several biotech start-ups that could benefit handsomely from such early insights into this pipeline of university-based innovation, I would call the company "Access Industries." Blavatnik does, and that's what he named it.

Along with Alan Garber's ascension to the interim role of president in 2024, another change occurred at Harvard's highest level:

a new member was added to the Corporation, the sometimes secretive group of trustees that governs the university and selects its own members. It has just twelve members plus the university president, and is ultimately responsible for all of Harvard's activities. With its roots dating back to 1650, it is the oldest corporation in the Western Hemisphere. The newly added Corporation member was Kenneth Frazier, who represented Merck as its general counsel and executive vice president during the Vioxx crisis, and later became the company's CEO. (He also sits on the board of ExxonMobil, which doesn't bode well for those trying to get Harvard to end investments by its $50 billion endowment in fossil fuel companies.) It does not seem likely that he will push for greater separation between the university and the pharmaceutical industry.

When some of the outside commitments by the leaders of our teaching hospitals first came to widespread public attention, the medical school and its affiliates set up a process of ultraorthodox scrutiny for all the rest of us. We faculty were warned that we had to report anything of value, of any size, that we received from any health-care-related company. If we went pro bono to an all-day scientific meeting sponsored by a drugmaker and lunch was served, we had to declare that lunch as a form of payment, to be reported on a national database. Because of concern about rampant payoffs by drug companies to doctors, as part of the Obamacare legislation the federal government established a website on which every pharmaceutical manufacturer must list every payment made to every physician (in cash or in kind), even small ones. It was originally referred to colloquially as "Dollars for Docs," but is now known simply as the "Open Payments" website (OpenPaymentsData.cms.gov). Some of my colleagues said they didn't want to be publicly shamed for receiving payments from a drug company if all they did was eat lunch at an all-day meeting. What should they do? "Don't have lunch," came the helpful advice from the hospital. "Or bring your own food in a bag."

What about interacting with scientists at companies who were designing clinical trials? Despite some tacky examples of a few of those interactions, these are often very useful colleague-to-colleague interchanges conducted with great integrity. Was it still okay to brainstorm with researchers at companies about ideas for how to best design a study of a new drug, or set up an experiment to test an idea for a new medication? “If you talk with them, it needs to be a formal paid consultancy run through the hospital’s Office for Interactions with Industry, and then it could be reported to the federal database,” my colleagues were told. “Even for just talking?” “Yes.”

“Can’t I just do it for free, and not go through all this?” “No,” came the answer. “That would be providing a service at below-market value, and would not be permissible.” Of course, careful scrutiny is needed in light of all the potential for abuse here. But it’s been striking to see all the pressure put on ground-level faculty by the medical school and its hospitals over these arrangements, while the leaders of our institutions were receiving astonishing sums to sit on corporate boards of directors—which seems far more impactful and potentially problematic.

Other Outside Entanglements

Similar issues arise when faculty and clinicians interact with the FDA, which relies on our expertise on the committees that advise it about drug approval decisions. Specialists in a given disease often conduct clinical trials for manufacturers, which makes sense, and they generally are paid for doing so, which also makes sense. Sometimes that payment is routed through researchers’ institutions, when it can help pay their salary but not augment it. Sometimes that payment is made separately, directly to the clinician. And sometimes additional perks come along with it, like paying for a professor’s postdoc or fellowship program, or lucrative speaking engagements. Such remuneration runs the gamut from totally fair compensation to exorbitant bribery, as we will see in the case of opioids (chapter 20).

When expertise is needed on an FDA advisory committee, for years the agency dealt with potential conflicts of interest through a perfunctory recitation at the start of the meeting stating the existence of those relationships, and that was it—as if just naming the conflict was enough to make it inoperative. After Vioxx was taken off the market because it tripled the risk of heart attack and stroke, some doctors surprisingly advocated for its return, arguing that it really worked better than other products for some patients. (There was no convincing evidence for this.) When the AdCom voted on the matter, there was a striking correlation between whether particular members did a lot of consulting for industry, and how they voted. The drug stayed off the market.

Around the time that Obamacare was being made into law, I was invited to join an Institute of Medicine panel trying to put together national "recommendations about recommendations." (The IOM is a federally designated body representing some of the most senior people in biomedical science and health care; it is now known as the National Academy of Medicine.) Many of us had been concerned about commercial influence on the development of guidance documents for the treatment of specific conditions, and that ties to industry could sometimes influence that advice. But defenders of loose standards argued, "Anyone who's any good consults for one drug company or another, so you have to tolerate these relationships. If an expert isn't a drug company consultant, you have to wonder what's wrong with them." As someone who's made it a policy not to accept industry consulting dollars, I remember thinking, What am I, chopped liver? But I phrased my response more diplomatically, noting that I had banned personal consulting arrangements with drugmakers in DoPE, most of us were considered pretty intelligent folks, and to my knowledge none of my faculty had fallen behind on their rent or mortgages, or died of starvation. Our IOM panel came up with a book of solid recommendations whose title said a lot about our mission: *Clinical Practice Guidelines We Can Trust.*

One way to handle the conflict-of-interest issue, especially for medications, is to require that anyone giving a talk disclose at its start any commercial affiliations that might relate to the topic; that has now become a universal expectation. This disclosure is useful and doesn't imply contamination of the lecture's content, any more than my lack of conflicts means that what I say is somehow truer. But increasingly, that simple requirement isn't taken seriously or is omitted entirely. Skipping this ought to be as objectionable as a speaker walking to the podium naked, but the practice is becoming so common (failure to disclose, not nudity) that it attracts little notice. Or the disclosure slide may be projected for a fraction of a second, rendering it unreadable. One neuroscientist colleague reviewed all the videotaped presentations from one international meeting and measured how long each disclosure slide was shown. The more financial ties a speaker had, the faster they were projected—often to the point of unintelligibility.

But worse still is making the disclosure process into a joke. At another international meeting, a doctor with extensive industry ties briefly put up the required slide, depicting consultancies for over a dozen drug companies. Then he added, "You will note that I work with a great many pharmaceutical manufacturers. If there is anyone in the audience representing a company for which I do not presently consult, please see me after the lecture."

Big Stakes

The U.S. now spends four and a half trillion dollars a year on health care, or close to 17 percent of our gross domestic product, making medicine one of the nation's largest business sectors. Pharmaceutical spending comprises about half a trillion of those dollars, with one added dimension: this spending is shaped by the preferences and decisions of the physicians who make them, rendering those people even more prone to subtle and not-so-subtle influence. The health-care systems that form the backbone of many medical schools' intellectual and fiscal operations are now far bigger than the universities that house them. For example, the Mass General Brigham system where I work is the state's largest employer; its annual budget of about $20 billion dwarfs that of our whole university. The number of faculty at Harvard Medical School is several times larger than the number at all the other Harvard schools combined.

This disproportion in part reflects the enormous value that society puts on health care, and the fact that medicine is one of the fastest-growing sectors of the American economy and of its universities. But such large sums inevitably carry the risk that our programs could become just another subpart of the nation's commercial enterprise, including our organizations that are nominally nonprofit. That intermingling of roles makes it harder to take the necessarily critical arm's-length view of what our institutions are doing—a key role for universities.

Academic medical centers and their faculty simultaneously serve as high-cost service providers and teachers and researchers. Why isn't there more concern that in virtually all medical schools, the faculty work for the companies (i.e., the teaching hospitals) and their industry partners that provide the very services and goods we're teaching about and studying? On one hand, that commingling is obvious and necessary, but shouldn't we rethink what effect it might be having on just *what* we're teaching and researching? What if a large oil refinery were the main base for all of a university's programs in earth science, geology, ecology, and energy policy? And if many of the faculty in these departments were supported by the refinery and the oil company that owned it? Or if the departments of dance and theater arts were funded or owned by TikTok? Would that have any effect on what the faculty study, and how students are taught?

CHAPTER 15

Making Medicines Affordable

Pharmaceutical companies now devote far more resources to lobbying than any other industry, having spent about $378 million a year on that activity in 2023—a full $140 million more than the second-place sector, the electronics industry. That money deploys armies of talented, well-paid influencers whose only job is to persuade policymakers at the federal and state levels to make scores of decisions that all push in the same direction: to make the world a more comfortable place for the $1.6-trillion-dollar-a-year global drug industry. The unsuspecting marks are not just members of Congress and the executive branch from both parties; they're also experienced bureaucrats at federal and state agencies who should know better. We physicians receive a different kind of expensive attention when we accept the stilted education proffered by industry-paid salespeople. Patients play a role, too, in their willingness to demand a drug they've seen in a commercial that directs them to "Ask your doctor if X is right for you."

Understanding how we got here makes it possible to reverse engineer our decades of drug policy missteps and begin some much-needed rethinking. Ranged against the armies of lobbyists and marketers and their allies, a small number of valiant, mostly outgunned groups around the country are working to change things. The work of my own programs, DoPE and Kesselheim's PORTAL, is wholly grant-supported; that allows us to cover our salaries and offer minimal salaries to our postdoctoral trainees, all of whom are MDs or PhDs or lawyers or pharmacists. For newly minted postdocs with four years of college followed by medical school or law school or a PhD program, at the time of this writing the NIH allows us to pay a salary of $61,000 per year. For colleagues with seven or more years of experience beyond their doctoral degree, that rises to $74,000 a year. By contrast, the starting salary at the consulting firm McKinsey & Company is between $100,000 and $140,000 for a bright kid fresh out of college. (That's the company that worked with Purdue Pharma to "turbocharge" the volume of prescriptions for their opioid products; see chapter 20.)

Swimming Upstream

Swimming upstream can work, though—for salmon and herring (see chapter 18) as well as iconoclasts in medicine. I learned that in helping to start the discipline of pharmacoepidemiology, which our more established colleagues looked down on because it wasn't really pharmacology and wasn't conventional epidemiology. Against the odds, our research has been funded by the NIH and FDA, of all places, as well as by philanthropies like the Commonwealth Fund and the Kaiser Permanente Health Policy Institute. Another source of support has been the philanthropist Al Engelberg, the lawyer who prospered by helping the generic drug industry to come into its own in the 1980s, and then spent the rest of his life giving away those millions to worthy causes, including PORTAL. A major pillar of support for our work, which has made it possible for us to serve as a contrarian voice in this space for so many years has been a foundation started by an unlikely benefactor, John Arnold. He was an energy futures trader at Enron, where he made a fortune before it collapsed, becoming the country's youngest billionaire in 2007. The following year, he and his wife, Laura, signed the Giving Pledge, committing to donate most of their assets to charity. For over a decade, they have spent the bulk of their time on their eponymous foundation, supporting work in fields from primary education to criminal justice. One of their greatest concerns has been curbing unaffordable drug prices; out of the $2.5 billion they've given away so far, their foundation has committed about $200 million to support many of the organizations described here that are working to make medications more affordable.

The Arnolds are evidence of the enormous impact that committed individuals can have. It also helps to be billionaires.

Armed with a better understanding of the history of all the nonrandom steps that created the exceptional economics of prescription drug pricing, we can now rethink each point at which our policies went astray and consider some specific repairs.

Fixing the Problem from the Eighteenth Century—Patent Reform

It's been about 235 years since George Washington signed the first patent in 1790 for a process to make potash, used in fertilizer. Our first-in-the-world system to protect innovation has not aged well in the way it's been applied to medications, but there are some practical ways we can fix it.

The drug industry's armies of smart and extremely well-paid patent attorneys have until recently always seemed to be a step ahead of the hardworking sheriffs at the Patent Office, as the feds seem forced to engage in endless games of intellectual property whack-a-mole. As at the FDA, many of the wrongheaded policies end up working in the interest of companies and against the needs of the public, so it's not surprising that they have been so durable. So, too, for Patent Office errors made in defining the expiration dates of patents: a recent PORTAL analysis calculated that hundreds of millions of dollars might be unnecessarily lost because of USPTO errors in defining the end date of patents on costly drugs. Creative scholars in the field, many of whom I've cited earlier, have proposed some solutions to these problems that could be implemented within the executive branch, while others might require commonsense legislative change, though that's often hard to come by in Congress:

- Stop funding the patent office by means of user fees paid by companies applying for patents. This is the same problem we've seen with the FDA's heavy reliance on user fees from the drug industry to pay its drug review staff. The nation ends up spending far more than it saves through such arrangements, when it later pays more than it should for poorly evaluated new drug products.

- Hire enough well-trained patent examiners and give them adequate time to make thoughtful decisions, rather than having to rush through complex issues of novelty, prior art, and other difficult determinations about potential billion-dollar products.
- Enforce the expectation based in the Constitution that a new patent should be issued only for products that are truly novel and nonobvious—not just minuscule manipulations that don't benefit people.
- Make it easier to challenge bad patents that are based on trivial changes. The creation of the Patent Trial and Appeal Board in 2012 was a good step in this direction.
- Make it harder for a manufacturer to tell the FDA that a product modification is so small that it doesn't require a new clinical review, and then go to the Patent Office to patent the same change as a meaningful innovation. Progress is being made to force companies to provide the same information to both the FDA and USPTO to make it harder to play them off against each other.
- Apply special scrutiny to drug patents that have been rejected by similar authorities in Europe and other countries; that should be a signal for skepticism here.
- Make it harder for an applicant to come back multiple times to reapply for a patent that was rejected—a practice more common in the U.S. than elsewhere.
- Enable generic manufacturers to more readily challenge frivolous patents that should have flunked the "nonobvious" and "novel" criteria. At present, such challenges succeed in about two-thirds of cases, but that consumes a lot of resources and time. And, of course, staving off a patent challenge can be very lucrative for the original manufacturer for as long as it continues, even if the patent is eventually thrown out.
- Prune back the thickets of problematic secondary and tertiary patents whose only pupose is to postpone the normal expiration of

an original monopoly protection. A convincing case for this was made in a recent court filing by several of us, led by PORTAL faculty Will Feldman and Kesselheim, concerning unaffordable inhalers for lung disease, and in ongoing work by our colleagues at I-MAK. In a major decision, the court agreed with us.

The Biden administration's Patent Office director had begun several promising reforms along these lines; she resigned a week after the 2024 election.

Fixing the Problem from 1980: Enforcing the Bayh-Dole Act Properly

Was it ever even true that promising discoveries made at the nation's universities with NIH support "withered on the vine" because the scientists who made them were too distractible to bring them to the public? Probably not. Fair attribution of responsibility and rewards can be hard, but we figure it out in many other industries. The smartphone combines thousands of separate innovations; each carries payments to the inventors and companies that created it. That movie you might watch this weekend on Amazon or Netflix may be based on a book by one person, inspired by a short story by someone else, adapted for a new medium with a screenplay by others, and filmed by a director funded by one or more producers. And then there are the actors and other professionals who also create the final product, as well as the streaming service or theater that provides access to it. Each plays a key role in moving from gleam-in-eye to finished production, and each gets a defined share of the proceeds. Our colleagues in Silicon Valley and Hollywood have figured out ways to partition revenues among all the sectors and players who make a final product possible. But in the world of medications, the drug company usually gets to keep ownership of a medication all to itself. How did that happen, and how can we fix it?

As it became clear how far the Bayh-Dole law had strayed from its original potential, many of us hoped that the two legislators who wrote it might weigh in on the problems it inadvertently created in offering nothing to the public even if taxpayers helped underwrite a drug's invention. But that was not to be. After he failed to score enough votes to win the 1996 presidential contest, Bob Dole left the Senate and became a paid spokesman for Pfizer, stiffly hawking Viagra on TV. Once he assumed that position he went soft on industry and never again took a hard line on drug prices, offering few penetrating insights on those effects of the law he had cowritten. His transition from elections to erections dashed hopes many of us had that the former member might become a missionary for drug affordability. Worse, he engorged the public debate in a 2002 letter to the *Washington Post* he cosigned with Senator Bayh, saying that their law's requirement that a publicly funded product must be made available to the public "on reasonable terms" was never meant to refer to its cost. The resulting system for privatizing publicly funded research that he helped erect seems likely to stand firm for years to come. The Trump administration's goal of shrinking the government likely means there won't be any happy endings on this in the foreseeable future.

In March 2022, Kesselheim and I wrote a piece in the *New England Journal of Medicine* with Al Engelberg. In it, we described the various legal strategies the executive branch could use to lower drug prices without any new legislation. First came the provisions of the Bayh-Dole Act allowing the government to take control of the patents on overpriced drugs whose development was publicly funded, if only the administration could see unaffordable prices as violating the "reasonable terms" provision. We also proposed using a lesser-known law enacted in 1910 known as 28 U.S. Code §1498, which allows the federal government to override patents if doing so is necessary for the public interest.

There is a precedent for that: shortly after 9/11, when it seemed that terrorists might use anthrax to wage biological warfare in the U.S., the medical community focused on ways to protect the nation. The best prevention and treatment would come from the antibiotic ciprofloxacin. But Bayer held the patent on it and demanded an extraordinarily high price, even in the face of a potential national health emergency. Working with Senator Chuck Schumer, Engelberg threatened Bayer with the government's use of its §1498 power to infringe their patent and allow generic manufacturers to make the drug at a fraction of the cost. Faced with that threat, the company reduced its price by 50 percent and agreed to commit half of its production to the government in case of an anthrax bioterrorism emergency. But in the decades since, the government never again used the threat of §1498 to address unaffordable medication prices.

In our *NEJM* article, we called on the then-president to issue "an executive order expressing the Biden administration's intention to take advantage of existing laws [to] pave the way for lowering the government's prescription-drug costs." Over the ensuing months, Kesselheim engaged in back-channel consultation with the White House and Senators Warren and Sanders. At the close of 2023, President Biden announced that he was changing course on federal passivity about the prices of NIH-funded discoveries. He undid Trump's decree that unaffordable prices could not be a rationale for implementing march-in rights, and said his administration was open to authorizing generic companies to make and distribute drugs developed with federal research funds if their prices were set unconscionably high. Reaction from the industry was predictable: "The Administration is sending us back to a time when government research sat on a shelf, not benefitting anyone." But what really had been sitting on the shelf was the government's legal authority to step in when private ownership rights stood in the way of a pressing public need—just as it had done with the doctrine of eminent domain in building the nation's railways and highways.

Biden also announced that he was implementing the Inflation Reduction Act provision that would force dozens of drug companies to pay back Medicare for their price increases that outstripped inflation. Beyond that, the new law also limited out-of-pocket costs for Medicare patients to just $2,000 per year, with insulin prices in that program capped at $35 per month. Together, these Biden initiatives did more to control the costs of unaffordable drugs than any other actions ever taken by the federal government. There were still some arrows left in the president's quiver yet to be shot, but the fate of all these reforms could be reversed by a swing to the right in Washington.

Fixing the Problem from 2003: Letting the Government Negotiate Prices

The IRA put a small crack in the 2003 deal that Billy Tauzin brokered between Congress and the pharmaceutical industry just before he left the former group to join the latter. Under its terms, by 2026, older patients will pay less for ten drugs for which Medicare can negotiate prices; more drugs would be added to that list annually. Viewed from the glass-half-full perspective, after twenty years the nation had finally broken the back of the special treatment that drugmakers had arranged in that initial legislation, and more negotiations would follow in the ensuing years. Seen with a glass-half-empty perspective, this would be only a small fraction of costly medications, while other industrialized countries do so routinely for *all* their drugs, year after year. The drug industry launched massive legal challenges on several fronts, which could delay the implementation for years or abort it altogether, and President Trump expressed interest in gutting one of his predecessor's signature achievements.

A different, more radical solution could rein in our unaffordably high drug prices, though it smacks of socialism. It would permit the government to refuse to cover medications it considers unfairly overpriced or poorly effective, and declare itself free of the obligation to pay for nearly every drug that is FDA-approved. Such a scheme would include many of the features of a drug-pricing system stacked in favor of patients instead of manufacturers:

- There would be a unitary payer with considerable clout, rather than the many fragmented payers in our current system.
- That body could choose from among products that offer the best patient benefit and value for the money.
- If several drugs met these criteria, it could use its negotiating power to get the best deals among them.
- Such a system would also employ the doctors writing the prescriptions, and own the pharmacies selling the drugs as well as the

hospitals that incur the benefits and harms that flow from good vs. bad prescribing.

- At federal expense, the system would deploy a nationwide team of impartial clinical educators to present the best non-commercial evidence to prescribers about drug choices.
- Medical care and medication coverage would be funded by the government and made available at no cost to patients.

This terrifying paradigm of socialist dystopia and government overreach is already in place and working just fine at the Veterans Health Administration. The largest integrated health-care organization in the country, the VA has for decades had an enlightened, effective, and patient-friendly approach to selecting and paying for medications. Perhaps shielded from industry and its lobbyists because these were medicines "for the vets," the VA is allowed to choose among similar drugs in a given class and pick those that work best and offer the best economic value. Having manufacturers of comparable drugs vie with each other on price to win those enormous federal contracts enables the VA to afford to cover nearly all the medication costs of the 9 million veterans it cares for. A recent analysis of VA drug expenditures showed that if Medicare were able to pay the same prices for the drugs it covers, it would save billions of dollars each year with no diminution in the quality of care. Thus, a marketplace-based free-enterprise system is alive and well in the heart of the country's only large program of socialized medicine—the one that serves those who have put their lives on the line to defend the nation and its way of life.

Exorcising the "Death Panels" and Embracing Cost-Effectiveness Analysis

Throughout the first part of my life as a doctor I'd often hear that "the U.S. health-care system is the best in the world!" I haven't heard that so much in the last decade or so. That's a good thing, because it can help get us over our infatuation with American exceptionalism and rethink some of the big problems we face, including drug costs. In reviewing drugs, prescribers, patients, and payers should expect evidence on what advantage a new medication brings to patients over existing treatments—even if the FDA can't legally demand this. If there isn't any, it might still be FDA-approved (too many legal hassles to prevent that), but it shouldn't cost more than similar older products until evidence is produced that it has some added benefit. Putting new medications through their paces in this way is also fairer to the drug industry, in a tough-love kind of way. If a company comes up with a treatment that offers an important advantage in survival or everyday health and shows this in well-conducted studies, it *should* command a higher price; that way we'll be less likely to reward and thus perpetuate mediocrity. As with the patent system, superiority should be rewarded in the marketplace, and unoriginal products should not.

We don't have to start from scratch on this. As we've seen, several European countries have established organizations to perform such analyses for new drugs that seek a place in their medical systems. Since virtually all advanced countries other than the U.S. provide health care as a right to all citizens, they've had to come up with a more data-driven way to figure out what things should cost. Going beyond our minimalist criterion of "It works better than placebo" and instead addressing the central question of "Compared to what?" is a much better approach than "It costs what it costs because that's what it costs." Such analyses could also empower government payers like Medicare and Medicaid to decline to purchase drugs that are extremely overpriced compared to alternatives.

Implementing these concepts fully won't be easy, especially at a time of conservative domination of the executive and legislative branches of government. Bernie Sanders visited PORTAL in 2024 to talk to us about medication policy while he was in town to give some lectures at Harvard. I asked him whether he thought the U.S. would ever adopt the idea of an independent body to determine reasonable prices for medications; he seemed skeptical. "In other countries the government regulates the pharmaceutical industry," he told me with a grin. "Here, it's the other way around."

Nonprofit Drug Companies?

A few groups have begun to connect the dots about the business model of some of the largest pharmaceutical companies that buy the research discoveries of other scientists and then hire contract research organizations to conduct the clinical trials necessary to prove effectiveness. The complex process of bringing a product through regulatory review can also be outsourced to some extent. Even the manufacture of the drugs themselves can be contracted out. This raises the question: For many medications, what do we really need the big drug companies to do? Might they have outsourced and disintermediated themselves to the edge of irrelevance?

Building on that idea, some new public interest organizations have started to perform many of the tasks that pharmaceutical companies have traditionally done. One of the most notable is Civica Rx, a not-for-profit generic drug company founded in 2018 by a network of health-care systems and hospitals, with additional funding provided by the ubiquitous John and Laura Arnold. Its goal is to ensure a steady supply of affordable, reliable generic medications to bring down the cost of older products like insulin, and to combat the crippling ongoing shortages of basic drugs—products that generic drugmakers often abandon when a low price makes them insufficiently profitable to manufacture and sell. Civica Rx describes its goals this way:

> Leading a movement for patients, not profits.
>
> Quality generic medicines.
>
> Game-changing affordable insulin.
>
> Medication prices based on the cost of manufacture—not shareholder return.

In 2023, California governor Gavin Newsom announced a $50 million deal with the company to produce low-cost insulin; the company is building its own manufacturing plant in Virginia.

That's a good development for older, established drugs, but what about therapies on the cutting edge of innovation? In 2014, Dr. Jennifer Doudna, who later won the Nobel Prize in Medicine for her research on gene-splicing, announced the creation of another nonprofit, the Innovative Genomics Institute, based at the University of California. Its mission is to bring gene-editing technology to applications for rare diseases unlikely to attract the interest of for-profit companies. Her goal, she said, was to bring down the cost of creating such new gene therapy treatments by a factor of ten. Her collaborator at IGI, Fyodor Urnov, stated it would be possible to create new gene therapies like those for sickle cell disease for a small fraction of the multimillion-dollars-per-treatment cost that for-profit companies are charging, as well as to target diseases that will never be economically attractive to big pharma. "We've built gene editing," he said. "It's versatile, it's widely used. There is an approved medicine, OK. Now, the next unsolvable challenge—which we will solve—is how to scale [it for] those who unfortunately have diseases with very low [or] nonexistent net present value." That is, conditions you can't make a lot of money treating.

Another new nonprofit on the far edge of innovative treatments is Odylia Therapeutics. It describes its origin and mission this way:

> Odylia was founded by Scott Dorfman, a successful entrepreneur and the father of two children with Usher syndrome, a rare genetic disease that affects vision and hearing, and Luk Vandenberghe, PhD, an innovator in the field of gene therapy. As a parent and business leader, Scott quickly recognized that the model used to support drug development is often based more on potential profits than on patient benefit, making many drugs to treat rare diseases unattractive candidates for commercial developers. The result is that many promising early-stage drugs never advance to clinical stage research. Scott and Luk saw a solution in utilizing an innovative nonprofit model to support rare disease drug development. . . . They founded Odylia with the sole mission to address the challenges keeping promising drugs from getting to patients who need them.

Getting Rid of Perverse Incentives That Raise Costs

At every step of the way, our heavily commercialized health-care system encourages the use of more expensive medications, even when more affordable products are available and work as well. Each problem is amenable to repair:

Incentives for Doctors

For physician-administered drugs like many treatments for cancer, a doctor can buy the medicine at a wholesale price and charge the health insurer markups that can generate hefty revenues each year. In some oncology practices, these markups became major sources of revenue in their own right. Why should the cost of a given medicine drive the margin collected for choosing it?

Incentives for Hospitals

The situation is even more out of control at many hospitals. "Safety-net" institutions were originally seen as those that care for poor patients; over thirty years ago Congress created a program to force drugmakers to provide such institutions with medications at a deep discount. As described by a medical school association that likes the plan:

> Congress created the 340B Drug Pricing Program in 1992 to protect safety-net hospitals from escalating drug prices by allowing them to purchase outpatient drugs at a discount from manufacturers. The program enables eligible hospitals to serve their communities by stretching scarce Federal resources as far as possible, reaching more eligible patients and providing more comprehensive services.

In reality, the 340B designation has been given to many enormous, often affluent medical centers (including my own) that use their discount drug prices to great advantage, though there is little clear evidence that the funds generated by buying low and selling high are actually spent on disadvantaged populations. Here, I'd have to agree with the position of the drug industry:

> The 340B program has strayed far from its safety net purpose. Instead, it has become less about patients and more about boosting the bottom lines of hospitals and for-profit pharmacies. How? Large hospitals buy deeply discounted 340B medicines and then turn around and charge both uninsured patients and insurance companies higher prices, pocketing the difference with little to no evidence they use that money to help patients.

If Congress can force drugmakers to offer discounts on their prices, maybe the best way to do so is to make sure that the benefits really do go to the care of the poor.

Incentives for Middlemen

Alone among the health-care systems of the world, the U.S. supports a massive additional layer of companies interposed between medication use and payment, the pharmacy benefit managers (PBMs). These companies have inserted themselves into the drug supply chain by offering to negotiate better prices on drugs, based on enormous pooled purchasing power. One component of the fee a PBM charges to an insurer or health-care system may be a percentage of the total drug expenditure it manages, so that's not a great incentive for lowering total medication costs. But the real mischief comes with secret behind-the-curtain deals, which is where most of the money leaks out. For many drug classes, several medications are more or less clinically interchangeable. So a PBM can take advantage of its middleman position by arranging to move market share within a drug class to the manufacturer offering the best rebates on the selling price. That sounds plausible, but it turns out that much of those rebates may not go to the patient buying the drug, or to the health insurer that hired the PBM, but to the PBM itself. And the more expensive a drug, the bigger the rebates can be; paradoxically, this can incentivize the use of costly products. We can't know who ends up with how much in these arrangements, since the amounts of the rebates and their destinations are not revealed. Trying to deflect blame for high drug costs, the pharmaceutical industry has charged that PBMs are the real culprits. (Of course, they both are.) By mid-2024, three separate federal investigations had produced scathing reports about the often-overlooked industry.

To address these scams, the billionaire entrepreneur Mark Cuban set up a new public benefit company, Cost Plus Drugs, to do this on an enormous scale. It buys generic drugs direct from the manufacturer, applies a straight 15 percent markup and a $5 pharmacy dispensing fee, and sends the medicine direct to consumers for a small additional shipping charge. The company's website strikingly illustrates how much can be saved by stripping away the often-exorbitant markups that PBMs sometimes charge. Its home page announces, "No Middlemen. No price games. Huge drug savings," followed by some examples. The first two are oral medications for cancer; the last is a widely used pill for diabetes:

- Imatinib (generic for Gleevec): $13.40. Retail price: $2,502.50
- Abiraterone (generic for Zytiga): $26.90. Retail price: $1,093.20
- Invokana (generic for canagliflozin): $245.92. Retail price: $676.14

In each case, the missing ingredient is the padding that health insurers and PBMs add to the cost charged to the patient. Amazon is also increasingly active in offering drugs online, delivered with the same alacrity it brought to books and everything else.

Hussain Lalani, a DoPE postdoc, published a report in one of the *JAMA* journals calculating how much Medicare could save if it simply used the Mark Cuban approach. Comparing the Cost Plus prices with what Medicare actually spent on a large group of generic medications, he calculated that the federal program could have spent $3.6 billion less *each year*—and that's only for the quarter of generic drugs that the Cuban company had available at the time. When a government coverage program costs more than a savvy private-sector arrangement, what's the point?

The Federal Trade Commission's PBM report accused some of these companies of price gouging, describing how "prescription drug middlemen profit at the expense of patients by inflating drug costs and squeezing Main Street pharmacies." The three largest PBMs process 80 percent of all the prescriptions Americans fill. Moreover, each of these PBMs are part of larger vertically integrated corporations that also own health insurance companies, mail-order pharmacy providers, or local drugstores, offering the opportunity for massive self-dealing. That, the FTC charged, enables some PBMs to drive patients to use the pharmacies within their corporate structure and then pay their affiliates much more for a given medication than is paid to rival drugstores for the same product. The agency report also called attention to subsidiary "group purchasing organizations" the PBM companies have created, often based in other countries, which can charge drug manufacturers "fees" in addition to rebates. This generates huge additional sums, which the PBM retains, but that aren't tracked and don't make it back to patients, health insurers, or anybody else. The FTC estimated that the excess revenues the PBMs extracted from the system earned them billions of dollars and increased health-care costs correspondingly. In one internal memo obtained by the FTC, a PBM executive wrote:

> We've created plan designs to aggressively steer customers to home delivery where the drug cost is ~200 [times] higher. The optics are not good. . . .

Despite this, many employers remain locked into the PBMs that their health insurance companies contract with, often because the PBMs are owned by the insurers themselves. The FTC report was preceded a few weeks earlier by an investigative report on the same topic by the *New York Times*. It documented how PBMs often push doctors and patients to use more costly drugs when perfectly equivalent products are far cheaper. Why? Because of the manufacturer-provided rebates the PBM collects on the more expensive product.

The article cited a consultant who observed that in the national conflagration of drug-cost escalation, PBMs serve the roles of both firefighter and arsonist.

The industry was not exactly thrown for a loop by the release of the FTC report: the stock price of one company drifted down very slightly, and those of two others—the two largest—actually rose the next day by over a percent each. Following the 2024 election, the activist head of the FTC was replaced by a more pro-corporation commissioner.

Ending Secrecy

Our current overly complicated system of prescription economics creates multiple confidential prices for the same brand-name drug, which are then modified in hard-to-define ways by rebates that are also hidden—ironically, all in the name of preserving the free-enterprise approach to medication purchases. The "price" of a given drug may be listed as its average wholesale price, or AWP, which many of us in the field understand isn't average, or wholesale, or really its price. (Insiders joke that AWP really stands for "ain't what's paid.") Then there's its WAC (wholesale acquisition cost), or the ASP (average sales price) used by Medicare for some of its programs, or the NADAC (National Average Drug Acquisition Cost, though it's not really an average) or U&C (the usual and customary price paid), and many more. These often-secret numbers also thwart those of us who try to study and improve the present system of what drugs really cost; interchanges like the following are common:

Our research team: This drug's price is indefensibly high.

Them (manufacturers, PBMs, sometimes state Medicaid programs, or the VA): That's not the real price. Big rebates mean that it's actually far lower.

Us: By how much?

Them: We can't tell you; it's a secret.

Would We Ever Accept a Headline Like This One?

GOVERNMENT PURCHASES NEW FIGHTER PLANES FROM DEFENSE CONTRACTOR

Neither the Pentagon nor the manufacturer will say what they cost.

Estimates for deal range into the tens of billions.

What can be done? Participation by government programs in secret pricing deals over drug prices could be made illegal. In the private sector, the labyrinth of secret rebates and the fees received by offshore group-purchasing originations could be defined as the kickbacks that they are and banned, as other kickbacks are in medicine. Other countries manage to run their health-care systems at lower cost and with better outcomes without relying on this utterly dispensable extra layer of complexity and skimming.

More Sensible Prescribing and Drug Taking: Humans Still Make the Choices

In the end, at least until the bots take over, drug-use decisions are still made by health-care professionals, and outside of institutional settings nearly all medicines are consumed voluntarily by patients. That means that the processes involved in prescribing and drug taking can lead to other ways to address our medication affordability problem; those are considered in a later chapter. Taken together, these measures could prune tens of billions of dollars off the nation's untenable drug expenditures. No matter what, stable or increased funding for the National Institutes of Health will still guarantee a steady flow of scientific advances that will inevitably be transformed into new medications: that holy process will move forward with or without the central participation of the pharmaceutical industry. Discovering things is what humans do, and we do it well.

Bloated

No discussion of medication costs would be complete without consideration of the transformative class of drugs known as GLP-1 agonists, the group that contains products like Ozempic and Wegovy and the related products that have rapidly joined them in the marketplace. As is well known to anyone who hasn't been living in a cave for the last few years, these drugs have proven remarkably effective for lowering blood sugar in patients with diabetes, as well as treating obesity. At present, after years of use in millions of people, they generally seem remarkably safe—so far. New uses include prevention of heart and kidney disease and perhaps treatment of obstructive sleep apnea and fatty liver disease. Some researchers believe that their capacity to reduce food craving—a brain effect on top of its gastrointestinal effect—might also be useful to help people who crave other things, such as alcohol or opioids or the chance to gamble; it is not yet clear where this research will lead. A long list of other conditions is also being studied.

The discoveries that would launch GLP-1-type drugs as one of the most important drug discoveries of the present century began in 1987 when researchers at the Royal Postgraduate Medical School in London first described their effects on glucose levels. In 1990, John Eng, a researcher at a VA hospital in the Bronx, built on NIH-funded studies and the work of researchers in Europe and extracted a promising GLP-type substance from the venom of the gila monster lizard, but he had trouble interesting pharmaceutical companies in its development. The VA chose not to patent the substance, since it didn't see it as relevant enough to the needs of veterans. Dr. Eng offered the product to drugmaker Eli Lilly, but the company decided not to move ahead on it. (Lilly paid $525 million a decade later for similar rights.)

In 2024, Jeffrey Flier, a researcher who would later become dean of Harvard Medical School, published two astonishing accounts of the work he and his colleagues were pursuing around 1990 on how GLP-1 compounds could be used to improve the care of patients with diabetes, long before that potential was widely understood. In those days, he was a full-time member of the Harvard faculty based at its Beth Israel Hospital, as I was; during the years he described he was head of the hospital's Diabetes Unit and then chief of its Division of Endocrinology, as well as running his own NIH-funded research lab. Nevertheless, he chose to pursue his work on the clinical potential of GLP-1 compounds by partnering with Pfizer and a small biotech company in a deal that paid him and his colleagues handsomely for ownership of their research on this approach and all rights to its commercialization. In exchange, the drugmaker acquired control of that work and its dissemination.

In those papers, Flier described his repeated trips to California and to Pfizer headquarters in Connecticut for meetings on those projects; during the same period, after a day of teaching, research, and patient care at the Beth Israel I often had a hard time making it home in time for a late dinner. He explained how he had gained key insights about the potential of the GLP-1 compounds by attending open scientific meetings at which academics and their trainees presented the findings of their work, even as his deal with Pfizer prevented him from fully reporting his own studies. Flier's 2024 accounts describe his group's groundbreaking studies from 1990, many years before the enormous clinical value of this approach was recognized:

> Remarkably, [our] team also presented data to our internal group, showing that GLP-1 slowed gastric emptying and reduced hunger. These observations were extensively discussed by our joint team, and both were indicators of the eventual efficacy of these agents against diabetes and obesity. Sadly, none of this definitive work was ever presented publicly or published, so its existence, until now, has been known only to those involved. The Pfizer approach, enshrined in the founding documents of the alliance [the contract with Flier and his colleagues], was to keep the findings confidential, and no one thought twice about this at the time. The role of publishing data was dramatically different in pharma than in the academic world in which the founders [Flier and his colleagues] had lived.

In a historic instance of mis-judgment, Pfizer then dropped its plans to develop this hugely important drug class, deciding that it had little commercial potential. But even after it aborted the program, Pfizer's contract with the academics blocked them from writing up their own findings for other scientists to see and potentially move the field forward. As Flier wrote, "None of our results were ever published, so apart from this account, they're only known to surviving participants, including me." It took about fifteen more years before this category of medicines came into clinical use; we can only wonder how much more rapidly this breakthrough field might have developed if Pfizer hadn't made the scientifically and economically disastrous decision to abort its support of this research—or if Flier and his colleagues had taken a less commercial path to further their studies, and had been free to present their important findings at open scientific meetings and in medical journals for other researchers to build on. It was poignant for me to read this late-life revelation from Flier and recall his summoning me to his office many years after these events once he had become dean, to chastise me for comments I had made about my concerns about problematic industry-academic ties (described more fully in chapter 17).

Two weeks after ex-Dean Flier published his 2024 accounts on his early insights about the potential of the GLP-1 drugs, the prestigious Lasker Awards for clinical research were announced; the timing was probably not a coincidence. Viewed as second only to the Nobel Prize as the highest accolade in medicine, the honor went to a trio of scientists whose work led to the introduction of these medications into clinical practice to treat diabetes, obesity, and a host of other additional conditions currently being studied. Two of the researchers were from the Massachusetts General Hospital and the Rockefeller University, and one was from the Danish drugmaker Novo Nordisk, for her pivotal work on modifying the compounds to make them clinically practical. All three had built on the published work of other scientists, and each had reported their findings in the open medical literature. The Lasker announcement also credited over a dozen other researchers who had made important contributions to the development of this world-changing medical breakthrough. Dr. Flier's name was not among them.

Based on this work, Novo developed its blockbuster products Ozempic and Wegovy, making it suddenly one of the largest companies in Europe. In an economic model quite different from that of other large drugmakers, the company is controlled by the Novo Nordisk Foundation, a charitable entity that the enormous sales of these drugs has transformed into the largest philanthropy in the world, worth more than $100 billion. The foundation awards over a billion dollars a year in grants "for research, innovation, treatment, education, humanitarian and social purposes"—quite different from the allocation of profits from U.S. drug companies such as Eli Lilly, the other dominant manufacturer of GLP-1 drugs. Decades after it abandoned development of this approach and despite its early opportunity to get there first, Pfizer is still working to establish a viable presence in this most profitable pharmaceutical sector of the century.

Additional Manufacturers Are Racing to Get into This Lucrative Market

We're considering the GLP drugs at this point for a simple reason. Their effectiveness in treating diabetes and obesity is both clear and impressive—no bogus surrogate end points or poorly controlled trials here. And despite extremely widespread use, there is not as yet much compelling evidence of widespread safety problems, though that could change with more pharmacoepidemiological observation. Absent those concerns, one of the most intriguing aspects of this drug class becomes its cost. In round numbers, the list price of most of the GLP drugs hovers around $1,000 per month, though rebates can bring that number down considerably. (Researchers at Yale have calculated that it costs only about $5 to make a month's supply of an Ozempic-type drug.) But even with a reduction of 50 percent from the list price, the sudden advent of a new and expensive drug class to treat conditions as common as diabetes and obesity and who knows what else is having a profound impact on health-care expenditures.

Senator Sanders, as chair of the Senate committee that oversees health matters, has become particularly upset about the economics here. In July 2024 he teamed up with President Biden to write an angry op-ed in *USA Today* asserting, "If Novo Nordisk and other pharmaceutical companies refuse to substantially lower prescription drug prices in our country and end their greed, we will do everything within our power to end it for them." The concern is understandable: if just half of the obese patients enrolled in Medicare or Medicaid took a drug like Wegovy, the two programs would have to come up with about $166 billion more per year—about the amount they spent on all retail prescription drugs in 2022.

The problem is of our own making, as we've seen above. Because we've allowed the drug industry to write the rules for drug expenditures, the price Americans pay for these medications is up to six times the amounts paid for the same drugs by people in Canada, Germany, or Novo's home country of Denmark. As a result, many state Medicaid programs have begun to refuse to cover these drugs for weight loss, paying for them only to treat diabetes. Some commercial health insurers have done the same or have saddled patients with onerous co-payments to discourage their use.

But even if we limited the use of these drugs to just diabetes and a few other clear-cut indications and avoid their use for weight loss—a policy that might be enforceable outside Beverly Hills or Manhattan's Upper East Side—the pricing structure we've let develop over decades would still require an outlay of billions of additional dollars. Will the risk of GLP drugs bankrupting Medicare and Medicaid and making private health insurance unaffordable be enough to motivate a rethinking of our "It costs whatever I want it to cost" drug pricing policy?

The nation dodged a bullet on this question with the Covid vaccine, showering manufacturers like Moderna and Pfizer with cash to make sure they'd be willing to make the shots available to every American who wanted them. But we can't keep doing that. As a thought experiment, what would happen if a drug company invented a vaccine that could safely and effectively prevent Alzheimer's disease? No such product exists, and none is close to being available. But if it were, and a manufacturer wanted a million dollars a dose, would our current industry-written payment rules mean that we'd just have to pay that amount or deny people such protection? Again, it would be like having to negotiate prices with the fire department while your house is burning down.

Trump's statement of his goals for the future of the massive Department of Health and Human Services in his second term reflected an odd scattershot vision for public health, saying that his administration would "ensure that everybody will be protected from harmful chemicals, pollutants, pesticides, pharmaceutical products, and food additives that have contributed to the overwhelming Health Crisis in this Country." Leaving aside how the drug industry may have felt about having its medications lumped in with pesticides and pollutants as a risk to the public, one can only wonder how this bizarre rethinking of the role of medications will impact the role the federal government will take in negotiating drug prices.

The U.S. was once capable of clearer thinking. After Pearl Harbor, when FDR needed to mount a vigorous military response, he didn't leave it up to the defense industry to name any price it wanted to manufacture battleships and planes and bullets. That would have been seen as un-American. We were all in the battle together, and some things were not considered suitable for profiteering. If only we could recapture a shred of that attitude now and rethink our no-limits approach to determining drug charges.

– PART FOUR –

Spreading the Word

CHAPTER 16

A Failure to Communicate

Pulling the Trigger

Once a drug has been shown to work and to be safe enough, and its price has been set for better or worse, the vital next step in its journey from lab to patient is for someone to decide whether to prescribe it. With thousands of drugs on the market, how do we doctors make that choice? At a deeper level, where does our knowledge come from, and how do we know what we know?

No prescription makes its way into any patient except through the hand or keyboard of a physician or another health-care professional. Artificial intelligence and the bots are waiting eagerly in the wings, but for now it's still mostly people who make the choices. With our armamentarium of treatment now so potent, many lives depend on getting those choices right. And since prescription drugs account for about half a trillion dollars a year in the U.S. and another trillion in the rest of the world, that makes those decisions economically potent as well. To shape those choices, the drug industry spends over $35 billion a year on promotion of various kinds. As a result, much of what many clinicians know about the medications we use comes from those sources. How accurate are they?

It shouldn't be surprising that if a drug company spends hundreds of millions of dollars to develop or buy the rights to a new drug, it will want to promote it in the most favorable light. The year after my poorly titled pharmacoepistemology lecture to the medical students I renamed the talk "The Social Construction of Medical Knowledge"; more students showed up. The next year I just described the topic as "What You Need to Know to Be a Better Prescriber When You Get to Take Care of Patients," and that was the most appealing title of all. But each description was about the same theme: understanding where knowledge about prescription drugs comes from, what gets studied and what doesn't, what is communicated and what isn't. Most medical students, doctors, patients, and policymakers seem to assume that there is a core body of information about effectiveness and risks that's just out there, that this knowledge gets extended by researchers in exactly the directions needed, and that the growing body of data thus accumulated is then transmitted to the world as is, without much filtering.

None of that is true.

Leaving aside the vital issue of what gets studied and what gets ignored about benefits, risks, and cost-effectiveness, those facts exist only as *potential information* until someone communicates them to clinicians and patients. But the law treats information about medications differently from that concerning most other goods, bringing together a heady mix of science, policy, corporate regulation, freedom of speech, and differing ideas about what constitutes the public good.

How We Know What We Know

Consider this list of some of the drugs approved by the FDA in one recent year. Read them aloud, from left to right:

Jaypirca	pirtobrutinib
Skyclarys	omaveloxolone
Zynyz	retifanlimab-dlwr
Elfabrio	pegunigalsidase alfa-iwxj
Inpefa	sotagliflozin
Izervay	avacincaptad pegol
Omvoh	mirikizumab-mrkz

The names on the left are the brand names concocted by a drug's manufacturer, usually after hiring a branding company that may charge hundreds of thousands of dollars for that service. The names in the right-hand column are the far-less-pronounceable generic names of the same drugs.

This list represents less than a seventh of the new drugs the FDA approved in just that year: a doctor's task of trying to keep straight the thousands of available choices keeps getting harder annually. Given how difficult the job is, and how lives depend on our getting this right, you might expect that there would be some kind of periodic requirement that prescribers keep current on the medications we use. Nope. To renew my medical license, I just have to self-attest that I spend fifty hours a year in some kind of educational activity, often "self-directed." The definition of that is very loose, and just showing up to doze or eat a donut in a darkened amphitheater during weekly grand rounds lectures will do the trick. Some professional societies, such as the American Board of Internal Medicine, do require passing a test of competency every few years to maintain certification, but that isn't true for all fields, and not all hospitals or health systems require such recertification. My own health-care system does make me prove annually that I know which fire extinguisher to use on different kinds of fires (I get that wrong every year), and how to deal with potentially violent patients or visitors (try not to let them get between you and the door), but not that I know how to prescribe medications properly.

Of course, patients have a compelling need for doctors to know about medications, but the nation isn't too effective at using our common resources to meet that public need. So in the bizarre commercial bazaar that American medicine has become, we just leave it to the marketplace to figure out what information gets disseminated and what doesn't. Clearly the drug industry has the most to gain from influencing prescribing, and it does so very effectively.

Most of the industry's eye-watering annual promotion budget is directed at us doctors, through ads in medical journals or on their sites when we go to read scientific papers, as well as sponsorship of courses and conferences. As a result, the drug industry is the most prominent funder of the continuing medical education that generates the credits we are all expected to accumulate to renew our licenses. Perhaps most effectively, manufacturers send sales reps directly into our offices to chat with us interactively about what we prescribe for specific conditions, in order to change our behavior to favor their companies' products.

All that promotion is really paid for by the public, since those expenditures are just added to the medicines' prices that we all pay one way or another. They are also deductible business expenses, reducing the companies' already-low tax burdens, so we get to bear their cost that way as well. Thus, it's not a stretch to say that the American people spend tens of billions of dollars a year to disseminate the companies' views about their products. Because we let it filter through the manufacturers first, we shouldn't be surprised at its content. But since it's basically our money, is this really the best way we can think of spending all those billions of dollars on communication about medications, or about health in general?

Freedom of Speech Isn't the Same for Everybody

The First Amendment guarantees that a government cannot limit statements made by individuals (and more recently, by companies), but this doesn't apply to the makers of prescription drugs. The law treats statements made by pharmaceutical companies much more stringently, requiring that everything a drug company says about the benefits and risks of its products has to conform to the FDA's views of their approved uses and harms. This is a higher standard than merely having to stick to the data. First is the obvious fact that a company can't promote a product that hasn't been approved for sale by the FDA. At one professional society meeting I attended, a company set up an enormous special exhibit booth to mark the launch of a new product it was about to bring to market. It would announce to the world the drug's catchy new brand name, its unpronounceable and easily forgotten generic name, and the uses that the FDA was expected to approve just before the meeting. But a last-minute glitch intervened and the approval date was delayed. All that the manufacturer was permitted to have in its huge dedicated display area was its corporate logo and some flowers. Lots and lots of flowers.

Once a drug is approved by the FDA for a particular use, only that use can be promoted to prescribers by the company. The manufacturer may believe that its product is helpful for other conditions as well: that a particular breast cancer drug may be good for other kinds of tumors, or that a medication for Crohn's disease will also work in ulcerative colitis, or that a treatment for chronic obstructive pulmonary disease could also help patients with asthma. There may even be large, well-conducted, randomized controlled trials demonstrating these beneficial effects are real. But if the FDA has not made its own determination of whether the drug works for those conditions, the company cannot promote it for those uses. In other sectors, the First Amendment protects all kinds of evidence-free speech by Americans who make demonstrably false statements, such as the idea that Barack Obama was born in Africa, or that Joe Biden lost the 2020 election. After all, the founders based the Bill of Rights on the idea that in a free society, people ought to be able to say or write anything they damn please. Their expectation was that an enlightened public would be best served by having all ideas available for its scrutiny, and that the people would eventually be able to choose the best ideas over less good ones.

But since the 1960s, that hasn't applied to manufacturers' statements about prescription drugs. We doctors are permitted to prescribe any approved drug for any purpose we want (including so-called off-label use), but drugmakers must limit their promotion only to conditions that the FDA has approved. The remarkable proliferation of drugs over the last sixty years perhaps justifies the instinct of those 1960s legislators that decisions about medications were so difficult and complicated that they should be protected from unrestrained free-speech marketeering. That is how the drug industry became one of the few groups in the country to which the freedom of speech protections of the First Amendment don't apply. That prohibition also extended almost until the end of the century to ban any promotional communication at all about drugs to patients, even for approved uses.

Pharmaceutical Exceptionalism

As we've seen, in evaluating a medication the FDA deploys multidisciplinary teams of physicians, pharmacists, pharmacologists, and statisticians who take months to carefully review terabytes of drug information, much of it arcane and some of it secret. And they usually but not always get it right. Given that, is it reasonable to ask frontline clinicians, no less patients, to "do their own research" and make their own efficacy-risk determinations about particular products? On the other hand, I can relate a bit to the skepticism of critics who despise this veneration of government expertise. It reminds me of the arguments made in the 1960s by defenders of the Vietnam War who took a stance uncomfortably similar to my current position about the FDA: The government, they'd argue, has access to all kinds of experts and nonpublic knowledge about the situation in Southeast Asia and what we need to do there. Do you really think you understand more than they do about whether we should continue or end the war? They must know what's best. Who do you think you are?

Regarding the Vietnam War, that argument turned out to be tragically wrong. But with medications, it's different. I've become a defender of the view that we should "Listen to the federal government. They sometimes know things you don't know," even though it makes me feel creepy sometimes.

A major expansion of drug communications began in 1997 when the government began to allow prescription drug manufacturers to advertise their products directly to consumers. The companies themselves had previously been willing to live with a ban, since they knew that doctors were the ones making the main choices among products, and entering the very expensive world of consumer advertising would pit them against the makers of cars, shampoo, and breakfast cereals, at enormous cost. But by the mid-1990s, cost-containing health maintenance organizations had started to limit doctors' prescribing options, so drugmakers realized it would help to enlist patients on their side to promote use of their costliest products. The official argument was that people had the right to participate in decisions about their medications, with the ubiquitous catchphrase "Ask your doctor if X is right for you." Every sick person could potentially become a drug sales rep. As a result, we now have $8 billion worth of commercials on television and in print media asking patients to weigh in on the right oncology drug for estrogen receptor-negative metastatic breast cancer, or hypertrophic amyloid cardiomyopathy. (Such drug commercials remain generally forbidden in every other advanced country except New Zealand.) Or consider this ad *for consumers* from Bristol Myers Squibb to promote a treatment for cancer:

> Opdivo (nivolumab) is a prescription medicine used in combination with Yervoy (ipilimumab) and 2 cycles of chemotherapy that includes platinum and another chemotherapy medicine, as a first treatment for adults with a type of advanced stage lung cancer (called non-small cell lung cancer) when your lung cancer has spread or grown, or comes back, and your tumor does not have an abnormal EGFR or ALK gene.

In short, everything a typical patient needs to make the best decision.

But why limit company statements to patients and doctors to just those that the FDA has certified as accurate? Libertarians and drown-government-in-the-bathtub activists have found common cause with the pharmaceutical industry in asking why drug companies shouldn't enjoy all the same free-speech rights as other American citizens and corporations. The idea began as a fringe concept, but has gathered steam under both Republican and Democratic administrations. In moving their agenda forward, conservative legal activists and drugmakers found a promising test case in the form of a small-time pharmaceutical sales rep at a little-known drug company promoting a minor medication. The drug was short on therapeutic importance but would become central as a free-speech precedent.

A Pivotal Case

Alfred Caronia was a frontline sales rep for a tiny drug company called Orphan Medical, Inc., incorporated in tax-friendly Ireland. Its winsome name came from the fact that its business model focused on marketing so-called orphan drugs—defined as those needed by fewer than two hundred thousand Americans. Caronia's job was to visit physicians and get them to use Xyrem, a product approved for use in patients with narcolepsy, an uncommon condition that causes sufferers to fall asleep suddenly and unpredictably. It is very rare, though it sometimes reached epidemic proportions among my classmates in medical school. Caronia did his job a bit too enthusiastically, telling the doctors he visited on sales calls that Xyrem was also useful for fibromyalgia, insomnia, and in children and the elderly. The first three uses were not FDA-approved, and the last was explicitly warned against in the drug's official labeling. This was not overhyping of just any medication: Xyrem had been a controlled substance and was notorious for its use as a date-rape drug. That raised the level of concern about its overuse and its potential criminality. Unfortunately for Mr. Caronia, one of his wide-ranging presentations was recorded as part of a federal sting operation; the unlucky sales rep was convicted of illegal promotion of a prescription drug.

He appealed the decision and it looked as if the appellate court would routinely side with the lower court on his conviction. But then the conservative Washington Legal Foundation joined in to help with Caronia's case, arguing that his First Amendment rights were being violated. In a surprise decision that threatened to upend the FDA's historic ability to regulate drugmakers' promotional claims, the Second Circuit Court of Appeals overturned his conviction on the grounds that it violated Mr. Caronia's freedom of speech. Kesselheim and I had worried about this possibility in a *New England Journal of Medicine* article in 2008; after the Caronia decision, we joined Michelle Mello, a professor of law at Stanford, in an essay in *JAMA* speculating that this could be the beginning of the end for the FDA's authority to limit the unfounded promotion of prescription drugs.

A longer article from our team appeared in *NEJM*; its title summed up the situation neatly: "Forbidden and Permitted Statements about Medications—Loosening the Rules."

Before his legal troubles, Caronia had recruited a psychiatrist, Dr. Peter Gleason, to give talks on Xyrem, a task for which Gleason was getting more than $100,000 a year. He advocated its use for chronic pain and bipolar disorder, among other uses that had not passed the FDA's evidentiary scrutiny (or anyone else's, for that matter). He argued that he was just a physician sharing his clinical experiences with his colleagues, as we doctors often do. Prosecutors saw it differently, arguing that his paid relationship with the drugmaker meant that he was acting as their sales agent, rendering his statements subject to FDA regulation. After one such talk in 2006, while waiting for a train, he was surrounded by federal agents and handcuffed.

"This is a gag, right?" he asked.

"No, it's not a gag," came the answer. He was hustled into a waiting car, taken to a nearby police station, and arrested.

Gleason faced loss of his license, prison time, and enormous fines. The drugmaker decided to cooperate with the authorities and would not help him. After years of legal wrangling, he pleaded guilty to a misdemeanor offense and his penalties were reduced to a $25 fine and probation. At the end of that period, impoverished by his legal battles and depressed, Gleason took his life in 2011, just over a year before the Second Circuit would vacate the conviction of his handler Caronia, and change everything.

Just Leave It at That?

These developments brought to mind the work of Thomas Hobbes, the seventeenth-century English political philosopher. In his book *Leviathan*, he argued that civilization requires citizens to willingly transfer some of their freedom to a sovereign who could use that power to organize society through the consent of the governed. Without such a social contract, Hobbes famously argued, we would all face lives that would be "solitary, poor, nasty, brutish, and short."

His vision of the Leviathan was not the sea dragon conjured in the Bible. Rather, it was a supreme ruler who would serve the people and overcome the anarchy of ungoverned society. The frontispiece of the 1651 edition of his book depicted the Leviathan as a hunky guy whose torso and arms are made up of over three hundred figures, representing the people who comprise his power, and for whose good he wields it. Hobbes's work has been seen as potentially justifying the rule of tyrants, but in a narrower sense his idea of trading off some liberty to live in a civilized society is relevant here.

Around the time of the Caronia controversy, I tried to relate all this to medication policy in an article in the *Annals of Internal Medicine* titled "In Opposition to Liberty: We Need a 'Sovereign' to Govern Drug Claims":

> As a prescriber, I have been willing to give up my freedom to prescribe any chemical I choose, and I am willing to have drug manufacturers give up some of their right to tell me whatever they may want me to hear. For all of us, including patients, to hand over some liberties to a Hobbesian sovereign such as the FDA offers a different kind of freedom—knowing that the medications we use are probably, at least as a first approximation, reasonably safe and have some evidence that they work. Rather than representing an infringement of companies' inherent rights as "citizens," maintaining our current standards for promotional statements can keep us from sinking back into an "all against all" state of poorly founded drug claims and understated risks.

Hobbes's vision of a government empowered by the governed helped inspire our Declaration of Independence and Constitution. But now, almost 365 years later, the latter document was being used to undermine a central aspect of medicine rooted in this "consent of the governed" idea: that people would agree to forego the right to ingest any chemical they want, and would willingly put the power to decide what works and what doesn't in the hands of a collectively chosen expert authority. That body would make those choices on behalf of all of us, and we would abide by its decisions.

Fear of Fighting

Why didn't the FDA move to contest the Caronia decision, which threatened its right to govern promotional drug claims? Apparently it feared it would lose the battle in the Supreme Court.

Hobbes made his case by referring to an unappealing "state of nature" that existed before consent-of-the-governed societies came together. Today, we have not one but two prescription drug "states of nature" to which we can compare our current situation. The first was prior to the early 1960s, before the FDA was given the authority to demand evidence that a product works in order for it to be sold. If the FDA were to lose its power to regulate the claims of drugmakers, we'd be back to those pre-1962 free-for-all days, with ineffective and dangerous products cluttering drugstore shelves and home medicine cabinets. Equally bad, there is also a different present-day pharmaceutical "state of nature" to see what a regulation-free pharmaceutical world would look like. It even comes with a built-in pun: the world of "natural" medicines or supplements, described earlier. We've seen how a company can depict its product as a dietary supplement and then promote it for everything from memory loss to arthritis with essentially no evidence, as long as it includes a tiny disclaimer that it isn't intended to treat anything, and that the FDA has not reviewed its claims.

If freed from the requirement that the FDA approve their promotional statements, prescription drugmakers could short-circuit the FDA's review of the totality of available data (including those secret proprietary files), and could present clinicians with cherry-picked studies that could make their product look good even if those studies were methodologically poor or didn't present a balanced picture of all the findings. I thought we had learned our lessons from the suppressed clinical trials that created such a scandal in the early 2000s. The travesty of a company ignoring the results of studies it didn't like had led to the reforms of the FDA Amendments Act of 2007 (see chapter 9), but memories in Washington are short.

A particular worry I developed in decades of closely reviewing medication evidence is the problem of "truthiness." That's the clever term coined by comedian Stephen Colbert to describe a statement that sort of sounds true but actually isn't. A poorly done clinical trial may pick an inappropriate comparison group or none at all, allowing sponsors to tout the "improvements" seen in patients given a new drug. Or an observational study using "real-world evidence" may fail to control for important confounders and yield an encouraging-sounding finding that's just wrong. Or a trial of a new cancer drug may feature its ability to prolong "progression-free survival" but not reveal that patients didn't actually live any longer. It takes an experienced analyst of medical data or a team of alert FDA scientists to pore over the details of the evidence to get this right. Remove those filters and the "truthiness" of some misleading drug claims could readily prevail.

The Caronia case left in limbo the crucial question of the FDA's authority over promotion. But a subsequent federal court decision upped the ante even further. Amarin Pharma, another aggressive little American start-up incorporated in tax-friendly Ireland, announced that it planned to promote a fish oil capsule (its only product) to prevent cardiovascular disease, based on controversial data. The available evidence suggested that its fish oil may or may not have been a little bit better than snake oil, but not by much. Amarin proactively sought an injunction that would block any future FDA attempt to stop them from making their planned claim. The court granted the injunction and the FDA meekly agreed to it in 2016.

In the years since, the FDA has not appealed the Caronia case to the U.S. Supreme Court and the deadline for doing so has passed, leaving the decision in force in some federal jurisdictions but not others. Of course, the court has become much more conservative since the Caronia decision; most observers agree that in the current anti-regulatory climate, an FDA appeal would likely lead to a high court decision that could strip the agency of much of its authority over claims made by drug companies and their agents. A PORTAL study found that in the years since Caronia, FDA actions against drugmakers over improper promotion have fallen considerably.

Xyrem is still not recommended for chronic pain, insomnia, Parkinson's disease, fibromyalgia, or other uses promoted by Al Caronia and the late Dr. Gleason. And the effectiveness of Amarin's fish oil capsule in preventing heart disease has met with even more skepticism; a 2022 analysis by Brigham cardiologists suggested that its apparent superiority over placebo in its single randomized trial may have been caused largely by the fact that the placebo chosen (against the advice of several experts) was capsules of mineral oil, which probably *increased* the risk of cardiac events in patients who took it, rather than a protective effect of the fish oil—sort of a Vioxx vs. naproxen issue, in reverse.

Freedom of Nonspeech

A different aspect of free-speech protections could soon emerge in relation to pharmaceuticals, this one a mirror image of the others. Just as the First Amendment forbids the government from preventing people from *making* statements, it also forbids "compelled speech" in which the government *requires* a person to state something. (And thanks to another Supreme Court decision, the rights of persons are now extended to corporations as well.) Like other drug manufacturers, Merck objected to the prospect that the Inflation Reduction Act would require it to agree to government-negotiated prices in Medicare. The company argued that making it sign such contracts would be a form of "compelled speech" prohibited by the First Amendment.

That argument is likely to fail in the courts, but another form of drug company "compelled speech" could have more widespread and strange implications. In a landmark 2023 decision (*303 Creative LLC v. Elenis*), the high court ruled that the government could not compel a company offering wedding websites to design one for a same-sex couple if it didn't want to, as that would represent compelled speech. What could that possibly have to do with communication about medications? In an article in the *New England Journal of Medicine*, I argued that a conservative court could also apply this logic to the FDA's requiring a company to make certain statements about the effects of its drugs. In the Vioxx case, what if Merck had said that the FDA's demand that it be more forthcoming about the drug's cardiac risks would represent "compelled speech"? After the wedding website decision, that seems less unthinkable.

A long shot? Maybe, but the court that dismantled voting rights and abortion rights, and to which the FDA still fears bringing a case about its regulatory authority, could do almost anything. It wouldn't be the first time that companies used the constitutional prohibition against compelled speech to block medically relevant statements. In one prior case, the FDA sought to have a cigarette manufacturer include graphic warnings on its packages depicting the diseases smoking can cause. No, you can't, said the D.C. District Court; that would be the government compelling speech by a company. In another case, San Francisco wanted to require that the makers of sugary soft drinks warn on their labels that excessive use could contribute to obesity, diabetes, and tooth decay. No, you can't, ruled the Ninth Circuit Court of Appeals. That could "chill protected commercial speech."

We will learn in the coming years whether an emboldened pharmaceutical industry can persuade an increasingly conservative Supreme Court that when the FDA requires them to list specific adverse events in a certain way, or constrains some descriptions of their products' benefits, that, too, represents government-compelled speech, violating a company's First Amendment rights. The ability of prescribers and patients to rely on the unbiased accuracy of those statements seems to rest on thinning ice.

Heading Backward

The Vioxx crisis of 2004 had led to important reforms in how we study adverse drug effects, and strengthened the FDA's authority to require their disclosure to the public. The Medicare drug pricing reforms of 2022 gave the federal government new powers to push back on high medication prices and negotiate with drugmakers on the cost of their products. But the legal developments of 2024—including the herring fishermen case that undercut the authority of federal agencies—will likely signal a shift in that momentum, weakening the influence of the federal government on several medication-related fronts; a further rightward drift in the other branches of government could accelerate that trend. These anti-regulatory impulses are now codified at the highest levels of government; and as any herring-man can tell you, a fish rots from the head down.

CHAPTER 17

Shaping the Prescribers of Tomorrow

Because nearly every prescription is the result of a clinical decision made by a physician or other health-care professional, medication use utterly depends on what we clinicians know, what we believe, and how we approach a given medical problem. All those choices are shaped by the years we spend in training: that molding is as vital as the papers we read later in our careers and the marketing to which we're exposed. That is why any consideration of medications would be incomplete without exploring how medical education determines what we doctors know and how we think.

For decades, there has been a quiet struggle over how we teach and socialize the prescribers of tomorrow—what they learn or don't learn, what's emphasized or isn't, how they understand pharmaceuticals, and all the other attitudes we as faculty inculcate. When do we turn to a drug, and when are other interventions more useful? *Which* drug? How do we balance conflicting evidence about medications? Which pharmaceutical policies will we favor, and which will we oppose? At elite schools, those effects extend far in space and time, since so many of our graduates go on to leadership positions in American medicine. That in turn influences how medication use and policy are taught elsewhere and how the next generations of leaders will think about these issues.

Acculturation and socialization are central to every educational setting, but particularly so in medicine. In my own student days, I recall being shown the same slide in at least three or four different courses. It was a black-and-white photograph of an enormous open ward of children inside iron lungs, the large cylindrical metal contraptions that kids with polio required to help them breathe. Only their little heads stuck out; alternating negative- and positive-pressure air was pumped into the clunky devices to simulate the effect of their own damaged breathing muscles. The invention kept thousands of children alive for the weeks or more it took for their own respiratory function to recover. I recall how the shiny metal of the machines in the picture contrasted with the starched white fabric of the nurses' uniforms and caps as they tended to the paralyzed kids in each apparatus. The first time I saw that photo I was struck by the ingeniousness of the invention, the compassion of the nurses who cared for the children, and the bravery of the youngsters encased in these confining lifesaving contraptions.

But that wasn't the reason we were shown that photo so many times. The iron lung, we were told, was a classic example of an "intermediate technology"—a not-very-satisfactory way to deal with a medical problem if you didn't have a good scientific solution—just a clinical finger stuck into a leaking biological dike. The actual moral of the story was that it wasn't until the development of the first polio vaccine that we could *really* deal with the condition adequately. Basic science and clinical research were needed to eradicate the disease altogether, a much more satisfactory solution than putting kids in metal cylinders to breathe for them.

A second slide I remember seeing in more than one lecture was of a famous 1891 painting, *The Doctor* by Sir Luke Fildes. It depicted a concerned physician sitting at the home bedside of a gravely sick boy, his anguished parents standing nearby. The doctor seemed to be staying with the patient to offer comfort in the face of a life-threatening illness for which no effective treatment was available. I was struck by his compassion and dedication, and assumed the painting was being presented to us as an example of the caring physician, the epitome of a committed doctor-patient relationship. Wrong again, Avorn. The description I recall hearing each time that slide was shown was how pathetic physicians were in those days before we had effective treatments like antibiotics. All that a doctor could do then was just sit at the bedside and hold the patient's hand, I remember being told. Now, with the advent of effective medications, that child could probably be cured quickly and up and around in no time. (The picture was put to a different use in another context; it was co-opted by the American Medical Association in 1949 in its campaign to block President Truman's plan for national health insurance. The doctors' organization circulated it widely, emblazoned with the text "KEEP POLITICS OUT OF THIS PICTURE." Truman's plan was defeated; near-universal coverage would have to wait about sixty more years for the arrival of Obamacare.)

Of course, both kinds of interpretation of the iron lung and sick child pictures are plausible—compassionate care, the need for more science. But why not both? Yet the science-focused one represented an orientation common at many medical schools throughout the country, especially during the era in which I trained. Sure, compassion is worthy, being there for the patient is commendable, but neither is as important as the science that can produce drugs or vaccines that can eliminate a disease altogether. That helps explain why my medical curriculum contained so much about molecular biology, genetics, and cellular infrastructure, and so little (actually, almost nothing in those days) about the doctor-patient relationship, epidemiology, preventive medicine, or health-care delivery. To hammer the issue home, we had several case-study teaching exercises that described complicated patients in whom the primary care physician (often described a bit contemptuously as the LMD, for "local medical doctor") had misunderstood what was going on and nearly killed the patient; the correct diagnosis and treatment were put in place only after referral to the academic medical center, where specialists saved the day.

To rethink those gaps, starting in 1969 in my first year of medical school, some classmates and I created a student-initiated course on all the topics we had expected to learn about as we became doctors but that weren't then in the standard Harvard Medical School curriculum: nutrition, alcoholism, human sexuality, the doctor-patient relationship, medical ethics, health economics, and many more. We brought in experts to lecture us about those overlooked subjects, and taught each other.

Early in those student years, I sought career advice from the HMS dean of students on how to pursue my interests, which already seemed at variance with the culture of the place. I explained that I wanted to study how doctors made clinical choices among interventions like prescriptions, what influenced that, and what could be done to make those decisions better. "Jerry, you're a smart fellow," the dean began, smiling. "You could be anything you want in medicine—an endocrinologist, even a cardiologist. Why would you want to spend your time on that Mickey Mouse soft-science bullshit crap?" Six decades later, I remember those last six words as vividly as if I heard them yesterday. Still trying to take that in, I asked if he thought I should spend an extra year to get a master's of public health degree at the Harvard School of Public Health next door, as some of my classmates were thinking of doing. "Don't bother," he replied quickly. "You'll learn all you need to know here. Once you have an MD from the Harvard Medical School, you won't need any other degrees." That provided a valuable lesson: that advice from anyone who refers to the place as *the* Harvard Medical School should be taken with several grains of salt. I've regretted the decision not to get an MPH ever since, and now encourage medical trainees to do so whenever they can. In fact, I think *all* medical students should learn the epidemiology, statistics, policy, and global health insights that are provided by MPH programs, whatever their career plans. Many years later, a special MPH track was created at Harvard to facilitate such exposure.

Sure, all of us would prefer a polio vaccine over an iron lung, or a healthy dose of antibiotic over an incurable infection; that goes without saying. But we don't have vaccines to ward off every illness, or magic bullets to cure every malady, and we never will. In the years since, I've often thought about the balance between those complementary aspects of medicine—not just in the education we offer, but also in how we deliver health care to people. That's what drew me, despite the dean's advice, to study how we deploy the discoveries we've made: turning pure science into treatments, the spirit of discovery made tangible in the form of new drugs. Those acculturation experiences built on one another, even though I was taught that *doing* basic science was one of the noblest (and Nobel-est) activities a medical trainee at Harvard could pursue; *studying* that process or *using* the resulting treatments, less so.

The same distinction came up again years later with the rise and fall of programs in geriatrics at Harvard, and it changed the course of my career. The 1980s saw the growth of a national movement to teach doctors how to care for older patients, with the hope that such training could one day have the same stature as programs in pediatrics. After all, the elderly were the fastest-growing demographic, with enormous and increasing medical needs; it was clear that the predictable and unprecedented aging of my own huge cohort of baby boomers would impact health care profoundly in the century to come. Particularly when it came to prescriptions, older patients weren't simply wrinkled middle-aged people, just as children were not just miniature adults, as our colleagues in pediatrics had taught us decades earlier. Older patients needed more prescription drugs, but aging often reduced the body's capacity to handle those drugs, and the multiplicity of medications compounded the risk of interactions and side effects. Worse, drug-induced symptoms like confusion, fatigue, or dizziness were often misinterpreted as signs of aging, and as a result not evaluated or managed correctly. Prescribing for this age group offered the opportunity to do a great deal of good, but also raised the risk of causing considerable harm.

Academic hospitals around the country began to set up clinical-training programs in the new specialty of geriatric medicine. In the early 1980s, Harvard established a Division on Aging to foster collaborations across its teaching hospitals, and I was one of its first members, focusing on the study of optimal medication use in the elderly. At one of our early meetings I proposed that the new program could also work with faculty and trainees from the sociology department on what it meant to live in an aging society, economists to discuss the major shifts in wealth, financial dependence, and medical care expenses that were occurring, anthropologists to study changes in families that would impact care. No, came the response. Let's stick to medicine for now. Maybe later. The sculpting process, for ideas and for people, was intense and unrelenting.

Dr. Eugene Braunwald, one of the most respected figures in American medicine, recruited me in 1992 to leave Harvard's Beth Israel Hospital in order to expand the growing geriatrics program at one of the medical school's other main teaching institutions, the Brigham and Women's Hospital, where he chaired its Department of Medicine. I brought several of my most talented colleagues with me. Under the leadership of Neil Resnick, our faculty in the Brigham's growing Gerontology Division worked on a variety of NIH research grants dealing with the care of elderly patients; we also trained fellows in Harvard's growing geriatrics fellowship program and provided clinical consultations for older patients within and outside the hospital. As with my previous training in the "newly invented" primary care internal medicine residency track, we seemed to be at the start of a welcome new era in medical education: the long-awaited rise of generalists caring for the whole patient rather than specific organ systems, in a world dominated by specialists.

As with primary care, things didn't go as expected.

The Brigham decided to end its geriatrics program in 1997; no clear reason was given. Some said the hospital didn't want to attract too many old people because they stayed longer as inpatients, and the reimbursement for their outpatient care was inadequate given how long those visits took. The same year, Harvard Medical School terminated its school-wide Division on Aging. Astonished colleagues quipped that the leaders of both institutions must have figured out that the population was getting younger, not older.

Faced with the dissolution of the programs that formed such an important part of my research on medication use in older patients, I set up an exit interview with Dr. Victor Dzau, who had succeeded Dr. Braunwald as chair of Harvard's Department of Medicine at the Brigham. To my surprise, he told me he wanted me to stay. A canny colleague said I should offer to remain only if I was given my own division to run. I asked for that, and he agreed. This was the birth of the Division of Pharmacoepidemiology and Pharmacoeconomics. We would examine how medications make it into the health-care system: how doctors and patients use them, what their "real-world" benefits and side effects are when studied in large populations, and their economic impact. "Most academic departments of medicine don't have a clinical division like this," Dr. Dzau said, "but I like your work, so let's do it." He had a similar conversation with Dr. Paul Farmer, the legendary late global health leader. The same year, he authorized Paul to create a new Division of Global Health, also in Harvard's Department of Medicine at the Brigham. I was honored to be in the same maverick category as Paul, whose work has inspired so many in medicine and global health policy.

Not long afterward, the Department of Medicine held a retreat for all the division chiefs to discuss our training programs. Farmer was overseas, as his work often required, and his program was represented by Jim Kim, his longtime and equally remarkable collaborator, who was less well known by the other chiefs. It was there that the quiet part was said out loud. A senior member of the department explained that the highest goal of the department's training programs should be to get people to go into laboratory research, drug development, or one of the clinical sub-specialties. "The problem we're having is that all these trainees want to grow up to be Paul Farmer," the senior professor explained to the group, probably failing to recognize Jim as co-chief of Paul's division. At the coffee break, Jim came up to me and whispered conspiratorially, "*I didn't realize that we were the problem!*"

In the eyes of some at the medical school and its teaching hospitals, we might have been. At the start of my career, the chairman of Harvard's Department of Medicine at the Beth Israel Hospital, where I had done my residency and where I was seeing my patients, had said I didn't really belong on the faculty there since my work didn't fit the usual mold, so I was exiled to the medical school's often-neglected Department of Social Medicine. (That Medicine chair and I had had a run-in while I was still a resident; I was organizing a meeting to discuss Medicaid cutbacks and resident working hours, which then numbered one hundred hours a week. He disapproved on both counts. "Jerry, Boston is a small town, medically," he told me one evening when he was making rounds and I was on call. "This is not the kind of behavior we like to see in our trainees if you ever want to get a job here.") Several of his successors at Beth Israel told me something similar—that what I did didn't really belong in a Harvard Department of Medicine.

When years later Dr. Dzau put me up for a professorship (I would have been content to stay an associate professor for the rest of my career), the medical school ruled that what I did wasn't really important science, and turned the promotion down, an action it rarely took. The decision was reversed years later, but the message had gotten through. Armed with that experience I'd later tell the young doctors I mentored, "Your work is what defines you, not what your institution calls you." When they became frustrated at the extremely high standards and long and sometimes obscure processes they had to endure to get promoted, I suggested they just replace the word "professor" in their minds with the word "poobah." "Tell yourself, 'I feel bad that I've been stuck at the rank of assistant poobah for so long. It's time they make me an associate poobah. Maybe one day I can become a full poobah.'" Doing that helps make the arbitrariness of the titles clearer. It's the work that matters.

I have to admit that in the decades since I first heard that remark about not wanting to turn out too many Paul Farmers, I've occasionally had a chance to rethink my visceral reaction to that statement. After all, the Brigham residency in internal medicine attracts some of the very best medical school graduates in the country. On some days, I can partly understand the perspective of the senior faculty member who had made that snarky comment. Paul was as close to a saint as anyone I'll ever meet; his work and his hands-on model of service inspired thousands and helped reshape our understanding of medical care in poor countries. Often Paul and his team would hike for hours through remote areas of Haiti or Rwanda to make sure a single patient was taking their medication as directed. But as described in Tracy Kidder's impressive book *Mountains Beyond Mountains,* even his acolytes occasionally wondered about the limitations of this utterly hands-on approach; one observed, "If Paul is the model, then we're fucked."

Some days I can channel the perspective of that skeptical senior Brigham scientist: he may have wondered whether instead of trekking alone through a remote part of a developing country, one of our residents might have instead become the person to take to the lab and eventually develop a new treatment for resistant tuberculosis, or make a key discovery about the biological basis of malaria that would pave the way to prevent it. I've managed to reconcile these opposing perspectives by thinking about what Dr. Braunwald said to me during my recruitment when I asked whether there would really be a secure place for geriatrics in a department of medicine as eminent and established as the Brigham's. "Of course," he reassured me. "Internal medicine here is like the Boston Symphony Orchestra; it needs a wide variety of instruments to perform at its best." He had no way of knowing that after his retirement they would fire much of the woodwinds section.

Reading the Room

I should have known the seas would be choppy if I persisted in the kind of medication-related research that some faculty objected to or just saw as silly, and my lighthouse-keeper acumen wasn't always equal to the task. As my dragged-out promotion process was unfolding Harvard held an event to commemorate a new endowed professorship, and a colleague asked me to give a talk on the problem of conflicts of interest in medication research and teaching. The auditorium was packed; I'm not a keen observer of sartorial style in myself or others, so I didn't notice that many of the people listening to me were far better dressed and more bejeweled than typical audiences on our medical campus. My talk seemed to have been well received, but soon afterward I got an angry email from the dean at that time, Jeff Flier (see chapter 15). He castigated me for my comments, and told me I had to come in to talk to him. I apparently hadn't realized that the stylish crowd to whom I gave my talk included many of the donors who had made the endowed chair possible, and several had flown in from New York for the event. The dean was not pleased that they were exposed to a lecture about messy issues of academic–drug industry relationships.

When I showed up for my appointment, I felt like a high school kid called in to talk to the principal after using a dirty word in class. The first thing I noticed was the elegant beige linen-like wallpaper that graced the dean's office. The last time I had been in that room was nearly thirty-five years earlier around 1970, when I was first impressed by the classiness of the same style of wallpaper. Back then, several of us medical students had held a sit-in in an earlier dean's office to protest his decision to join the board of directors of the pharmaceutical company Bristol Myers Squibb: it seemed incongruous to us for a medical school dean to sit on the corporate board of a drug manufacturer. Fresh from our college years in the late 1960s, the best response seemed to be to stage a sit-in. We succeeded in creating a little turbulence, and the dean agreed to withdraw from the drugmaker's board. Waiting to see Flier, I reflected on how much standards had changed in the ensuing thirty-five years, even if the dean's wallpaper looked the same.

Dean Flier began our conversation by mentioning *Powerful Medicines*, which had recently been published by Knopf. He compared it to two other books by HMS faculty that came out around the same time, both of which were strident attacks on the pharmaceutical industry. The dean said that my book was the least bad of the lot, but that he wasn't happy about any of them. You need to understand, he explained, that the pharmaceutical industry is our ally. Many of these people are scientists just like us, he went on, and science is what they care about. As evidence, he added that he had recently been given an award by Bristol Myers Squibb for his research on diabetes. He had no reason to know why I had last been in that office three decades earlier (or at least I didn't think he did; the high school specter of a bad deed going onto your permanent record dies hard). But the irony wasn't lost on me.

Dean Flier went on to explain that drug companies have to live within the confines of the marketplace, which provided them with the necessary discipline. You may like the idea of government control, he explained, but that's because you like the government that's in power now. (I didn't; it was the Bush administration, and a cruel and unnecessary war was raging in Iraq. But that was beside the point.) He said there could come a time when there would be a government in charge that I wouldn't like as much, so that's why it was important that the government not be too powerful. I remember thinking, *Holy cow! The dean sounds like a libertarian!* How does he square that with the hundreds of millions of dollars the medical school and our hospitals get from the feds every year?

It would be about twenty years before Dean Flier published his revelatory 2024 account of his own abortive misadventure with industry-sponsored research (see chapter 15). But I left that meeting with him a bit shaken, having learned two lessons. The first was that it's risky to be a critic of the drug industry in an institution that is so close to it, both ideologically and financially. The second was that I should check out the attire of an audience before giving future talks at the medical school. It turned out that wouldn't be necessary: with each passing year I've received fewer invitations to lecture the medical students, residents, or anyone else there. It seems that the more insights I have to pass on, the fewer chances I get to do so. Giving a talk to trainees doesn't just let faculty share their knowledge: it's also a way to model values and a career path, interest young people in one's research, and begin relationships that can take on a life of their own. That's how I met Kesselheim and other key members of DoPE to begin years of fruitful collaboration, so not getting to do that is a problem.

By 2016, Jeff Flier had retired as dean and was replaced by George Daley. Early in his deanship, he gave a State of the School speech to alumni to outline his agenda. One youngish alumna raised her hand to say that as a student she hadn't learned enough practical information about prescription drugs and how to use them, even though she now does so all day long. Was he planning on doing something about that? She echoed a persistent complaint I had heard since my own student days. That concern was behind my creation several years ago of a new twenty-five-student medical school elective called "Medications and Evidence." We'd teach the students about how to evaluate the medical literature, and have them read drug-related papers critically and then discuss their methods and implications in detail with us in small groups: how well a study was done, any shortcomings in its approach or conclusions, what it means for practice. These were some of our most popular sessions. At the end of the course, I'd ask the students how often they had done that kind of critical reading of papers in their prior years at HMS. Most said they hadn't, which was troubling. Of all the facts we try to cram into students' heads about medications, many will be out of date by the time they hit their stride in practice. But the ability to carefully read a research paper about drug effects and understand whether it should change one's practice or not—that's a skill that doesn't change, and will remain relevant and useful to them until they retire. (Our Medications and Evidence course is not currently being offered.)

I was eager to hear Dean Daley's response to the alumna's question. We realize, he began, that this is an area in which we need to strengthen the Harvard medical curriculum. We are fortunate, he went on, that we have many talented people in our environment who can help us teach that. (My heart leapt; maybe our moment had come.) That is why, he continued, we will be reaching out to the many smart people in the pharmaceutical and biotech industry in the greater Boston area to help us do a better job in teaching our medical students about drugs. My heart sank.

A Bold New Beginning

Given this history, I wasn't sure what to expect when I was asked soon afterward to come to a meeting about a new initiative HMS was starting in "regulatory science"—the study of decisions made by governmental bodies like the FDA in dealing with issues in their domain. The planning would be headed up by Peter Sorger, an accomplished non-physician basic scientist. That wasn't surprising: basic science was the lens through which the medical school viewed most issues. Still, along with my colleagues at DoPE, I was excited that there would be an initiative out of the dean's office that could bring together faculty from clinical medicine, pharmacology, policy, epidemiology, statistics, along with biochemistry and other basic sciences, to study how drugs are evaluated and regulated.

The initial organizing meetings seemed filled with promise. Always a victim of my interdisciplinary passions, I said how exciting it would be to also bring in people from other parts of the university: political scientists, economists, ethicists, historians like Jeremy Greene in my division, who had gotten a doctorate from Harvard's History of Science Department along with his medical degree; he had been working with me since he was an undergraduate and was becoming an expert on the history of the pharmaceutical industry. Not so fast, I was told; we need to start this out as a project based in the medical school. There was a vague suspicion of departments in other parts of the university, even (actually, especially) the School of Public Health. The initial planning for the regulatory science initiative didn't even bring in hospital-based faculty with expertise in designing and running clinical trials, a core area for such a program. Political scientists and ethicists? That would be way too far a stretch at that point.

Several of our early-planning meetings were attended by Josh Boger, the brilliant non-physician CEO of Vertex Pharmaceuticals. Several of those early meetings were chaired by Bill Chin, an accomplished physician-scientist who was the HMS executive dean for research; before that, he had spent nearly a decade at the pharmaceutical manufacturer Eli Lilly. (At a medical school symposium on careers in the drug industry, someone had mentioned how commonly people went from academia to pharma and back again. "Yes, there's a lot of human trafficking going on," Bill had said, not mindful of the more common meaning of that term.)

At one of those planning meetings, Chin had to leave and asked Boger to chair the meeting in his absence. Several of us looked surprised, so Bill decided it would be more appropriate for an actual faculty member to fill that role. It soon became clear that much of the seed funding for the new regulatory science program was being provided by Boger. He was one of the largest donors to Harvard Medical School and served as chair of its Board of Fellows, a group composed of many wealthy donors. At subsequent meetings when we were considering small seed grants to faculty for various regulatory science projects, more than once someone would ask, "Would that be okay with Josh?"

The blurring of boundaries between companies and researchers can also have effects on non-physician trainees earning doctorates in fields like biochemistry or cell biology. Over the years, several graduate students have mentioned to me that they longed for the "basic" in "basic science." As one said,

> It used to be you'd find a faculty mentor studying a really interesting fundamental question that excited you, and sign up to work in their lab. Now people look for mentors whose research might lead to a marketable drug. You hook up with them and hope they'll hit the jackpot and spin off a start-up company you can be part of.

For the emerging Reg Sci program, most everyone felt that Aaron Kesselheim would be the most likely person to lead the effort once it got up and running. With his medical, law, and public health degrees and his clinical training as an internist at the Brigham, he had become one of the nation's most respected experts in the study of drug regulation. He was publishing major research studies on that topic in top journals at such a clip that he had become one of the most cited scholars in law and medicine in the country. In establishing our division's PORTAL unit, he had built a widely respected research program on the policies and outcomes of drug-regulatory decisions. Hardly anyone else at Harvard was doing regulatory science work of that high quality and volume, or at all. To no one's surprise, he was soon named codirector of the emerging Harvard Medical School Program in Regulatory Science.

That didn't last long. About a year later, a mid-level administrator called on behalf of Professor Sorger to tell Aaron that he was being terminated as codirector of the new regulatory science program. No reason was given for this unexpected decision, but Aaron and I worried that it might have been because some of our research together was seen as critical of the pharmaceutical industry.

Taking the Initiative

Aaron was surprised and saddened by his dismissal from that role; I was just saddened, having experienced something similar with another new Harvard program. A few years earlier, as the work in DoPE was prospering, I requested permission to set up a new university-wide program that would be called the Interfaculty Initiative on Medications and Society, or MedSoc for short. Drew Faust was the university's president then and she was eager to facilitate such programs that would cut across Harvard's notoriously rigid departmental lines. We have too many walls here, she said, and not enough bridges. It seemed natural to expand the study of medication use to that kind of interdisciplinary inquiry, bringing together political scientists, historians, doctors, economists, and business researchers, among others. I enlisted the help of respected colleagues in other parts of the university whom I had known for years: Arthur Kleinman in the Anthropology Department was also a physician, and studied the relationship between culture and healing; Dan Carpenter in the Government Department was writing what would become the classic book on the political science of the FDA's regulatory performance; Richard Hamermesh was a professor of management practice at Harvard Business School with an interest in emerging biotechnology products. They agreed to join me in shaping the new interfaculty initiative, along with Jeremy Greene in my division.

I even had some external grant funding I could bring to the project, that had its origins in a strange phone call:

> "Hi, Dr. Avorn. You don't know me, and I'm not a doctor, but I've read some of your papers and like them a lot."
>
> "Thanks very much."
>
> "I'd like to come in and talk to you about them. I have some interesting ideas about how your work might relate to the meds I take for my bipolar condition."
>
> "Sorry, I can't do that; I just don't have enough time. Plus, I can't get involved in individual patients' prescriptions if I'm not their doctor."
>
> "We really ought to get together. I'm the guy who started CVS."
>
> "When can you come by?"

The caller was Ralph Hoagland, an entrepreneurial genius who was by then well into retirement. In 1963 he founded a chain initially called Consumer Value Stores; he had long ago sold the pharmacy chain, but retained an active interest in the use of medications. "I don't work there anymore, but I still know some of the folks who run it."

It seemed like a long shot, but in a research environment where the only funds to run our programs and pay anyone's salary, including my own, were what we brought in ourselves, it seemed a chance worth taking. My DoPE colleagues Will Shrank and Niteesh Choudhry and I took a trip to nearby Woonsocket, Rhode Island, CVS's corporate home. Our research interests in how patients filled their prescriptions and why they didn't struck a chord with the CVS executives that Ralph had set us up with. After several more trips to Woonsocket, the company agreed to fund a series of studies we wanted to do, with a budget of several hundred thousand dollars a year, no strings attached. That seemed like a good possible nest egg for the future MedSoc work.

The next step in building the new cross-cutting Harvard endeavor was to meet with Steve Hyman, the university provost; I needed his blessing to get the project off the ground. He understood the interdisciplinary nature of what I proposed and said it would be a natural for the new interfaculty initiatives agenda. He gave me his approval and provided a very small annual budget to support some logistical help, dinner meetings, conferences, and so forth. Surprisingly, he then brought up the issue of naming rights for our not-yet-existing program. I had mentioned that DoPE had gotten some funding from CVS for our research on patients' adherence to their medicines, which could help cover the cost of some of the work I envisioned for MedSoc.

"This wouldn't be called the CVS Center on Medications and Society, would it?" Hyman asked. "Because that wouldn't be allowed under university policies. You know, if Shell Oil gave us millions of dollars to set up a program to study energy, we wouldn't want to call it the Shell Center on Energy."

"No, of course not," I said. "The thought never crossed my mind." Hyman thanked me for my efforts in creating the new activity, and said he'd be eager to hear how its work progressed.

A next step was to meet with Professor Steve Kosslyn, the dean of social sciences who had also served as chair of the psychology department. This would help us build ties to the graduate school of the Faculty of Arts and Sciences, which the university describes as the "historic heart of Harvard." (It has since been renamed the Harvard Kenneth C. Griffin Graduate School of Arts and Sciences, following a gift of $300 million from the conservative businessman.) Our session with Professor Kosslyn was a bit bumpy. We met late in the afternoon; Kosslyn looked tired and seemed a little defensive about this academic border-crossing adventure. I assumed he had spent the day being hassled by other professors who wanted something from him. I thought of the adage an associate dean at the medical school once shared with me: "A dean is to faculty as a fire hydrant is to a dog." But we weren't asking for anything; we just wanted to provide him with a heads-up.

"We think medication use could be a great focal point for research and teaching from many different perspectives," I said enthusiastically. "Economics, policy, history, pharmacology, ethics, medicine, and so on. We could even design a course around that approach."

"Oh, you mean the whole 'universe in a grain of sand' thing?" he asked, quoting the early nineteenth-century English poet William Blake. "Taking one topic and looking at it from several different disciplines? Yeah, we used to do that more; we're not into it so much now."

Jeremy Greene tried to get the conversation back on track. "We want MedSoc to offer a space where people from different fields and different parts of the university can come together to talk about how their perspectives relate to medications," he said.

The dean blanched. "*Space?!*" he asked. "You want space? Do you have any idea how tight space is on all our campuses? Don't ask me for that!" Jeremy rushed to point out that he was referring to intellectual space, not square feet. The dean was visibly relieved.

MedSoc went on for a year or two. We brought together speakers from many of the university's schools and disciplines, people who wouldn't normally be in conversations together or even meet one another. Some of them were advocates of the current system of medication research and payment, some were foes of it, some couldn't care less about that. But a community was developing across the university; the interchange among doctors, social scientists, business school faculty, and others was bracing. I got permission to set up an email address for our little community, @medsoc.harvard.edu, to help bring people together free of any divisional domains, and moved all my correspondence to it. We were finding our footing, and there was talk of offering an interdisciplinary freshman seminar. (One colleague said cynically that wouldn't be a problem, since the criterion for being allowed to offer a freshman seminar at Harvard College was that you had to have a pulse rate over forty.)

Then the rug was pulled out. I got a memo from a mid-level administrator in the Office of the Provost saying that our tiny annual budget was being cut to zero. Belt-tightening, and all. That was a surprise, since it seemed like a very small amount for an institution that at the time had about a $30 billion endowment. (Our budget was just a few minutes' worth of interest income on that investment, I calculated sadly.) All right, I responded, I'll use some grant funding from DoPE to fund MedSoc's tiny budget; we'll make it work. No, you don't understand, came the reply. Even if it costs us nothing, the Interfaculty Initiative on Medications and Society has to come to an end. It's no longer authorized by the Office of the Provost as an interfaculty initiative. As a twist of the knife, the @medsoc.harvard.edu email address that we were using also had to go.

I never managed to get a clear answer from the Office of the Provost about why any of this happened. Colleagues from around the world who wrote to me at my MedSoc email address got a bounceback message that the recipient was unknown to the university. "I thought you had left Harvard," one of them said, after tracking me down at my hospital email address. In a sense, I had.

As I rethink my tumultuous career at Harvard, some days I feel as if I've developed Stockholm syndrome—not the fervor to win a Nobel Prize that motivates many of my colleagues, but the transformation that sometimes occurs in prisoners who end up identifying with the values of their captors. Occasionally I wonder whether upstream-swimming faculty like Kesselheim and me may not really belong at Harvard. As some of our mainstream colleagues would point out, if you take the hundred-year view—which a nearly four-centuries-old institution does get to do—maybe what really matters the most is making the key scientific breakthroughs, the ones that will transform the way we treat human illness for many decades to come. Cure-finding over hand-holding.

Viewed from the perspective of the next hundred years of sick people, maybe our petty concerns about drug approval criteria, costs, and side effects could be seen as pathetically shortsighted. By contrast, learning about the very mechanisms of sickness and health—*how biology works, for God's sake*—is eternal. According to that view, the good drugs that such research makes possible will go on forever, or until even more cutting-edge research comes up with even better treatments. The bad drugs will eventually fall by the wayside, even if they should have been abandoned sooner. But the basic biological discoveries our scientist colleagues make will be true in ten years, in a hundred years. They will be true in America, they will be true in Europe, they will be mostly true in China and Africa, as long as racial differences are studied and defined.

According to that perspective, if some approved drugs don't really work, over enough years people will eventually figure that out. If people can't pay for those drugs, that's a local and transient business problem, according to this view—a concern of politics, not science. Sneaky patenting strategies may keep drugs expensive far longer than they should, but eventually cheaper generics or biosimilars will probably come along at some point, even if takes more years of unaffordable drug bills. Really bad side effects will eventually get figured out, even if it takes more time than it ought to. But developing fundamental insights into biology—that's kissing the face of the eternal.

In the Years That Followed

Today, the Harvard medical curriculum is not as devoid of the "social science crap" the dean of students had warned me about when I was starting out: there are now brief lectures and even some small-group electives covering several of the topics we had to figure out for ourselves in our student-initiated courses of the 1970s. But until those modest changes, several generations of graduates including my own came away with a narrowed understanding of what medicine is about. And we went on to help shape the world of American health care with that mindset.

Unlike the late MedSoc, other interdisciplinary drug-related programs at Harvard continue to thrive, some of them copiously funded by grants from pharmaceutical companies or their executives, though that isn't always reflected in their titles. I thought of my original talk with the provost about Harvard's rules for naming programs. Shell Center, indeed.

Here are follow-ups on some of the people involved in the rise and fall of Harvard's short-lived Interfaculty Initiative on Medications and Society:

- Bill Chin, the executive dean for research at HMS, left Harvard in 2013 to become chief medical officer of PhRMA, the drug industry trade group, where he also served as its executive vice president for science and regulatory affairs.
- Jeremy Greene, the wide-ranging historian-internist who helped me start MedSoc, was backed strongly by me and his other mentor, Paul Farmer, for academic advancement at Harvard, but we were told by senior faculty that his future would be brighter elsewhere. He left for Johns Hopkins several years after the demise of MedSoc and is now the William H. Welch Professor of Medicine there, and chair of its eminent Department of the History of Medicine.
- Peter Sorger remains the Otto Krayer Professor of Systems Biology at Harvard and leads its Therapeutics Initiative. A company he

cofounded based on his research, Merrimack Pharmaceuticals, sold the rights to a drug for pancreatic cancer to a French drugmaker in 2017 for $575 million. In 2022, Merrimack received an additional $225 million payment when clinical trials showed the drug's effectiveness.

- Josh Boger continues to be one of the most generous donors to Harvard Medical School, as do other pharma executives and their companies. Boger retired as CEO of Vertex Pharmaceuticals in 2009. His net worth, based mostly on ownership of Vertex stock, was estimated at $284 million in 2024.
- Aaron Kesselheim remains one of the nation's most published and cited scholars in law, medicine, and drug policy, and was elected to the prestigious National Academy of Medicine in 2020. He continues to run PORTAL in our division, and has built it into one of the world's most respected programs studying drug regulation; he also teaches FDA policy at Yale Law School. He and most people in our group have little contact with the Harvard Program on Regulatory Science.
- Social Science dean Steve Kosslyn was named in a 2019 review of Harvard's ties to sex offender Jeffrey Epstein, which found that Kosslyn had advocated for Epstein's unconventional acceptance as a visiting fellow in the psychology department without acknowledging that Epstein had made a $200,000 gift to his program. Usually, visiting fellows are scholars with advanced degrees, but Epstein had not completed college; he was given an office on campus, but seems to have done very little work as a fellow. Kosslyn left Harvard in 2011.
- Jim Kim, co-chief with Paul Farmer of the Harvard-Brigham Global Health Equity programs *("I didn't realize that we were the problem!")* left Harvard to become the president of Dartmouth College and then went on to head the World Bank.
- In December 2023, Leonard Blavatnik announced he was suspending his hundreds of millions of dollars in donations to Harvard, angered at the congressional testimony of the university's then-president on combating anti-Semitism on campus, and Harvard's performance on that issue.

The cultures of universities are shaped bit by bit, year after year, the way a sculptor working in clay will add an additional part here and take a little off there until a piece is finished. But unlike clay sculptures, universities are never truly finished. The shaping goes on continuously, endlessly forming and re-forming (though rarely reforming) the contours of the institution, responding to external forces and inner imperatives. Those values are communicated to students and faculty and influence their work; that's one of the key functions of a university. In the present context, that helps determine how medical students and faculty come to think about medications, what research and programs matter, which values are promoted and which are marginalized, and the role of all the diverse actors in our complicated system of drug development, policy, and use. What our students hear and who teaches them can influence how they will think about these matters for the rest of their professional lives, and how they will go on to train others.

Of course, all organizations, including corporations, constantly reassess their values, goals, and incentives, and how they should be transmitted. But companies have a consistent North Star guiding their journey—the mission to maximize profit. That's not a value judgment, it's just a fact. Universities are more complicated creatures: our agendas are guided by less easily measured imperatives: creating new knowledge, teaching the next generation, serving as an arena for public discourse on vital issues of the day. Medical schools and their clinical affiliates add two more dimensions: training and socializing young doctors and caring for sick people. Those goals are not always perfectly congruent. (There's a joke about a teaching hospital research scientist who said, "This would be a great place to work if it weren't for all the students and patients!")

Somehow, we need to align those often-competing tasks; we get it right often, but not always. Traditionally, universities and academic medical centers would just try not to go broke in the process, since there does have to be some fiscal component of the agenda or—we're constantly told—everything would grind to a halt. This used to be an afterthought, a necessary evil, but it's not that now. At Harvard, perhaps it's no accident that the governing body that ultimately controls the university is called the Corporation. How large that fiscal imperative looms in academic medicine, and how its incentives are communicated, is a source of concern. Many of us chose to work at universities and their academic medical centers because we expected them to be very different from companies that have to focus on maximizing revenue. That is changing.

CHAPTER 18

Better Signals

Many patients seem to believe that we doctors know most of the key facts about the drugs we use, and that we somehow make optimal choices among the alternatives on that basis. But we've seen that there's just too much information out there for any clinician to absorb and digest, even if we all had the time and analytic savvy to do so—which we don't. Drugmakers understand this, and pick the information they want us to be aware of, package it engagingly with pictures, headlines, and big graphs, and present it to us in ways that are skillfully designed to influence what we prescribe. Most effectively, they also transmit these messages to us interactively, through appealing sales agents (known as "detailers") who come to doctors' offices and chat with us about our medication choices.

Those conversersations enable a skilled detailer to understand *why* we make the prescribing decisions we do; they already knew *what* we prescribe, because their companies purchase that detailed data from virtually every pharmacy in the country. But knowing *how* we make our decisions and what lies behind those preferences enables them to wield the persuasion trifecta known as KAP: understanding our Knowledge, Attitudes, and Practices. Getting a handle on that, preferably through in-person conversation, is the most powerful way to change what we do and nudge it toward greater use of their company's products. Those casual-seeming conversations are actually finely honed Kabuki based on lengthy, sophisticated sales training. Back in medical school, I was struck by the mismatch between the elegant principles of pharmacology we were being taught in our classrooms, and the more chaotic, less evidence-based medication use that was so evident in typical practice settings.

Later on, I wondered what would happen if we could take the very effective adult learning and behavior-change principles used by the drug companies, but use them instead to promote better prescribing based only on the best evidence. Because the sales reps are called detailers and I was trying to do this from a medical school base, I named the approach "academic detailing." But to know if the idea worked, I'd have to test it in a randomized controlled trial—just as we do for new medications. Too many neat-sounding health services improvement ideas have a lot in common with those ineffective drug treatments that were so popular before we began to test medicines in randomized trials to find out what actually worked: they seem like good ideas, but aren't effective. So two years out of my residency, in 1979, I applied for a small grant from the federal government and trained a cadre of nurses and pharmacists to become the first "academic detailers." We focused on three areas of typically bad prescribing: overuse of antibiotics for viral upper respiratory infections; the management of pain; and treating older patients who have memory problems. (Sadly, over forty years later these are still common areas of poor medication use.) We also trained our outreach educators in "un-salesmanship 101": how to establish a relationship with doctors, how to understand why they were doing what they were doing, and how to persuade them to change their practices.

Good Evidence Doesn't Disseminate Itself: Public-Interest Marketing

Then I convinced four state Medicaid programs to ship me all their paid pharmacy claims data so we could know which doctors to target—these were much simpler times when it came to privacy. That was the origin of what I later called "interventional pharmacoepidemiology"—using population-based data from health-care systems to identify areas for improvement, roll out programs to achieve the desired change, and then examine the same data sources to measure their impact. In that first study, we randomly allocated 435 doctors to be offered the new program or serve as controls. The idea worked:

physicians took to the program gladly, and the intervention reduced problematic prescribing by 14 percent. We published our results in *NEJM*. My colleague Steve Soumerai, whom I hired as one of the project's first research assistants, later did his doctoral dissertation at the Harvard School of Public Health on a benefit-cost analysis of the program. It found that the approach saved Medicaid two dollars for every dollar it cost to offer the program—not surprising, since many of the drugs we targeted were both inappropriate and expensive.

I followed that first experiment with another randomized trial in nursing homes, using academic detailing to convince doctors and nurses to stop overusing sedating medications in these vulnerable patients. That worked, too. We didn't just reduce overuse of the problematic drugs: in patients who had been taking antipsychotic medications, we found that in the homes randomized to our educational program, their memory function improved compared to similar patients in the control homes. The magnitude of that effect was impressive, and better than that seen with some of the latest intravenous drugs promoted to treat Alzheimer's disease. It wasn't that we had intervened in their neuropathology; we had simply lifted the burden of unnecessary over-sedation, and that made a clinically important difference. That study was published in *NEJM* as well. We went on to conduct another randomized trial of academic detailing to improve antibiotic use at the Brigham; it was led by Dan Solomon, of our prophetic Vioxx–heart attack study. It worked there as well. Studies replicating the academic detailing approach in other U.S. centers and abroad began to appear in the medical literature; systematic reviews of several dozen randomized trials of the method have concluded that it really works.

Meanwhile, I was expanding my research program's large collection of data tapes from health insurers, built on the anonymized pharmacy records of the prescriptions they had paid for. That would later become a key platform for our work studying medication use and outcomes, especially in older patients. It began with data from the four Medicaid programs that participated in the first academic detailing randomized trial, and then just kept going. Pennsylvania attracted my interest, since it had an unusual program that paid for the drug expenses of its older citizens with funding supplied by its state lottery, known as the Pharmaceutical Assistance Contract for the Elderly, or PACE. It began in 1983, more than twenty years before Medicare started paying for medications. I began to get regular shipments of detailed but anonymized filled-prescription data from Tom Snedden, who had been running the PACE program from its earliest days and still does, having shepherded it through nine governors.

In 2004 a new Pennsylvania governor, Ed Rendell, noticed that through PACE, Medicaid, and other programs, the state was spending around $3 billion a year on prescription drugs. He asked his senior officials whether there was some way the state could be getting a better deal on such a large expenditure. Snedden said he knew a doctor at Harvard he had been sending PACE pharmacy claims to for his epidemiological research. Tom was aware that in another part of my life I had developed a way to improve prescribing by sending people to doctors' offices to teach them about the drugs they prescribed. Rendell authorized him to see if we could do a program like that in Pennsylvania.

Scaling It Up

Until then, my work on improving prescribing had been done on a research basis only. I had offered advice to colleagues elsewhere who had read my original papers and wanted to set up their own programs based on that work: Australia wanted to set up a continent-wide academic detailing activity of its own, and the enormous Kaiser and Veterans Affairs health systems were eager to establish such programs as well. But this was the first time I'd have a chance to build a large operational academic detailing program of my own. Working with a state government to do this made perfect sense: after all, if governments build roads and provide public education, why not also fund programs to help doctors take better care of their patients?

"I think we can get approval from the governor to implement academic detailing throughout Pennsylvania," Snedden told me. "How much do you think it would cost to do that?" Channeling my mercantile ancestors, I asked, "How much do you have?" "Could you do something for about a million dollars a year?" Having absolutely no idea, I answered, "Sure!"

Guidance from Fish

Running the program through Harvard or the Brigham proved infeasible because of their rigid bureaucracies and high overhead rates (the hospital currently adds on an additional 79 percent of a project's budget for such charges on most government grants). It seemed best to set up a separate nonprofit organization, but what would we call it? In New England, each spring the herring unerringly return from the ocean to the rivers and streams in which they originally hatched—unless they are caught first by herring fishermen like the plaintiffs whose litigation helped curtail the authority of federal agencies, as described in chapter 8. Like salmon, herring somehow know exactly where to go to spawn, even after years in the open sea. This requires them to swim upstream vigorously, paddling against the current, jumping over rapids, defying gravity. Then, after starting off a new generation to begin the cycle afresh, they die.

That ardent swimming upstream felt a bit like what we were trying to do in bringing more evidence-based training to our colleagues in the face of a torrent of promotional messages. (The part about dying in the process resonated less.) I looked up the name of the genus of these spunky little creatures; it was "Alosa"—fine name for our new counter-current nonprofit.

"Going upstream" can mean much more than just going against the fire-hose flow of drug promotion. It's also about getting further up the chain of events that culminates in a prescription decision—for example, thinking about the progression of an illness like chronic obstructive lung disease: what factors caused it and led to a patient's current clinical state, and what can be done to address those prior issues, whether they are smoking or poor adherence to prescribed medications. The "upstream" concept also helps me fit together our frontline educational work with other activities in our division, particularly in PORTAL: What led to this drug being approved in the first place? If a drug is unaffordable to many patients, how did that happen? What can be done to make *those* upstream forces work better? Further, we all attribute our intentions and actions to our own personal goals and strategies, but might each of us also be guided at some primal level by the same kind of passionate drive that motivates the swim-upstream behavior of herring and other creatures?

Growing Fame

Word of Alosa's man-bites-dog approach spread, and a few inquiries from the press began to come in. A reporter from the *Wall Street Journal* was interested in our work and wrote an article that became a front-page story in March, 2006: "As Drug Bill Soars, Some Doctors Get an 'Unsales' Pitch—Harvard Professor Helps Team." Around the same time, the *New York Times* ran an unrelated story on its front page describing how pharmaceutical companies liked to hire former cheerleaders to work as salespeople, since they were perky and engaging. The comic geniuses who produced *The Daily Show* saw both articles and put them together in brilliant synergy, to create a segment that began with a conversation with a former Miss Florida who had been hired by a pharmaceutical company to work as a sales rep. The show sent a correspondent to interview her; he was smitten by her beauty, though not by her abundant pharmacological knowledge.

> "What can I bring you—lunch? Dinner?" she asks him in her best sales-rep mode. "You can beat me to the ground with a flaming cat," he responds. "The answer is yes." He arranges for a series of "seminars" with her in a fancy restaurant, over wine. "She taught me that you can never be too healthy," he recounts. "That's why I'm now on Lipitor, Zyrtec, Nexium, Celebrex, and Wellbutrin. And I've had an erection for over 96 hours."

Then the *Daily Show* correspondent visited me in Boston to talk about our work; I was the staid professor who used boring "generics goons" to go out and teach doctors about evidence-based prescribing, putting the benevolent pharmaceutical industry in grave jeopardy. The *Daily Show* segment conveyed what we were doing and why far more effectively than many of our journal articles did. It may represent some of my most influential impact.

Alosa has continued to grow since those early days. Thanks to its state lottery, Pennsylvania's Department of Aging has continued to support our work there, and some of our most experienced academic detailers have now passed their twentieth year of interacting with the doctors they visit. Other backers came forward, including the Centers for Disease Control, the federal Agency for Healthcare Research and Quality, and the insurer Aetna. By 2014, pain management and opioid use had become one of the most challenging areas in need of better evidence-based education for health professionals. It had become clear that the very way that doctors understood the concept of pain and its treatment had been distorted by drugmakers that had hacked into the cognitive programming of medical professionals and our institutions, as discussed below in chapter 20.

What was needed was a user-friendly interactive explanation of how to manage pain without reliance on opioids, and how best to identify and treat patients who had become opioid dependent. We would use the same kind of in-office interactions that opioid manufacturers like Purdue Pharma had used to persuade doctors that these medications weren't really that addictive or problematic. To help develop our materials, I turned to Brian Bateman, who had begun working with me when he was starting his training in anesthesiology at the Massachusetts General Hospital. We developed "de-marketing" materials about managing pain without resorting to narcotics, and how to care for patients with opioid-use disorder (what we used to call addiction). Even though the opioid epidemic was raging, there was still no clear place one could turn for an evidence-based guide on how to treat pain without over-using opioids. Brian led our effort in reviewing the literature and crafting these materials, coming up with excellent evidence-based practical recommendations. We put them into a clear, readily understood format for use by our academic detailers when they went into the field—initially in Pennsylvania, and later around the country. The creation of that material, along with a lengthy, amply footnoted evidence document, were supervised by Alosa's Ellen Dancel, who holds a doctorate in pharmacy as well as a master's degree in pharmacoepidemiology. With the help of a talented graphic designer, she transforms our materials, which sometimes start out excessively wonky, into materials that are as engaging and compelling as any pharmaceutical promotional piece. (Internally, we call our twelve-page summaries "un-ads.") A year and a half after we built the program, the Centers for Disease Control issued its 2016 guidelines, which made pretty much the same points, but in a much less engaging way. The CDC has now identified academic detailing as a proven approach to helping doctors prescribe better and has funded much of this work by programs on the ground in several states.

As interest in our approach to academic detailing increased, Alosa grew. We hired Paul Fanikos to manage our increasing field staff of educators. He, too, was a pharmacist by training, but had the added advantage of having managed a team of field representatives for a large pharmaceutical company. Like Paul, some of the most talented people on the Alosa team used to work for drug companies. They have the skills of interactivity and salesmanship that we sought, but we chose only those who also had solid clinical training in nursing or pharmacy, and a commitment to put those skills to work for "the other side." As with all of our clinical education materials, we put everything on the Alosa website for people to use at no charge for any non-commercial purpose.

Once word of what we were doing spread, we began to get requests from around the country to help teach doctors about other clinical issues for which standard methods of communication hadn't reached their goals. The topics that welled up from the health-care system have been quite varied: Shelby County in Tennessee, where Memphis is located, was seeing an upswing in congenital syphilis: babies were being born to pregnant women who had the disease, but had not been diagnosed. The consequences for the child could be dire, yet the problem could be completely prevented by testing the mother for the condition before delivery and giving her penicillin. So we mounted a program of educational outreach to bring that message to doctors there who cared for pregnant women. Public health officials in Washington asked us to develop and disseminate programs to encourage the use of pre-exposure prophylaxis (PrEP) for HIV-positive patients—an effective and woefully under-used way of preventing infection. Additional topics Alosa has taken on include educational outreach on other common clinical topics for which practice doesn't always line up with the best recommendations, including heart failure, atrial fibrillation, diabetes, chronic lung disease, depression, and insomnia. (Current materials, along with information for patients, is available at no cost at AlosaHealth.org.)

I've done all my academic detailing work pro bono; the biggest reward was getting to work with young doctors at the Brigham who were sharp clinicians and were also drawn to the upstream work we were doing. One was Mike Fischer, who sought me out when he was a resident. He joined DoPE as a faculty member and we applied for federal funding to create a National Resource Center for Academic Detailing (NaRCAD) to provide free help to programs around the country and the world on how to set up this kind of educational outreach program, as well as train people on how to do it. With the help of its director, Bevin Amira, we put all those materials as well on the web for anyone to use at no charge at NaRCAD.org.

As our academic detailing programs grew, in 2018 I got a call from Dan Knecht, a doctor at the large health insurer Aetna. He said the company wanted to be a good corporate citizen and do what it could to address the opioid epidemic, and he had heard about our academic detailing work. I asked him a dozen different ways whether there was any hidden company agenda, or whether the clinical content would remain totally in our hands; he answered every question as I had hoped. That began an ongoing relationship between Alosa and Aetna that has continued for years, with the company supporting our little nonprofit to set up academic detailing outreach programs in about ten states since the collaboration began; it asked nothing in return.

If I Knew Then . . .

It's now over forty-five years since I wrote that first grant application at the start of my career, proposing the idea of academic detailing and how to evaluate it. I guess I expected at the time that if the concept worked, by the 2020s it would be in widespread use to improve the quality of prescribing and contain its costs all over the health-care system, even paying for itself through reduced use of overpriced drugs and better clinical outcomes. Yes, the approach has proliferated, with many impressive success stories beyond Alosa and NaRCAD. Programs have sprung up throughout the country and the world to provide this kind of educational outreach to prescribers. But many of them are funded by year-to-year, hand-to-mouth funding that, like ours, is vulnerable to ending at any moment. The largest such program in the U.S. is the very effective one run by the Veterans Affairs health system, employing about a hundred academic detailers in all fifty states. Kaiser Permanente also maintains its own active academic detailing program. Both programs are integrated health-care systems—for the most part they employ their doctors, own their pharmacies, pay for the drugs, and run the hospitals in which patients are cared for. That helps to line up incentives favoring evidence-based, cost-effective prescribing, with an eye toward optimizing care and preventing bad outcomes for patients down the road.

That contrasts sharply with the more limited vision that dominates health care in most of the U.S. system, which is hampered by fragmentation of each of these segments as health insurers, PBMs, physicians, and hospitals each try to maximize their own fiscal advantage. In those nonintegrated (or perhaps dis-integrated) parts of the health-care enterprise, the whole is much less than the sum of its parts. I've spoken to large insurers about supporting educational outreach programs to improve medication use in a given region, and gotten answers like this: "Our market share is just 21 percent in that area. If we paid to teach doctors how to prescribe better that would benefit all the other insurers, too, on our dime. We don't like free riders." What about putting together a consortium of payers? I've tried;

it makes coming up with a peace plan for the Middle East look easy in comparison. The problem is particularly galling when the reluctance to join in also comes from publicly funded programs like Medicare and Medicaid, or ostensibly nonprofit insurers like Blue Cross programs, that should know better.

Sometimes the genius of American enterprise has led to "carve-outs" of some types of coverage, in which a separate insurer manages and pays for just one aspect of care. For our purposes that would be the drug benefit, but other brilliant carve-outs make mental health or hospice care clinically and economically separate services, peeled away from a patient's main coverage and run separately. I once spoke about academic detailing to a senior manager of a group of accountable care organizations, which are designed to consolidate medical care into coherent groups of practitioners with compatible clinical and economic incentives. Might they want to help their doctors use medications better and save money through more cost-effective prescribing *and* better outcomes? Not necessarily, came the reply. "We carve out our drug benefit to an outside program, so the people in charge of paying for medications are different from the people in charge of prescribing." It was a solution right up there with King Solomon's baby-splitting idea.

That constricted perspective can have a time dimension as well. I've spoken to people in charge of drug use at some large health insurers and tried to convince them that increasing the use of effective, underused medications could reduce disease in the future. When I started out, it was still-expensive products like statins to reduce heart attack and stroke, or drugs for osteoporosis that prevent hip fractures. More recently, it would be excellent but expensive drugs like Sovaldi that cure hepatitis C infection (see chapter 12), or drugs like Ozempic for diabetes that also reduce heart failure hospitalization, other cardiac disease, and kidney failure. "Yes, they're great products," would come the reply. "But we need to manage our rising drug spend on a quarter-by-quarter basis, and that's how my performance is judged. Besides, the 'churn rate' for our customers is around 25 percent a year: they get another employer who has a different insurer, or they lose their job and have to go on Medicaid, lots of reasons. So a quarter of these people are gone each year. And those events you're talking about preventing? Most of them would happen when the person is older and on Medicare; why should I spend a lot now to save the government money years down the road?" I recalled the "all against all" state of nature that Hobbes warned us about. Such meet-my-own-needs considerations are less relevant for integrated-care systems like the VA and Kaiser, where everything is mostly under the same tent, both economically and clinically, and the churn rate is lower.

In sharp contrast, drug manufacturers can afford to shower doctors and patients with a copious stream of information lauding their products. Each member of their audiences, whether professionals or patients, may be connected to a different health-care organization or insurer, but all are potential customers. And the companies' only motivation is laser-focused in a golem sort of way: *increase product revenues.* By contrast, doctors, patients, payers all have multiple interests: providing or getting good care, avoiding hospitalization, saving or making money, and a dozen more. But the shining clarity of the pharmaceutical industry's agenda is unidimensional: they just want to sell more of their drugs—as much of them as possible. The mixed goals and motivations of everyone else in our conflicted, ambivalent, often well-meaning, confused, and embattled health-care system may be all over the map, but drugmakers just want one thing.

So where do we go from here in improving communication about drugs? Some legislative fixes are as obvious as they are unlikely. Could we ban the pharmaceutical spam known as direct-to-consumer advertising, which nearly every other advanced nation manages to do without as they run effective and far more affordable health-care systems? Much as we'd all like to be able to turn on the TV without having to watch commercials about eczema or psoriasis, or being asked to ponder the best treatment for specific forms of metastatic cancer, such a ban isn't likely to happen. Besides the pharmaceutical industry, which wants to maintain its own direct highway into our brains, the media companies on which they lavish well over $5 billion a year wouldn't accept such a prohibition. The nation lived comfortably with a ban on assault rifles until 2004, when it expired, just as we managed to live without drug ads targeting consumers until that ban ended in 1997. Now it seems we can't find our way back to those saner times on either front.

On the prescriber side, could we require doctors to confirm our knowledge of current medications before renewing our medical licenses? And expect the same before we are permitted to charge payers like Medicare for our services? Not likely. Our own professional lobbies would come out swinging, wailing about infringing our rights, and block such attempts at the state or federal level. I assume those lobbyists would be fine with the prospect that the Uber driver who takes them across town doesn't have a valid driver's license, or that the meat in the hamburger they eat for dinner was never inspected by the Department of Agriculture.

On a more positive and practical note, we can begin to think about how we can provide prescribers with the best drug information in a more voluntary way, to help us in making the best medication choices; that ought to be a public good. In my ideal world, the emerging evidence—new clinical trials, economic analyses, observational studies of drug use and outcomes—would be reviewed by groups that function like the health technology assessment organizations in many other countries. They would be nonprofit entities whose members are free of any commercial entanglements and would continuously review the practice-relevant evidence base. There would have to be an implementation arm as well: its output could resemble the rigorous evidence documents with scores of references that we produce at Alosa, along with the shorter and more engaging heavily illustrated brief summaries.

Given all the pressures under which we've seen the FDA frequently buckle, none of the output of these organizations should be generated by the government, although some arm's-length federal funding could be offered to qualifying groups. But the content itself could be generated by any of several nonprofit evidence-synthesis organizations, each with strict prohibitions on conflicts of interest by those who do the work and a ban on any kind of industry funding. As someone who practiced primary care for many years, I'd want to see that content be made available to every front-line health-care professional, to help the system work better for all. If the nation can afford to pay tens of billions of dollars a year for the drug industry to "educate" clinicians and patients, why not redirect a fraction of that enormous amount of communication expense to pay for the creation and provision of unbiased content? It could be funded by a small tax on pharmaceutical company profits—a tiny fraction of all the government dollars that are poured into the industry's coffers.

But generating these evidence syntheses would just be the first step. We know that simply summarizing the evidence and issuing guidelines often doesn't change prescribing. And when it comes to medications that can cost hundreds of thousands of dollars a year and may (or may not) have enormous impacts on health, it should be in the interest of *some* entity to make sure we all get accurate information from a source that is independent of the people selling the product. We also need to deal with *under*-prescribing: inadequate treatment of atrial fibrillation, osteoporosis, diabetes, hypertension, obesity. The purpose of educational outreach is to *optimize* medication use, not just reduce it. If we move further into embracing nonprofit integrated health-care systems like the VA and Kaiser, those groups could look deep into their information systems and identify physicians who could benefit from educational interventions focusing on their own personal patterns of medication underuse, overuse, or misuse, running programs of their own, through the concept of "interventional pharmacoepidemiology." There is so much we could do to match everyday prescribing to the best available current evidence; but even where they exist, such activities, even our own, often rely on year-to-year, hand-to-mouth funding. Our atomized, golemized, bottom-line-focused health-care system isn't yet ready to take on this issue seriously.

There was a time when I was much younger (that is, before the elections of November 2024) that I thought the federal government would one day rise to the occasion and support publicly funded non-commercial medication information for prescribers and perhaps even for patients—exactly as it assumes responsibility for other public goods like roads, clean air and water, and national defense. But a shift to the right with an impressive electoral mandate that led to control over the executive branch and both houses of Congress, along with a compliant Supreme Court, forced a rethink of the likelihood of such a pro bono solution. Yet there may be a silver lining here: if the nation degrades its reliance on the evidence required to approve new medications and further lightens up its vigilance about drug safety, just as other parts of the Department of Health and Human Services back away from containing drug costs, perhaps health-care systems themselves will have to enter these arenas to generate and disseminate this vital information.

– PART FIVE –

Mind-Altering Examples

Medicine is a social science and politics is nothing else but medicine on a large scale.

—Rudolf Virchow, nineteenth-century German physician and pathologist

CHAPTER 19

Acid Redux: The Death and Rebirth of Psychedelics

Drugs like LSD, MDMA (ecstasy), and psilocybin strikingly illustrate how the same molecule can play very different roles in medicine and in society depending on how it's handled or mishandled. The first two drugs have been around for over eighty years; the third, for thousands. Over that time they have each been variously seen as sacraments, oddities, recreational substances, and crimes. And in the last decade they have been transformed into some of the most promising medicines we may have to treat a variety of psychiatric illnesses, from depression to addiction to PTSD. Some of them could become prescription drugs before long, and the group as a whole is projected to become a new multibillion-dollar extension of the pharmaceutical industry.

In the 1960s, research on hallucinogens came under a dense cloud of suspicion. Some of the problems began with Timothy Leary's outside-the-box experiments with LSD and psilocybin while he was a member of the Harvard faculty early in that pivotal decade; his trajectory through the world of psychedelics helped define many of the legal and cultural peaks and valleys of these drugs for years to come. I had a chance to interview him for the college radio station when he visited the Columbia campus in 1969 to promote his book *High Priest*—a work advocating for his vision that we all needed to turn on, tune in, and drop out. He came across as charismatic, affable, and a little goofy, with a casual relationship with regulations and the law. He was all over the place—having recently founded the League for Spiritual Discovery as a religious movement, he ran for governor of California against the incumbent Ronald Reagan, and then joined John Lennon and Yoko Ono in their "bed-in" to protest the war in Vietnam.

Around the time of our interview Leary had been arrested in Texas for possession of cannabis in violation of the Marihuana Tax Act of 1937; he was fined $30,000, sentenced to thirty years in prison, and required to undergo psychiatric treatment. He brought his conviction (and his convictions) to the U.S. Supreme Court and later won on constitutional grounds, in one of the more interesting drug cases the high court has ever reviewed. After we met, Leary was again caught with a small amount of marijuana in California and sentenced to twenty years in prison. He escaped from jail with the help of the Weather Underground, an ultraradical group some of whose members had helped occupy several buildings on our campus the prior year. They transported him to Algeria to stay with Eldridge Cleaver, a Black militant that our group of editors at the *Columbia Daily Spectator* had foolishly endorsed for president in the 1968 election, since we refused to back either Richard Nixon or Hubert Humphrey because of their stands on the Vietnam War. Leary's stay in Algeria didn't work out well, and he was eventually extradited to the U.S. and jailed in Folsom Prison in a cell near that of Charles Manson. Does all this sound like some kind of a fever-dream mash-up? No; it was just the sixties.

An Evolving Field

When I arrived at Harvard for medical school a few years later, large swaths of its psychiatry department were dominated by psychoanalysts who had little use for the emerging field of psychopharmacology that we were learning about in our preclinical lectures. This was disconcerting, because that was the field I then planned to enter. Marijuana was still an illegal substance classified by the government as a narcotic in the same forensic category as heroin, and its mere possession could lead to years in prison. Recreational doses and potency weren't predictable, so smoking a joint or some hashish from an unknown dealer could result in anything from a sensation of "I'm not feeling high at all; I'm gonna get my money back from the bastard who sold me this shit!" to "I'm not sure I can stand up look at my hand it has all these funny lines on it is it normal to feel your breathing this much everything is everything I can talk to God," with the former mindset sometimes transitioning to the latter surprisingly quickly.

In my second year of medical school a few of us sublet a big house in Brookline, a leafy suburb adjacent to Boston, to set up a commune. Since it was the 1970s and the house had a large basement, one of our friends set up shop there for some chemistry experiments he was doing. He was inspired by the work of a Harvard dropout, Alexander "Sasha" Shulgin, who became the hero of underground organic chemists because of his capacity to synthesize new mind-altering molecules faster than the Drug Enforcement Administration could illegalize them. Our friend used the basement productively to synthesize a variety of chemicals related to MDMA (3,4-methylenedioxymethamphetamine), better known now as ecstasy. It wasn't declared illegal until 1985, so in 1970 to '71, experimenting with it could be viewed as a legitimate part of our medical training; ingesting mind-altering substances once in a while seemed an appropriate extracurricular extension of our pharmacology courses.

The two sides of my split-screen medical school experience in psychopharmacology merged transiently during an elective in neuropharmacology, in which the professor showed us a slide of one MDMA-like molecule and stated that its ingestion by humans produced a state of extreme stress and paranoia that could resemble psychosis. "Not necessarily," I blurted out, but decided not to elaborate. As we'll see below, that substance has shown promise in helping patients with post-traumatic stress disorder, and is today also being studied for the treatment of depression, eating disorders, and end-of-life care as well.

The medical school permitted monthlong rotations to places that offered clinical experiences not readily available at the Harvard teaching hospitals, though most such requests were met with initial skepticism. ("What could any place offer that we don't have here?")

I asked for permission to go to a state mental hospital in Maryland, and it was eventually granted.

Dr. Pahnke: What else happened during the day?

The patient: I died.

Dr. Pahnke: What was that like?

The patient: Beautiful. It sounds vindictive, but it was beautiful.

Dr. Pahnke: How can that be?

The patient: I don't know, I felt like I was dying. . . . I don't know how I came back.

Dr. Pahnke: What does it feel like to die?

The patient: You're just like the thin air, that's it. You have no pain, no fear.

Dr. Pahnke: Did that scare you?

The patient: No. No fear at all, very relaxed. If it's unusual, maybe it's me; I don't know. Is it?

Dr. Pahnke: What?

The patient: Unusual to feel that way?

Dr. Pahnke: That it's relaxed to die? Other people have said the same.

Like many mental institutions, Spring Grove State Hospital in Catonsville, Maryland, was laid out as a series of small buildings scattered across a bucolic campus; it didn't look like the site of some of the world's most important experiments in mind-altering research. I went there to learn about experiments in which doctors were giving LSD to terminal patients to ease their transition from life. My main mentor was Dr. Stanislav Grof, a Czech-born psychiatrist interested in the capacity of those drugs to put people in touch with the unity of all beings and their place in the universe. Some of his key collaborators in that work were Drs. Walter Pahnke and Bill Richards.

One of my jobs at Spring Grove was to review dozens of hours of videotaped LSD sessions with dying patients, to try to learn what could be gleaned from this trove of rare clinical experience. I was first struck by how unremarkable the patients were. They came from no particular walk of life, their religious orientations varied from devout believers in Christianity to no obvious belief at all; none of the interviews I saw was with people interested in Eastern mysticism or the occult. All had terminal cancer that had proven resistant to all available treatments. The LSD sessions themselves were conducted only after patients had undergone several pre-drug therapy sessions to talk about their hopes, fears, and expectations.

In the early 1970s, the idea that the process of dying was something to pay attention to was a novel concept in medicine. Elisabeth Kübler-Ross had published her classic book, *On Death and Dying*, a few years earlier, but dealing with the end of life was still ignored in much of medical education then. If a patient was near death it meant there were no treatments left to try, except pain relief. Paying attention to a patient who was dying—thinking of that word as a verb and not as an adjective—just wasn't something we learned much about. In those days, the most common treatments for cancer were often-lethal radiation, toxic intravenous drugs, or surgery that was sometimes mutilative. We would monitor patients' vital signs and lab tests carefully, but rarely talk with them about the imminent prospect of their death. On rounds, if nothing was working, the visits by the clinical team became shorter and more awkward; sometimes, once it was clear we had little to offer medically, we might pass by the room without entering. If there were any discussions about care, they'd be narrowly linear: Should the doctor attempt to lengthen the patient's life, or perhaps shorten it? In the 1970s, medicine was not yet ready to ask more creative questions or to consider what rights patients had in deciding the shape that their last weeks would take.

Set and Setting

Treatment sessions at Spring Grove were rooted in the core concept of "set and setting"—the patient's expectations about the treatment, and the environment in which it occurred. This concern with the *context* of a drug's use and not merely its pharmacology was based on the key insight that the effect of a psychoactive medication isn't predicted only by its chemical structure, but also by how that chemical interacts with a patient's orientation to it, and the circumstances under which it's given. Unlike medications for cholesterol and blood sugar, the effects of psychoactive drugs can't be totally summed up by chemical data alone. Those issues were to return vividly to center stage in the 2020s in the battle to get MDMA approved by the FDA to treat post-traumatic stress disorder.

The "set and setting" concept was based in part on ingenious experiments by the Columbia social psychologist Stanley Schachter and his student Jerome Singer in the early 1960s, at a time when ethical standards for experiments on humans were looser. In those key studies, they injected volunteers with placebo or with adrenaline, the body's naturally produced substance that causes our fight-or-flight response. Study staff told volunteers they were being given a vitamin; some were told what to expect in terms of side effects, and some were not. The subjects were then put in a room with another supposed subject, who was actually an experimental confederate; the shills were instructed to act in either a euphoric or a hostile manner. The researchers discovered that subjects' perceptions of the effects of the "vitamin" were heavily shaped by what they were told to expect about its effects, and by the mood of their companions as its effects set in.

Based in part on these insights, at Spring Grove the pre- and post-drug therapy sessions became a vital part of the LSD treatments. The preparatory work that Drs. Grof, Pahnke, and Richards provided didn't come from any particular theological orientation: if a patient was a devout Catholic, the therapist would work with that; if the patient was an atheist, the conversation would take a different form. But despite this variable prework, once they were given LSD, patients often reported similar experiences of shedding the burden of their bodies and being reborn into a different level of existence; the experience often left them with insights and equanimity that lasted long after the drug session was over. These findings were common in the early clinical research on psychedelics and are now being rediscovered as this work picks up momentum again today. Many of the patients' experiences reminded me of the contents of *The Tibetan Book of the Dead*, a cult classic of the 1960s that was said to have originally been written as a guide for the soul after the end of life, but was read by many of us as a road map for acid trips.

The names we've given to these drugs say a lot about how we think of them. The few times I heard them mentioned in medical school, they were referred to as "psychotomimetics"—substances that simulated psychosis. Or they might be termed hallucinogens; some acidhead friends criticized the idea that these drugs made you see things that weren't real, arguing that they actually enabled you to see things that were the Most Real of All. A more positive early name was "entheogens." It never caught on, but was appealing because it was based on the idea that there is an internal (*en*) sense of godliness (*theo*) that all of us carry, which can be awakened (*gen*) by these drugs. A term used mostly for MDMA was "empathogen," since it wasn't technically a conventional psychedelic, but seemed to have a special property of generating empathy. (I find the idea that empathy may have a neurochemical correlate to be deeply amazing.) The current term, "psychedelics," combines the roots for mind (*psyche*) and manifestation (*delos*).

I wondered whether the frequent rebirth experiences that patients reported in their psychedelic sessions at Spring Grove represented a rehashing of concepts that had been presented to them in their predrug therapy sessions, or whether they were getting in touch with insights inherent in their own brains. The latter seemed more likely, given the similarity of these accounts historically across cultures and millennia. And if that's so, what might be the place of these medicines in the care of patients facing death? That therapeutic potential was brought home to me powerfully during my month at Spring Grove by a patient whom we'll call Mr. Case, a middle-aged laborer with only a basic education and a fundamentalist Christian belief. He was dying of metastatic lung cancer, and despite all the pre-drug counseling sessions, he seemed to believe that the "treatment" was supposed to manage his pain. The day after his LSD treatment, Dr. Grof asked him to describe what he went through:

> *Mr. Case:* I was in a junkyard. Everything got thrown together: skeletons, cans, whatever. Then everything got burned, destroyed, by a big ball of fire. . . . I felt I was going in it, too. I felt all my bones was in amongst all those other things. Like you said, you had to let it bypass you, or let it know it didn't get the best of you.
>
> *Dr. Grof:* Some of these feelings are new, aren't they? I didn't hear you talking like this before.
>
> *Mr. Case:* This is through this [experience]. This is what I feel through all this other stuff that was going through me . . . that you'll be living, in other words that your soul will be living, your soul will be with you all the time, but yet you don't know what you'll be on the next earth.
>
> *Dr. Grof:* Do you feel that you will live in another form?
>
> *Mr. Case:* I feel that way, yes. . . . I feel I'm living through God, that's the way I'd put it, if you can understand that right.

Another Spring Grove cancer patient was a fifty-one-year-old homeless alcoholic who described his LSD experience this way:

> Now I found myself not as a person but as what I can only describe as my soul or spirit. I was part of everything ugly dirty and filthy. I traveled through intestines, garbage, dung, in an out of the rectum and anything else you can imagine. . . . It seems I became part of everything, good or bad. I didn't think I would ever get out of this. Next, I was going down through a lot of misery and gloom. The further down I went, the worse it got. I was going down something like a black vein [that] got smaller the further down I went. The closer I got to the end of it, the more

afraid I became. I saw a vulture which I took as Death, or the Devil. When I got to the end, I was too terrified to look at it for fear of what I might see. . . .

After seeing all these horrible things, I came up to the beautiful and the wonderful. I continued to go higher, passing among billions and millions of new spirits like myself. I felt a very, very small part of the whole thing. There seemed a small place above and beyond everything else, and I found myself being drawn to this place. After getting to this peak, I found who I thought was God. We were on the same level, looking down at his greatness. Something made me feel he wanted me to exchange positions with him. This I didn't want to do because I felt unworthy. He insisted, so we made the change. It was a wonderful feeling to be there with him, far beyond any of the ambitions of any astronaut—peaceful and wonderful. . . .

I reached my arm toward [Jesus] and I started to rise up to him. As I got closer to him, I began taking on his appearance. Something seemed to be holding me down, but I wanted so much to go to him. I looked down and my body seemed to be tearing apart from my feet up. I kept reaching for him. The closer I got to him, the less there was of me. This was a little terrifying, but I wanted to go to him. Finally, when I got to him, I became him. I was Jesus and he was me. We were one.

I remember thinking, They're never gonna believe this back in Boston.

LSD was the main focus of the work at Spring Grove, but other modalities played peripheral roles. One woman walked around the campus teaching people "toning"—how to chant a particular frequency that was just the right pitch to enable your body/mind to vibrate in tune with the rest of the universe. Then there was the sensory deprivation tank, a small pod filled with warm water in which one could float in complete darkness in order to feel at one with the planet. Of course, a main goal of mine was to access some pharmaceutical-grade hallucinogen to try. The Maryland team still had a supply of Delysid, the trade name of the LSD that the Swiss pharmaceutical maker Sandoz had been making until it stopped production several years earlier. (This was one of the only times I have strongly preferred a branded drug over its generic equivalent.) I wish I could include here my own adventure of hallucinatory oneness with the universe. But all that I can recall happening that day is that I vibrated intensely for several hours, with essentially no cognitive content at all. The miscellaneous homemade compounds I was able to access in Boston were much more satisfying.

Since the Enlightenment, the West has steadily narrowed its view of the broad spectrum of consciousness, focusing on the pure light of science to the exclusion of the more subtle and exotic colors beyond. Rationality has given us penicillin, lasers, and computers in exchange for the kingdom within. Death suffered a parallel disfigurement: we find it hard even to imagine what medieval writers might have meant by *ars moriendi*—the art of dying. The end of life moved from the province of philosophy and theology to that of medicine, and we clinicians can certainly claim better survival rates than our predecessors. What priest could measure up to a well-placed defibrillator, what minister or rabbi or imam could infuse the breath of life with the efficacy of a mechanical ventilator? We can even raise the dead if we get there fast enough. But in the process, we've turned death into what is sometimes just another mass-produced, impersonal commodity controlled by expert technocrat providers rather than by the patient.

Life after LSD

I came back from Spring Grove open to considering a career similar to those of Stan Grof, Bill Richards, or Walter Pahnke—embracing what would surely be the exploding world of psychedelic research. But not long after my return to Boston, a sad truth became evident. Rather than being the vanguard of a new era in mental health, the Spring Grove experiments turned out to be the last dying embers of a field that would soon be completely extinguished. The Maryland team found that their LSD research had been made illegal, and the federal government saw to it that no similar work went on anywhere in the U.S. over the next thirty-five years. It was a victim of the nation's aggressive War on Drugs declared by President Nixon. To me, the ban resembled the medieval Church's ban on the dissection of human bodies, out of its fear that what might be learned was too high a price to pay for delving into the mysteries of the body God had given to man. That set the study of anatomy and physiology back a few centuries.

A wide range of psychoactive substances got caught in the tightening legal dragnet: marijuana, LSD, psilocybin, mescaline, cocaine, heroin—despite the tremendous differences across these products from a pharmacological, clinical, and societal perspective. A darker explanation of Nixon's zeal was that the War on Drugs fulfilled a larger political purpose at a time when the nation was embroiled in an unpopular real war in Vietnam that we were losing. A journalist interviewed John Ehrlichman, Nixon's chief domestic policy adviser, and reported this statement:

> The Nixon campaign in 1968, and the Nixon White House after that, had two enemies: the antiwar left and black people. You understand what I'm saying? We knew we couldn't make it illegal to be either against the war or black, but by getting the public to associate the hippies with marijuana and blacks with heroin, and then criminalizing both heavily, we could disrupt those communities. We could arrest their leaders, raid their homes, break up their meetings, and vilify them night after night on the evening news. Did we know we were lying about the drugs? Of course we did.

Nixon's office taping system recorded this statement he made to his aide Bob Haldeman, three years before that system would precipitate his resignation:

> You know, it's a funny thing: every one of the bastards that are out for legalizing marijuana is Jewish. What the Christ is the mat-

ter with the Jews, Bob, what is the matter with them? I suppose it's because most of them are psychiatrists, you know, there's so many, all the greatest psychiatrists are Jewish.

Thus began decades of insane drug policy in the U.S.

Breaking the Spell

After nearly a half century of prohibition (which worked about as well as when the nation used it to try and stamp out alcohol use in the 1920s), the story did seem to be headed toward a happier ending in the current decade, with the resurgence of research on a wide variety of uses of psychedelic drugs to treat a variety of problems. In the interim, my own practice and research had gone in a different direction—internal medicine rather than psychiatry, and then pharmacoepidemiology and research on the approval, effectiveness, and safety of conventional medications. Then, more than forty years after my stay at Spring Grove, I learned about the renaissance of psychedelic research and saw how its trajectory had come to intersect in some remarkable ways with the seemingly different work I had been doing in the intervening decades.

Rick Doblin, who was only nine years old when Timothy Leary was thrown out of Harvard over his LSD studies, decided early on to commit his life to making it possible for psychedelic research and clinical care to move forward legally. Rick's full vision extended well beyond the decriminalization of marijuana or the funding of controlled clinical trials to study psychedelics in mental illness. His ultimate long-term goal has been nothing less than the transformation of human consciousness and society through the greater availability and widespread use of mind-altering substances of many kinds. To address what? Everything.

Rick realized that such a grand undertaking would have to be approached systematically in well-defined steps. Leary had believed that society would be transformed by millions of people spontaneously turning on with acid, tuning in to some universal cosmic message, and then leaving society as we currently knew it . . . for what, he was less specific. Leary, Ken Kesey, and other psychedelic revolutionaries of the 1960s believed that widespread enlightenment would be best achieved by dosing enormous numbers of people with hallucinogens, sometimes whether they asked for it or not. By contrast, Doblin decided that a useful way to help bring access to psychedelics to America would be to get a doctoral degree in public policy from Harvard's Kennedy School of Government, which he did in 2001. His dissertation was on the regulation of medical uses of psychedelics and marijuana.

In 1986, Rick had founded MAPS, the Multidisciplinary Association for Psychedelic Studies, to be the nonprofit vehicle through which this work could go forward. By the time we met, Rick had pulled off the previously unthinkable accomplishment of getting the Food and Drug Administration to approve a controlled clinical trial in which subjects would be randomly allocated to receive either MDMA or a comparison treatment, to learn whether the drug could be effective in managing PTSD.

When we met, we had much to discuss about my years of work on legal prescription medications: how they are discovered and developed, how we measure their effectiveness and their safety, how that work is supported, who owns the resulting products, how new medicines are evaluated, what FDA requires for approval, how medications are paid for, and how we can measure their cost-effectiveness. These were exactly the issues that were now coming to a head around psychedelics.

Paying for Enlightenment

But what about funding? Running a clinical trial is costly, and the substances that Rick and MAPS were interested in were too old to be patented, eliminating interest from a pharmaceutical company that could own the product and in exchange support the studies needed to win FDA approval. Psychedelic research, which I had always seen as part of the hippie-lefty anti-establishment counterculture, turned out also to be a cherished cause of conservatives, including some on the far right, perhaps because their libertarian values did not condone the government's limiting the menu of chemicals that citizens could ingest. They included Rebekah Mercer, the extreme conservative who was a longtime donor to various ultra-right causes, as well as the children of one of the Koch brothers. Scions of more moderate Republican families were also involved. A young Rockefeller had become interested in the growing psychedelic therapy enterprise as a student at HMS, but died tragically soon thereafter in a plane crash. His family continued to generously support the field to which he had been so committed.

Even if the goal was to make these substances available at cost, somebody would have to pay for the expensive clinical experiments and daunting regulatory advocacy required to pass the necessary legal hurdles at the FDA. Since Doblin had constituted MAPS as a nonprofit, he sought to cover the costs of clinical trials and regulatory combat through philanthropy, and he managed to raise over $140 million to support the research agenda. Those emerging studies were now confronting all the issues my program in DoPE had been working on for years concerning more mundane drugs: approval, safety, cost, ownership, and proper prescribing.

Building a Community

In New England, people interested in the resurgence of this work came together to form the Boston Psychedelic Research Group (BPRG); before Covid, we met in person on Sunday afternoons every few months. Speakers from around the country and the world came to describe their research and experiences: patients who had participated in studies of depression reported how their sessions enabled them to feel normal for the first time in years. We heard about a program that brought ex–Navy SEALs to Mexico for psychedelic care of their PTSD, and a project in the Middle East in which Israelis and Palestinians took ayahuasca together and sang Hebrew and Arabic songs.

At each session Rick would report on the status of MAPS projects: ongoing battles with the FDA on clinical trial design, the difficulty of raising the enormous funds needed to mount those studies, the growing tension between the nonprofit MAPS and the growing number of for-profit companies moving into what was seen as a new psychedelic market that would one day be worth billions of dollars. He described a presentation he had made at Burning Man on the future of the field: "It was the shortest talk I ever gave, maybe because I was totally naked." He recounted his struggles with the FDA to convince them that the approval of MDMA, if and when it happened, would have to require its use with a trained psychedelic therapist. The FDA, working from their standard playbook, wanted that to be a doctor. Rick pointed out that it was more important for therapists to understand psychedelic care, whether or not they were physicians. And some MDs would be useless in that role, even if they had a license to prescribe anything.

At the end of one of the group's meetings, a young woman rushed up to Doblin to show him a photo on her smartphone. He beamed: "How adorable!" he said. "You must be so proud!" "I am!" she replied. A baby? A kitten? I peered over at the image; it showed the mushrooms she had grown at home. Once a drug category comprises substances that people can produce in their own houses, the regulatory landscape changes forever.

More formal clinical research on psychedelic drugs was now proceeding globally on several fronts at respected institutions including Johns Hopkins, New York University and, eventually, Harvard. Some reports of clinical benefits were starting to appear in peer-reviewed medical journals. The psychedelics would now have to address questions similar to the ones we've considered above for every other drug on the market—and a few unique ones. With the guidance of an all-star science team and the backing of his affluent financial supporters, Rick and his colleagues had designed a study of MDMA to treat PTSD intended to meet the stringent criteria of a typical controlled clinical trial submitted to the FDA. If successful, this would be a major milestone on the road toward making these substances widely available for clinical use.

But MDMA wasn't like any other drug. Because set and setting were so important, Rick felt strongly that psychotherapy would have to be an essential part of the whole treatment, including preparatory sessions, accompaniment of patients during their three drug sessions, and then consolidation sessions afterward to process the insights and help the patient use them to manage their symptoms later on—just as in the Spring Grove LSD sessions I had observed.

In a trial submitted for FDA approval, patients with moderate or severe PTSD were to be randomized to MDMA or placebo treatment, and also undergo the same number and intensity of psychotherapy sessions—even though we've seen how the agency sometimes gives pharmaceutical companies a pass on such rigorous comparisons for less controversial drugs. Such randomization and blinding are easy for cholesterol pills, nearly impossible for psychedelics. At best, as we've seen, neither the patient nor the doctor should know which treatment was administered, to avoid the well-understood problem of placebo effect. This is even more important when the outcome studied involves mental health, whether it is crippling anxiety or the terror that can come with confronting death. But it's far more difficult here.

From the outset, it was clear there could be problems with the ideal double-blind placebo-controlled concept. If study subjects experienced being hurled into the fiery pit of hell, or saw the colors of the music they were listening to, or met God, they'd probably suspect they had been administered the real thing. (Interestingly, a few trial subjects did report having mystical experiences even though they were in the placebo group.) And any therapist working with them during those sessions would be very likely to know which group the patient was in.

Might the answer be an active placebo, a comparison drug that produced some noticeable effect to which patients could be randomized without their knowing which group they were in? Some early studies used a "body" drug that had no known psychoactive properties, but caused a slightly elevated heart rate, skin tingling, and occasionally itching—reminiscent of those early Schachter and Singer experiments. Others considered using a far-lower dose of the active drug for the control group, given at a level unlikely to produce any therapeutic effect, that would not be mistaken for a mere sugar pill. That seemed like a good idea until it turned out that for many subjects, the cardiovascular effects and fuzzy-headedness that low-dose MDMA can cause might actually be dysphoric—that is, create a feeling of malaise that could put the full dose MDMA treatment into an unfairly favorable light in comparison.

In close consultation with the FDA, the study team decided to go with a conventional dummy placebo. Assessing the severity of a patient's PTSD symptoms would be done with a standard widely used scale administered by a rater who didn't know which group a patient had been assigned to. As for blinding of the subjects and therapists, they wouldn't be told which group they were in—but we've seen the obvious limitations of that approach.

By early 2020, members of the PTSD research team had a growing sense of optimism that things would go well in the trial. Even isolated examples of improvement in patients who had been crippled for years by their affliction seemed compelling—not good enough evidence by itself to warrant approval, of course, but encouraging. When the data were unblinded, the results seemed to show convincingly that the new treatment worked.

The possible success of the PTSD trial brought into sharper focus the difference between the groups working on the nonprofit testing and dissemination of psychedelic therapy, versus the groups with a commercially oriented for-profit orientation. But even the latter groups didn't resemble Merck or Pfizer. Some saw the for-profit corporate model as a necessary evil, a means to an end for underwriting the very high cost of clinical trials without having to rely on charitable contributions. Others saw it differently. Cannabis had recently morphed from the illegal fuzzy sacrament of the 1960s counterculture to one of the hottest new investments of the early 2000s, with successful new companies springing up around the world and new exchange-traded funds with ticker symbols like TOKE, WEED, and YOLO making it possible to invest in groups of these stocks.

For those like Doblin on one end of this commercial spectrum, promoting greater access to psychedelics was a vital step in transforming human consciousness. For those on the other end, with estimates of the future worth of the psychedelic industry ranging into ten figures, it was just another hot new start-up idea, like internet-linked exercise bikes or a novel dating app. Unlike new drugs for obesity or cancer, some of these were compounds you could grow yourself or any smart chemistry major could synthesize. Drugs like peyote, psilocybin, mescaline, and ayahuasca were plant-based ingredients that Indigenous people had been cultivating and using for millennia. How would that mesh with the approach that for-profit drug companies were accustomed to? For some, the answer was the same one that pharma companies had used for years—make small tweaks to the molecule so the Patent Office would consider it a brand-new substance and grant it years of market exclusivity. That would entice investors to invest in a company that could control the new substance, charge whatever they wanted for it, market it aggressively, and provide the millions of dollars needed to mount the clinical trials needed to gain FDA approval and the patent monopoly that would come with it. Would the new drug work better than the existing substances? Maybe, maybe not. But you could *own* it.

Impending Success?

By the end of 2020 and leading into 2021, anecdotal reports within the MDMA-PTSD study community kept suggesting that things were looking good. Even with a smaller than required study sample necessitated by the intrusion of Covid, the results still seemed to show that MDMA had an impressive effect in treating PTSD. Anecdotal evidence of long-tormented patients who started to feel dramatically better were impressive, but, of course, not the stuff of rigorous randomized trial results. Another question arose: Would the FDA approve just the molecule, or the molecule-plus therapy combination that was so central to its effectiveness?

Then would come the economics questions, very similar to the ones we've considered earlier. If the drug entered the medical marketplace, what would be its selling price and its cost-effectiveness? What benefit would be obtained at what expense? The molecule had first been synthesized decades earlier and was a pretty simple structure that an adept entry-level chemist could concoct without too much difficulty—as we learned in the basement of our commune back in my medical student days. In fact, Rick had told me during one of our first conversations that he had a large white block of pure MDMA he had been given many years earlier; in principle, he could have shaved some powder off it as needed, weighed it carefully, and used that for the research. But understandably the FDA expected a very different approach, with the drug synthesized under rigorous conditions that met standards of GMP, or good manufacturing practices. This necessary step consumed months of additional work, and hundreds of thousands of dollars.

Making the drug to government standards was only a small part of the cost of the treatments. How would the expense of the vital preparatory and follow-up psychotherapy be folded into the price of the medicine? This was a new kind of drug-cost problem, and answering the "Does it work?" question would be intimately linked to that. Would the FDA approve just the chemical, or the chemical only in combination with psychedelic psychotherapy? And would the mandated therapy have to be provided by MDs, or not? Or by people with special training in guiding experiences like these? Who would certify that? MAPS? Would that be another kind of monopoly?

It wasn't just about the molecule anymore.

Although Doblin hoped for a day when these substances could be freely available to people for many purposes, the last thing he wanted at this stage was to enable any physician in the U.S. to hand a patient a prescription for MDMA, maybe suggest that they bone up on some Buddhism and take it with a friend around, and leave it at that. The predictable horror stories that would ensue could set the entire field back even further than Timothy Leary had.

A great deal of evidence had accumulated that by following clear protocols, non-physicians could prescribe some medications at least as well as MDs, including antibiotics, drugs for diabetes and hypertension, even opioids. In many states, a defined set of drugs can be prescribed by nurses, pharmacists, and other health-care professionals. And for psychedelics, it was clear that many doctors, including psychiatrists, had no clue how to use them appropriately. How could they? At the same time, thousands of successful underground psychedelic sessions were being conducted by non-physician psychologists, social workers, and experienced guides who had no formal clinical credentials at all. How would FDA regulate *that?*

What's the Price of Sanity?

An FDA-mandated combination of pills and skills would heavily impact the cost of MDMA use—something that would have to be addressed by payers after the hoped-for government approval. The chemical would cost pennies to produce, but the super-specialized therapy would be much more costly. Increasingly, insurers in and outside of government were demanding assessment of the cost-effectiveness of drugs (see chapter 13). If MDMA worked in this setting, how to put an economic value on being freed of PTSD versus being crippled by it?

The decision on mandated therapy sessions would be a key driver of whether the treatment would be seen as cost-effective by insurance companies. Rick knew of my interest in the cost-effectiveness of medications, and asked me to help his colleagues think about such analyses in the MDMA-PTSD case. Both the cost part and the effectiveness would be a challenge to quantify: the former would have everything to do with the credentialing of treatment guides, and the length and number of sessions with the patient. The latter posed an even thornier challenge. The problem reminded me of an editorial I was asked to write for the journal *Circulation* when new blood thinners like Eliquis were being introduced into practice; they were expensive, but also seemed to work better than the existing treatment. I titled it "Cost-Effectiveness Analysis of the New Anticoagulants: Simple, Except for the Cost and Effectiveness Parts." Same problem here.

Sure, some things could be measured easily, like days lost from work, the cost of mental health services consumed or averted, life-years lost in patients who committed suicide, the cost of hospital care for what is sometimes (and horribly) called "incomplete suicides," and so forth. But so much of the tragedy of severe chronic PTSD manifests as daily misery, fear of engaging in everyday activities, the pervasive and often overwhelming sense that one's life truly sucks—even if none of these feelings ever leads to a suicide attempt or mental hospitalization. If MDMA could alleviate that, it would be vital to measure it. But how? I provided some "quality of life" input to a cost-effectiveness researcher who was making a brave attempt to get these numbers on paper pending the drug's approval, for all the insurers who would want to see them before deciding whether and how much to pay for these treatments if they were ever approved. It's an evolving science.

More Clinical Trial Challenges

The design and implementation of the MDMA-PTSD clinical trial ended up presenting daunting difficulties. Paradoxically, the drug had been granted special "breakthrough" status by the FDA, meaning that it held promise as an effective new approach to a condition that had few good treatment options. At the same time, it remained on the government's list of Class I substances, a designation reserved for illegal drugs like heroin that were seen as having no legitimate medical use. Many of the issues that came up in the trial were extreme versions of concerns we've considered above for more conventional medications:

- Does it work?
- What does "work" mean in this context, anyway?
- How to accomplish double-blinding if subjects in one group are given a drug that produces a dramatic mind-altering experience, and the control group is randomized to placebo?
- Even if the corporation that funds and conducts the study is a nonprofit, how can the reported findings be insulated from its enthusiasm about the product?

- How to define and standardize the psychotherapy sessions that precede, accompany, and follow the MDMA sessions, since they are such an integral part of the treatment?
- If the drug-plus-therapy regimen is approved, how would the therapy part be regulated?
- What adverse events should be monitored? Aside from the obvious ones, like cardiac problems, should euphoria be counted as a potentially problematic side effect? (This turned out to be a bigger issue than you'd expect.)

Rick Doblin and his colleagues at MAPS worked closely with FDA officials and some of the nation's most respected names in psychiatric research to try and address these issues. The study's lead investigator was Jennifer Mitchell, a professor in the departments of neurology and psychiatry and behavioral sciences at the University of California, San Francisco. Since MDMA-based care is an art as well as a science, the trial had to recruit psychotherapists with MDMA experience, which, of course, is still illegal, requiring the team to identify clinicians and patients in multiple countries. Part of the study had to be conducted in the midst of the Covid pandemic, making enrollment even more difficult. In the end, for its main study the team screened 324 people and identified 121 who had long-standing severe or moderate PTSD; most had failed all previous attempts at treatment. Consenting subjects were randomized to receive MDMA plus psychotherapy, or placebo plus psychotherapy. MAPS put the manual for its eclectic psychotherapy component on its website for anyone to use at no cost.

During 2022 and 2023, at the periodic BPRG meetings—now mostly on Zoom—we'd continue to hear success stories—patients who had been crippled by PTSD for years following sexual assault, military service, or childhood abuse and were now dramatically better. But encouraging anecdotes are still anecdotes. Though the intensive psychotherapy sessions on their own probably did some good, it was no surprise which treatment many of the most improved patients had received. After their three drug sessions, the severity of subjects' PTSD was evaluated as planned by a blinded evaluator using the field's most widely used rating scale. When the data were tabulated, the subjects randomized to get MDMA and psychotherapy appeared to do much better than those randomized to placebo plus psychotherapy. The difference was becoming significant both clinically and statistically, and seemed to show an effect much greater than that achieved previously by the most commonly used drug treatment, SSRI antidepressants. Professor Mitchell and the team published the results in the respected journal *Nature Medicine* in September 2023. It was the most compelling randomized trial of any psychedelic drug ever performed, and it seemed likely to launch not just MDMA but the whole category into the medical mainstream. All those years of effort seemed likely to vindicate Doblin's four-decade campaign to make these medications available to the world as a proven component of medical care.

As this was moving ahead, Rick gave one of his periodic Zoom updates to the BPRG group. He was not his usually ebullient self as he announced that the nonprofit MAPS was spinning off its clinical development work to a rebranded entity that would be named Lykos Therapeutics. (That's Greek for "wolf.") As a public benefit corporation, Lykos could earn a profit, but was not legally required to maximize return to shareholders the way that conventional corporations were (see golems, page 85).

Despite his prodigious success in raising philanthropic funding, Rick sadly explained to the group that more money would be needed to conduct the costly clinical trials that FDA approval and commercialization of the drug would ultimately require. Lykos would be the official sponsor to bring the trial findings to the FDA for approval. Rick stepped aside as leader of that effort, but remained a member of the Lykos board. In early January 2024, Lykos announced that it had succeeded in obtaining over $100 million in an oversubscribed round of Series A funding.

A Near-Death Experience

Then, within a few months everything started to unravel. At several BPRG meetings, I had witnessed the evangelistic enthusiasm of many

MDMA practitioners about the benefits this radically new approach could provide to people suffering intensely from mental illness. But as the clinical trial evidence was pored over by the FDA and the scientific community following publication of the paper in *Nature Medicine*, charges emerged that the zeal of some researchers may have created pressure to misinterpret or underreport negative developments. One harsh critic put it bluntly: "MAPS is an MDMA therapy cult." In March 2024 the normally dispassionate Institute for Clinical and Economic Review issued a draft report expressing "substantial concerns about the validity of the results" of the MAPS-supported PTSD research. Part of the concern was based on the "functional unblinding" that resulted because subjects were usually aware of whether they had gotten MDMA or a sugar pill, even though that would have been hard to prevent. Worse, other aspects of data handling seemed to range from amateurish to allegedly deceptive. An ICER colleague told me that even after years of argumentative discussions of many high-profile new drugs, the hearing about MDMA "was the most contentious meeting we've ever had." Separately, other reports related charges of alleged "boundary-crossing" interactions between therapists and patients.

In late April, the FDA received a citizen petition with over seventy signatories representing former MAPS/Lykos employees, study subjects, clinicians, researchers, and others charging that "evidence from multiple sources indicates that the sponsor has engaged in a pattern of systematic and deliberate omission of adverse events from the public record while minimizing documented harms." Others depicted what might charitably be called a cavalier approach to data capture and analysis. The citizen petition concluded with a warning that seemed calculated to strike fear into the heart of FDA officials considering approval of the drug:

> The FDA must take action to ensure that this does not amount to another regulatory scandal like the opioid crisis, where widespread harm retroactively illuminated substantial regulatory failures. If the FDA again prioritizes industry interests over public health, the outcome could mirror the trajectory of OxyCon-

> tin, which was also once promoted as a wonder drug offering relief from chronic suffering. If an unsafe therapeutic adjunct is sanctioned by the FDA, the resulting harm could result in corrective restrictions that ultimately limit MDMA's potential utility as a therapeutic.

The reference to opioids had another dimension: the FDA had instructed MAPS/Lykos to track feelings of euphoria experienced by patients in both groups, so it could monitor the risk that MDMA might prove so enjoyable that it could pose a risk of overuse after the trial ended; that explains the agency's definition of euphoria as an adverse effect. Unfortunately, this requirement was not communicated to the study staff promptly or clearly, and was ignored in many instances. That was one of several bad rookie mistakes—when the FDA tells you to monitor something in a preapproval trial, you'd better do it.

By the time the FDA advisory committee met in early June, the prognosis had turned from optimistic to anxious. Despite the impressive data in Professor Mitchell's peer-reviewed journal report, and apart from the striking anecdotes of remarkable improvement that clinicians had reported, too many negatives were piling up: the missing data, the stories of patients encouraged to report positive results and downplay negative ones to help make this new treatment widely available, the flouting of the FDA's requirement to track euphoria as a potential risk, less-than-rigorous data handling at some study sites, the allegations of isolated irregular relationships between therapists and patients during treatment. The benefit-risk balance for the agency seemed to shift over approving a party drug whose chemical name ended in "-amphetamine" to treat severe mental illness. It all was beginning to look too problematic for the committee to endorse.

There was also the complicated regulatory issue posed by the other component of the treatment. MAPS/Lykos was deeply committed to the idea that the medication be given along with a meaningful psychotherapy engagement, but how would that work if the combined treatment were approved? Would these have to be MAPS-certified psychedelic counselors? Would these people have to be physicians, the usual intermediaries the FDA empowered to use approved treatments? Or others? The agency had expertise in regulating drugs, not psychotherapy.

A Downward Spiral

By the time the advisory committee voted, the concerns had piled up, diminishing the hope that this could be the first impressive treatment for PTSD cleared by the FDA. By a vote of 10–1, the outside committee recommended against approving MDMA for the treatment of PTSD, citing the irregularities it saw in the conduct of the key trials. The FDA did indeed follow that advice when it made its final determination in August, declaring that the evidence Lykos had submitted was not sufficient to warrant approval. It detailed its concerns in what is known as a "Complete Response Letter." Despite its positive-sounding title, that's the name for the document the FDA sends to a drug's sponsor when it rejects a new application. In keeping with its policy and apparently in deference to a drug sponsor's ownership of its own trial data, the FDA doesn't disclose the contents of such Complete Response Letters to the public—not a great way to move science forward.

The reasons for the rejection were thought to be similar to those that had been cited in the ICER review and during the dismal advisory committee hearing. Doblin felt betrayed by the agency: it had given MDMA "breakthrough" status as a drug that had important potential to meet a serious unmet medical need; that meant that the FDA was supposed to work closely with the sponsor on the trial design, providing the study team with ongoing "special protocol assessment" consultation to review all aspects of the research—including the obvious and predictable problem of double-blinding with a drug like ecstasy. Why hadn't the regulators expressed more concern about this key issue much earlier? Rick accused the FDA of "changing the goalposts" to make approval harder even after its criteria had been agreed upon.

I found myself thinking about other goalpost-moving decisions the agency had made in the opposite direction, to make approvals easier. There were many: switching the ineffective Alzheimer's treatment Aduhelm to an accelerated approval pathway once it failed to show a convincing clinical benefit; accepting a gene therapy for muscular dystrophy even after it flunked its main agreed-upon patient outcome measure; requiring an advisory committee to come back a second time to approve an ineffective drug for ALS after the committee had rejected it. As for the magnitude of the drug's benefit, we've seen how the FDA had spent years greenlighting drugs for cancer on the basis of surrogate measures like imaging changes that were never followed up with concrete proof of patient benefit. What about the "functional un-blinding" of clinicians and patients as to who got which treatment? A concern, of course, but one that may have been impossible to avoid here—and that should have been clear from the outset. But it didn't pose a problem for any of the three intravenous Alzheimer's drugs, each of which caused infusion reactions in about a quarter of patients; wouldn't that have been a clue as to who was in the treatment or placebo group? And data from PORTAL and other groups made clear that the agency had long become comfortable dispensing with the need for concurrent control groups in assessments of new drugs for cancer and other hard-to-treat conditions.

I recalled other drugs whose sponsors hid important side effects (antidepressants in children), used differential follow-up to make a product look better than it was (Celebrex and Vioxx), and suppressed trial results they didn't like (most of the SSRI antidepressants), letting a company's goals—generally commercial rather than countercultural—skew the evidence about a treatment's clinical worth. As for the magnitude of the supposed effect, if the MDMA trial data were to be believed (and unfortunately that had become a very big if), its effectiveness seemed at least as impressive as that of the new Alzheimer's drugs, or Johnson & Johnson's nose-spray antidepressant, for which the sponsor and the agency had to do some data-dredging to find studies impressive enough to warrant approval.

Clearly, there were substantial problems with many important aspects of the MAPS/Lykos trial of MDMA as it was implemented;

these would likely have been disqualifying in their own right, despite any altruistic motivation that may have driven them. If we're going to get things right in measuring the safety and effectiveness of any drug, the research has to be done carefully—even obsessively—and without bias or sloppiness.

It became apparent after the decision that the FDA would now require new clinical trials to address all of these issues, which would take several years and cost many more millions of dollars. A key unresolved question going forward would come back to the old "set and setting" question. Would future applications ask the FDA to approve MDMA simply as a chemical compound, or in combination with psychotherapy to potentiate its benefit? The latter had been a key aspect of the MAPS/Lykos approach, but dealing with that had been difficult for an agency accustomed to regulating chemicals, not counseling.

The week that followed the FDA rejection was a painful one for MDMA advocates. Lykos laid off three-quarters of its staff, and Rick Doblin left his position on its board. Its parent organization MAPS let go a third of its own staff. Lykos brought on the former Johnson & Johnson executive who had spearheaded the company's nose-spray antidepressant. Three papers that included MAPS-affiliated authors, including Doblin, were retracted by the journal *Psychopharmacology* because they contained data from a study site in Canada where accusations had been made of sexual misconduct connected to its MDMA research—a problem the authors had not disclosed to the journal. (These data appeared to be separate from the Phase III clinical trial reports submitted to the FDA.)

With official approval of MDMA now years off at best, people suffering from severe PTSD and other psychiatric symptoms who wanted to access it would have to seek such help elsewhere—and there were no great alternatives. Many patients expressed anguish similar to what we saw decades earlier when AIDS activists and cancer patients argued that the FDA was coming between them and the drugs that might save their lives. State referenda were introduced in Massachusetts, California, and Colorado to facilitate access to a variety of banned psychedelic substances. A 2024 Massachusetts ballot initiative would have allowed people to grow their own naturally occurring psychedelics like psilocybin and mescaline, but that wouldn't cover the synthetic MDMA. The "natural psychedelics" would be de-criminalized, with their purchase and supervised use permitted at licensed facilities, potentially setting up a framework for access to some of these drugs even in the absence of FDA approval. Details of the plan would be fleshed out by a to-be-named panel of mental health professionals and consumers. The measure lost, 57 percent to 43 percent. Colorado and Oregon had previously decriminalized some of these drugs, with varying results. I found myself rethinking the virtues of the "right to try" position, and in an unaccustomed way, seeing its merits compared to the "FDA knows best" side of the argument.

Underground clinical use of MDMA and other banned substances continues to proliferate, often with the help of effective but unregulated therapists. Perhaps some informal community rating service will emerge to evaluate these people, sort of like a mental health TripAdvisor. While facilitating use of these medicines still brings with it the risk of federal criminal penalties, if states step in to create safe spaces in which these drugs can be used legally, the riskiness of that possibility could recede. (In addition to Colorado's permissive laws, the city of Denver has ruled that enforcement of regulations banning such use has been relegated to its lowest priority level.)

During the same summer that the MAPS/Lykos research on MDMA was heading for a cliff, across the Atlantic the Dutch Committee on MDMA presented its own lengthy report, "MDMA: Beyond Ecstasy" to that nation's Minister of Medical Care. It noted that the Netherlands had one of the world's highest rates of ecstasy use (about 4 percent of the population) but did not have a problem of abuse. It concluded that the drug did seem to be clinically useful for people with PTSD, and expressed concern over the severity of their suffering and their lack of good treatment options. Since it was unlikely that any regulatory body in the Netherlands or Europe would approve MDMA in the foreseeable future, the committee recommended that it be administered unofficially by qualified therapists in specialized settings, with the nation's mental health professionals providing guidance about its appropriate use. Results would be monitored by observational research studies.

What a sane country.

As the MAPS-MDMA drug approval process unraveled, I felt terrible for Rick Doblin, who in the 1980s committed his career to bringing psychedelics into the mainstream of American health care and everyday life, with a goal of nothing less than transforming human consciousness. After all those years of tireless fundraising and advocacy for his nonprofit, it turned out that the challenges and cost of bringing this new drug to market might not be a match for the best intentions, smartest advisers, and most generous philanthropic support. For this simple, decades-old, unpatentable molecule that now had a checkered regulatory history, how many new investors would seek to make it widely available and affordable, especially if they wouldn't be able to later cash in on a government-granted monopoly if the drug were approved? Still, the pioneering path that MAPS opened is now being trod by many other groups around the world studying a growing variety of mind-expanding substances. The for-profit company Compass Pathways was making headway on its clinical trials of the proprietary (and therefore patentable) version of psilocybin it had created, for which it was seeking formal approval. As venture capitalists like to say, it's often the second mouse that gets the cheese.

The MDMA-PTSD controversies certainly will not mean the end of the new modern era of psychedelic research; there's now just too much evidence out there that these chemicals are the best thing to come along in psychopharmacology in generations. In their methodological missteps, the MAPS/Lykos studies will provide a vital lesson for all future research in this complex and demanding area, which will be the better for it. Many of us who've gotten a glimpse of the alternative reality these drugs reveal understand that this isn't a vision you can choose to unsee. I expect that eventually MDMA and other psychedelics will be accepted treatments for the crippling illness of

PTSD as well as many other conditions, but this episode was a big setback.

The federal government isn't likely to support this potentially controversial research itself, even though it spent millions on funding late-stage clinical studies of less controversial treatments, like the trials that helped bring the Covid vaccine and hepatitis C cures to market. Despite the major setback for MDMA, the movement is probably unstoppable. As those dying patients at Spring Grove taught me in the 1970s, sometimes it takes a near-death experience to help you get on with your life.

The indefatigable sense of optimism in the subculture of psychedelic research provided a bittersweet reminder of the similar sense of enthusiasm I first felt in Maryland as a medical student, right before the government shut all that research down. It's poignant to reflect that apart from a few modern studies that put people into MRI scanners while they're tripping, all the clinical research that is now going on could have been performed with technology that was available in the 1970s—or, for that matter, as early as the 1940s, when a Swiss chemist first synthesized LSD—or a thousand years ago, when Indigenous people routinely used mind-altering substances like ayahuasca or peyote or psilocybin. We can only wonder how much more we would know today, and how much more human suffering could have been alleviated, if we had been able to avoid those long years of mindless prohibition.

CHAPTER 20

Pain, Killers

Despite the color and high drama of the psychedelics, opioids are the drug group that has had the most widespread societal impact over the last thirty years. Those continuing effects are rooted in the very same dimensions discussed in the first part of the book: we got it wrong in assessing their effectiveness, we got it wrong in predicting their risks, we fell victim to distorted messaging that was designed to increase product sales rather than communicate the truth, and we wasted billions of dollars on overpriced prescriptions that were more hazardous than their manufacturers would admit. These mistakes built on one another to give the U.S. the highest per capita level of prescribed opioid use in the world, the worst rate of overdose deaths, and enormous expenditures to address a problem of our own creation—one that we still can't fix. For people suffering from addiction, opioids are dangerous because they get into your head, cloud your thinking, and cause you to make bad decisions. That is exactly what their manufacturers did to the FDA, to clinicians, and ultimately to patients. Rethinking each of these mistakes can help clarify what we can do about the problem now.

How We Got Efficacy Wrong

Opioids are truly great analgesics, as anyone who has had to take them for severe short-term pain know. Because of their fearsome addictive potential, we try to reserve their use for major conditions like broken bones or significant surgery. But that's a limited commercial market. As is now widely known, to pave the way for their more extensive use the manufacturer of OxyContin, Purdue Pharma, had to accomplish several goals: persuade doctors that it's fine to use it for smaller self-limited problems like sprained ankles and for long-lasting conditions like low back pain, and it's not really that addictive. I became immersed in the surprising shortfall in our knowledge about these drugs during the opioid epidemic, when my colleagues and I at Alosa were developing our educational materials to help doctors care for pain better without relying so much on addictive drugs. Committed to actual evidence rather than hype or conventional wisdom, I asked our lead physician on this work, Brian Bateman, to review all the published clinical trials of chronic pain treatments, to see how other medications stacked up against narcotics. He spent hours searching the medical literature and came back with the reply "There just aren't any good long-term trials out there on that." How could this be? Chronic pain is one of the most common problems we have faced in medicine for thousands of years, and the drugs we use to treat it have been around for decades (e.g., the NSAIDs), or over a century (aspirin), or even millennia (e.g., the opioids). No one had studied this? But the FDA had authorized OxyContin for use in chronic pain, and its manufacturer was hyping that to the skies. How did that happen?

As we've seen, with thousands of drugs on the market we doctors rely on FDA approval and the facts described in its official labeling documents to guide our prescribing—just as that wording also defines what a company can and can't say in its promotion. The FDA laid the groundwork for our epidemic of overuse by endorsing the claim that addictive drugs like OxyContin are suitable to treat chronic pain, even though there were no long-term trials to show whether this was true. The approval of that use opened the door wide for Purdue's sales force to market Oxy to doctors for that lucrative purpose. Years later, as the enormity of this overuse was becoming clear, several groups representing patients who had become addicted to prescription opioids asked the FDA to rescind its authorization for chronic use, which would have belatedly helped limit the ability of Purdue and other pharmaceutical companies to make those claims. The FDA refused, and instead approved a Purdue-generated statement that the drug could be used "for the management of moderate to severe pain when a continuous, around the clock analgesic is needed for an extended period of time." That sure sounds like a recommendation for chronic use to me. Former FDA commissioner David Kessler described the label change as a "blank check" for the company to overpromote its use; opioid researcher Andrew Kolodny called the agency's decision-making on this "the worst medical regulatory failure in U.S. history."

Because the FDA didn't require it, hardly any large-scale clinical trial studies were done on how well these drugs work with extended use. In earlier chapters we've heard companies lament how hard it is to do studies of rarely used drugs that treat unusual conditions. But long-lasting pain is one of the most common conditions in all of medicine, and opioids have been the most widely used drugs to treat it: this was no orphan disease problem. If the FDA had required such studies before giving Purdue permission to advertise this profitable use, that research would have been done. But it didn't, so it wasn't.

That was another consequence of letting manufacturers define the clinical research agenda rather than funding the studies patients and doctors most need. Researchers at Johns Hopkins reviewed the clinical trial evidence on opioids submitted to the FDA *after* the approval of OxyContin and found the agency and the industry hadn't learned their lesson—the median duration of more recent studies of "chronic" pain was under three months. That doesn't look like the profile of the long-term pain patients I've cared for.

At Alosa, we kept searching each year as we continuously updated our materials. It wasn't until 2018 that we found the first large randomized trial addressing the question. It was conducted by doctors at the Veterans Health Administration, who apparently were as frustrated as we were about the lack of solid evidence on this question. They had the particular burden of having to treat thousands of veterans with chronic pain like Mike Humeston, whom we met in connection with Vioxx. Worse, unlike Mike many vets had also developed addiction problems from their prescribed drugs. Published in *JAMA*, the landmark study was called the SPACE trial, for "Strategies for Prescribing Analgesics—Comparative Effectiveness," and was funded by the VA itself. The researchers randomly allocated

240 vets with chronic hip, knee, or back pain to take either opioids or NSAIDs like Advil plus acetaminophen (Tylenol). After twelve months, pain relief was significantly *better* in the non-opioid group, and adverse drug effects were significantly *worse* in the opioid group. The better relief in the NSAID group wasn't a surprise; in addition to controlling pain, those drugs also reduce inflammation, a key component of many kinds of pain.

Instead of 2018, it would have been good to have had these study results in 2008, or 1998, or 1988, or any decade at all before that. As a prescriber, I certainly would have wanted to see those results back then. Even before there were NSAIDs, the same sort of trial could have been conducted at any point since the early 1900s, when aspirin came into widespread use.

How We Got Safety Wrong

In late 2023, the FDA published a self-serving sixty-page timeline defending all its activities related to "substance use." On the first page it described its 1995 approval of OxyContin, parroting the manufacturer's incorrect claim of its reduced potential for misuse:

> At the time of approval, FDA believed the controlled-release formulation of OxyContin would result in less abuse potential, since the drug would be absorbed slowly and there would not be an immediate "rush" or high that would promote abuse.

Even though precisely the opposite turned out to be true, the agency also let the company put that bogus concept into its official label, allowing it to promote the idea widely, stating without much compelling evidence that delayed absorption was "believed to reduce the abuse liability." To the contrary, the high doses of oxycodone packed into OxyContin's patented "time-release capsules" made it much easier to just crush them in a liquid and inject it, for a high similar to that provided by heroin. Purdue's formulation actually made the drug *easier* to misuse. But the drugmaker still had to get doctors over the time-honored concern, based on more than a century of clinical observation, that opioids were habit-forming; that required undoing our understanding of their risks. This assault on the evidence was so well crafted that it must have been based on carefully conducted focus groups with scores of clinicians to get into prescribers' heads, understand our concerns, and get around them.

The FDA could have readily learned about the emerging overuse as the opioid epidemic was gaining steam by looking at large databases of actual prescribing patterns and outcomes, the approach taken for years by my DoPE research group and by several other groups around the country (see chapter 9). It could have used these databases to track how much the drug was being prescribed for what purposes, how long people were taking it, how many of them had medical complications like overdose and death, and so forth. But the FDA was not then into doing that kind of post-approval population surveillance, and didn't see it as part of their job. It was weak on looking at patterns of use and outcomes once a drug was on the market, remaining fixated on the randomized controlled trials submitted by manufacturers to win approval, even though it sometimes didn't require randomization or control groups for those studies, or dispensed with the need for data altogether, as it did here.

How We Got Communication Wrong

Like other prescribers, by the mid-1990s I was being taught about a new public health threat most of us hadn't heard about before: the massive undertreatment of pain in America. Papers, opinion pieces, and guidelines began to appear in medical journals explaining that American physicians were badly under-medicating pain. The messages were patterned after warnings about other undiagnosed and undertreated medical problems we were neglecting: high blood pressure, elevated cholesterol, osteoporosis. Once we were sensitized to those issues, we learned that we could make new diagnoses and prescribe medicines designed to help our patients. The "undertreated pain" movement touched every corner of health care. On every office encounter and at each visit with a hospitalized patient, we were told that pain was so important that we had to think of it as "the fifth vital sign," along with blood pressure, temperature, pulse, and respiratory rate. Experts at the American Pain Society advocated for that approach, and even copyrighted the term "Pain: The 5th Vital Sign." We did not know at the time that the society was receiving a million dollars from Purdue, or that key members of their leadership were also well paid consultants to the company, or that the doctor who chaired the society's committee advocating more opioid use would later join Purdue to become its vice president for health policy.

A now-ubiquitous smiley face/frowning face infographic began to appear in every exam room so we could point to it and ask patients on every encounter what their level of pain was, from none to "the worst pain ever." Overenthusiastic health assistants asked about it even if the patient was just in for a blood pressure check. More attention to the new fifth vital sign was encouraged by the powerful Joint Commission on the Accreditation of Hospitals, which we later learned was receiving grants from Purdue to educate health-care professionals about pain care. The powerful American Hospital Association decreed that adequate management of pain would henceforth be a key quality measure and encouraged the use of the pictograms in routine encounters. The goal seemed to be for every patient to be virtually pain-free all the time. If they weren't, the implication was, we weren't doing our jobs right. And, of course, the modern way to manage pain of all kinds was to be less hung up by old-fashioned worries about the opioids and use them far more liberally, since it turned out they were much safer and risk-free than we had been taught!

Pressed for even a shred of evidence that opioids are not very habit-forming, spokespeople and sales reps would refer to "the Jick paper in the *New England Journal of Medicine*," which purportedly had shown that addiction was really very uncommon in patients given opioids. It was a study, we were told, of large numbers of people taking these drugs for pain, and it had documented that hardly any of them had a problem getting off them. That sounded pretty good unless you actually read "the Jick paper." Hershel Jick worked in the early days of pharmacoepidemiology running a project called the Boston Collaborative Drug Surveillance Program. He would send nurses to hospitals to collect information on what inpatients were taking and what adverse effects they were experiencing. Much of his work was funded by the pharmaceutical industry. It turned out that his "study" was not really a paper at all. It was merely a one-paragraph, five-sentence, non-peer-reviewed letter to the editor of *NEJM* in 1980 titled "Addiction Rare in Patients Treated with Narcotics." In it, he and a colleague reported that in reviewing their files of patients who were given opioids while hospitalized, they didn't find much documentation that many had become addicts. The report was widely used by Purdue and is spokespeople as proof that drugs like OxyContin were not habit-forming.

A follow-up letter to the *NEJM* in 2017 by a team of Canadian researchers cleverly analyzed all 608 references that were later made to the Jick letter in subsequent papers. They found a big jump in citations of it starting in 1995, fifteen years after it came out, the year that Purdue marketed OxyContin. Nearly three-quarters of those citing the Jick letter depicted it as presenting evidence that addiction was an uncommon risk in patients given opioids. The Canadian authors concluded,

> We believe that this citation pattern contributed to the North American opioid crisis by helping to shape a narrative that allayed prescribers' concerns about the risk of addiction associated with long-term opioid therapy.

The *NEJM* editors have now taken the unusual step of adding a special disclaimer to the original Jick letter as it now appears in their online archives: "For reasons of public health, readers should be aware that this letter has been heavily and uncritically cited as evidence that addiction is rare with opioid therapy."

Increasing the Dose

In 2019, I was called by a team of journalists from the *Financial Times* and Boston's public television station WGBH. They told me they were thinking about doing a program on problematic prescribing and opioids, and knew I had an interest in those areas; could they come by to talk? They said they couldn't provide much more explanation. On arriving they set up a large monitor in the DoPE conference room and explained that they wanted to show me a video and get my reactions to it. It depicted an unremarkable-looking middle-aged man; he said he had worked for an unnamed drug company and recounted how he sought to meet his company's very high sales goals for its products. "The only way I knew of to get there was to bribe doctors," he said, straight-faced. He described a program of "physician education" that came across like a grotesque imitation of the worst industry-funded continuing education programs. Speakers weren't chosen for their expertise, but on the basis of how much of the company's product they prescribed. They got $1,200 or $1,500 for each talk they gave to their peers, often over dinner in a nice restaurant. "No one cared if anybody showed up to the programs, or if the doctor even spoke," the man on screen said, explaining that these were really bribes for prescribing a lot of product. The firm maintained a spreadsheet noting how many dollars each doctor wrote in prescriptions and how much each was paid in speaker's fees, to keep track of the return on its educational investment. One doctor wrote $1.2 million in prescriptions and was paid $86,000 for his "teaching."

The thought crossed my mind that this might have been a crude attempt at satire, with an actor hired to portray a ruthless pharma executive in a ham-handed, over-the-top parody.

"Is this guy real?" I asked.

"Absolutely," came the reply. "We interviewed him a little while ago, but promised not to let anyone view the tape until his sentencing was completed," adding that I was one of the first people to see it. He was Alec Burlakoff, who had been the vice president of sales at Insys, a high-flying Arizona start-up that sold only one product, called Subsys. Approved by the FDA in 2012, it was fentanyl formulated into a mist form; it could be sprayed into the mouth to provide a rapid drug effect, since it was absorbed immediately without having to travel through the GI tract. (The mist-ification mystification allowed Insys to patent their version of the drug, even though fentanyl itself had been around since 1968.) That formulation produced an instant "rush" almost like an injection directly into the brain, making it one of the most addictive products imaginable. (The FDA also approved a fentanyl lollipop for use in "breakthrough pain" for cancer patients. I was reluctant to approve it when it came before the Brigham's formulary committee, because I was concerned about the risk of a possible lethal overdose if a child ever got hold of one. But the oncologists said it would be mainly for in-hospital use under rigorous supervision; it was understandably approved.) Using a super-fast-acting high-potency narcotic for carefully selected cancer patients with unbearable pain can be justified. But apparently oblivious to the consequences of its earlier decisions, the FDA failed to keep adequate track of how Subsys was actually being used. (How approved drugs are prescribed isn't our responsibility, the agency seemed to say; that's up to the doctors.) Its inadequate surveillance was documented in a scathing *JAMA* paper by researchers at Johns Hopkins.

Free of any effective oversight, Insys sought to address its problem that the drug's very narrow approved use wouldn't meet the company's ambitious financial goals. So it transformed Subsys into a favored product of pain specialists whose practices included many people addicted to narcotics. As head of the company's salesforce, Burlakoff told his staff to drive around to find such "pill mills," which were often located in strip malls. "Doctors with patients in the parking lot sitting on the floor drinking Mountain Dew [waiting for the clinic to open]—those were the ones you wanted to engage with." He explained that once clinicians became committed prescribers, the company's strategy was to persuade them to keep increasing the dose, known as titration, since higher doses were much more profitable, even though they were also far more addictive. Salespeople were evaluated and rewarded based on the actual doses prescribed by the doctors they saw: "If the doctor's not escalating the dose quickly," he said, "then we have an issue." Of course, that is the exact opposite of what we encourage practitioners to do with opioids.

To achieve the company's goals, Burlakoff encouraged relationships between sales reps and prescribers: "Sex with a doctor or chartering a private jet to take several docs to Cancun, Mexico? It's been done." The people hired for this work generally didn't have any background in the pharmaceutical industry or any aspect of science: one was an ex-firefighter, another an ex–pro football player, another a former *Playboy* model. The sales manager in charge of the entire Midwest was a former exotic dancer at a gentlemen's club in Florida. As Burlakoff explained in his videotaped interview:

> I wasn't nearly as concerned [with their backgrounds] as I was assessing whether or not they had what I call, unfortunately, a killer instinct. Almost no conscience. . . . I didn't think about the patients, the people suffering, the addiction, the deaths. I imagined that I was selling a widget.

To motivate the sales force, the company sponsored contests to see who could get their doctors to increase doses the most. To illustrate that, the journalists who brought me the taped interview put on a slick music video made in 2015 of guys dancing around on the rooftop of an office building. Some wore baggy pants and hoodies and huge gold necklaces; others were in formal wear, and Burlakoff himself wore a whole-body costume made to look like the product's fentanyl spray dispenser. They moved jerkily to a peppy rap lyric urging the detailing team to get their doctors to keep increasing what they prescribed:

> I love titration and it's not a problem; I got new patients and I got a lot of 'em.

This overpromotion of a uniquely addictive and overprescribed opioid went on for years; neither the FDA nor the Drug Enforcement Administration nor state authorities seemed aware of or able to deal with its grotesque overuse. Wall Street loved the company's stock, which soared and made its founder and CEO, John Kapoor, a billionaire. His company became the country's top initial public offering the first year it was traded publicly. After seeing the videos and regaining my equilibrium, I discussed the issues with the documentary makers and offered some perspective on their project. The program aired in 2020.

Dr. Kapoor and Insys were finally brought down not by doctors or public health authorities, but by journalists, short sellers, and government lawyers. The U.S. attorney based in Boston charged him and key Insys staff under federal racketeering laws; insurance fraud was a key element of the case, since the company had set up a special division tasked with lying to insurers about whether patients filling the prescriptions actually had cancer. Most of them didn't.

Fast-Forward

Subsequent events have had the elements of a Greek tragedy, as well as a human one:

- In 2007, Purdue Pharma, maker of OxyContin, pleaded guilty to a widespread campaign to mislead doctors, regulators, and the public about the addictive potential of their product. The company was forced to pay $600 million—a lot, but not the largest pharmaceutical settlements ever. Three of its executives also pleaded guilty as individuals, for an additional $34.5 million. Some have charged that much of our opioid epidemic stems from a problem at the southern border. It does, but not the one with Mexico; it's Stamford, on the southern border of Connecticut, where Purdue's corporate offices are based.
- Dozens of participants in the health-care system, including drugmakers, wholesalers, and pharmacies, have been sued for damages over their roles in creating America's opioid crisis. While some cases are still being litigated, the nationwide settlement is expected to exceed $50 billion. The funds are to be used to ameliorate the consequences of the nation's rampant overuse of these drugs. A 2024 Supreme Court decision blocked the component of the settlement involving the Sackler family, owners of Purdue Pharma, putting much of the settlement package on hold.
- A year and a half after Alosa produced our recommendations for pain management that Bateman had created, in 2016 the Centers for Disease Control came out with guidelines that said about the same thing.

- A 2017 presidential commission concluded that the FDA's mishandling of the evaluation, approval, and use of such medications was an important cause of the nation's opioid crisis.
- In 2021, Janet Woodcock was one of three top contenders to fill the long-vacant job of FDA commissioner and was heavily favored by the drug industry. But twenty-eight groups accused her of presiding over a major regulatory disaster, stating, "In its opioid decision-making, Dr. Woodcock and the division she supervised consistently put the interests of opioid manufacturers ahead of public health, often overruling its own scientific advisors and ignoring the pleas of public health groups, state Attorneys General, and outraged victims of the opioid crisis." Her role in overseeing the approval of OxyContin and other opioids ended her chances to become commissioner.
- As we've seen, Woodcock went on to play a key role in the FDA's approval of Aduhelm for Alzheimer's disease (see chapter 2), and then helped drive the agency's approval of several clinically ineffective drugs for muscular dystrophy (see chapter 3). She retired in 2024 after thirty-eight years at the agency.
- The CDC estimates that since 1999, a million Americans have died of drug overdoses. That number remained stubbornly high, approximating 100,000 new deaths a year. The good news is that harm reduction approaches (see below) and better education of clinicians may have begun to dent that number.
- Dr. John Kapoor was convicted in 2019 of bribing doctors to prescribe Subsys and defrauding insurers to pay for it; he was sentenced to five and a half years in prison. He served only two years and was released in 2023.
- Alec Burlakoff pleaded guilty to one count of racketeering conspiracy, and cooperated with the government; he was jailed for twenty-six months. He's now out and working as a sales trainer and coach; his LinkedIn profile notes that he offers consultation on training and compliance systems for sales professionals. In it, he notes that he "hired and led a sales team that resulted in [Insys] being named the #1 IPO in the country," adding, "Profound attention from federal authorities and the judicial system have made me wiser."

In helping to develop Alosa's materials on pain management further, I've come to understand better that the right question for prescribers is not whether a patient is completely pain free, but whether that pain is interfering with their functional capacity. Setting the right expectations is key. If someone with pain is asked to fill out a pictogram and led to believe that they ought to be at the level of the smiliest face on the chart, they will have an unrealistic understanding of their need for medications. By contrast, it's much better to explain after a tooth extraction or a normal vaginal birth or a bad sprain, "You're going to hurt for a few days. Aspirin or an NSAID, along with some acetaminophen (Tylenol) will make you feel better. Then the pain will go away." Physical pain, while, of course, important, can also be accompanied by other contributors to the total experience of discomfort, such as psychological pain ("Does this mean my disease is getting worse?") or spiritual pain ("Why is this happening to me?"). Each component may require a different kind of intervention, and that's not always a pill.

Fixing the Communication

In our educational outreach programs to reduce opioid overuse, why use a person-intensive approach like academic detailing when other methods are cheaper? It turns out that although they are cheap, reproachful letters to physicians who are heavy prescribers often don't work very well. Confronted with such a letter, most physicians become defensive and feel, "I was there in the room trying to help a patient in pain. Who are you to tell me what to do, you pointy-headed cubicle-bound bureaucratic idiot?" Requiring a doctor to get special permission to exceed a certain number of pills by calling a 1-800-DROPDEAD telephone number is demeaning and inflexible. What's missing from these approaches is what academic detailing does best: responding to a particular physician's knowledge, beliefs, and attitudes, showing empathy for both the prescriber and the patient in pain, and offering workable alternatives to overusing opioids. We don't want to be told that we're misbehaving as prescribers; we want help caring for the patient. These points are worth considering one at a time.

- **Understanding where they're coming from:** Some doctors will need to learn more about the pharmacology of addiction, some will need to talk about their feelings about this kind of care ("Addicts should just have more willpower"), others will need to appreciate that patients who are opioid-dependent often got that way because of drugs we prescribed for them. If the educator doesn't ask, they can't know about a given prescriber's beliefs and attitudes.
- **Empathy:** Most people in medicine chose that path to help people who are suffering; a patient sitting in front of you describing their pain is one of the most poignant examples of this. In Alosa's programs, if the initial conversation reveals that a practitioner thinks opioid overuse is a moral failing of the patient, or a problem of simply needing more willpower, we try to address this knowledge deficit. In some respects, opioids are like antibiotics: getting a prescription for them, even when it isn't needed, enables the patient to feel that the healer is trying to meet their needs. It's sort of "a dose of the doctor."

There's also a darker side to this. A patient who has been taking opioids steadily for a few weeks, either because of an ill-advised prescription for a back sprain, or (more appropriately) after a major surgical procedure, may be neurochemically changed. Steady use of opioids even for a limited period can alter receptors in the brain to the point where abrupt cessation of the drug can actually precipitate withdrawal symptoms. Besides providing a compelling reason for not starting an opioid regimen that isn't really necessary, understanding this also has important implications for stopping opioids. You can't just tell the patient to suddenly get used to living without them.

I learned this firsthand in a compelling way after having a knee replacement. Initial recovery from this invasive procedure can be quite painful, but my symptoms were held in check by a necessary opioid regimen my surgeon prescribed. Without the painkillers, I had trouble doing any physical therapy, or even moving around the house. After several refills the intense pain persisted, but my doctor's assistant informed me that I couldn't have any more controlled substances because I had reached the end of the permitted number of pills.

Such "physician extenders" can make health care more efficient, but because of their more limited training they usually have to follow a strict written protocol to guide their decisions. More pain medicine for me wasn't on the protocol; just tough it out with Motrin and Tylenol. I got anxious and demanding, then frantic; the assistant was unyielding, saying that he had to follow the instructions he was given. The more he remained firm in his refusal to renew my opioids, the more I wanted to tear out his eyeballs. I realized I had temporarily come to inhabit the brain of a drug-dependent person in acute withdrawal; I remembered reading about the panicky sense of doom that addicts experienced when they couldn't get a fix.

Fortunately, I was able to page my colleague the surgeon to tell him I *really* had to have more drug. He had done thousands of joint replacements and had seen this all before. "No problem," he said soothingly. "Sometimes people can get a little too cautious about these things; happy to give you a new prescription. I used to write for a hundred pills at a time, but they've gotten more strict lately. How many do you want?" Within hours, my murderous rage disappeared and I felt fine; before long I was able to taper my opioids to zero. That first-person experience transformed my understanding of "taking people off opioids"; it was a dramatic illustration of the need to walk in a patient's shoes. For an instant I had the odd idea that it might help for every doctor who prescribes opioids to be given enough of them to reach this state of neurochemical derangement, so we could better understand what it's like to tell a patient they can't have any more narcotic. But that would be a hard thing to get past an ethics review board.

Harm reduction: The health-care system has now managed to swing from mindless overuse of opioids to unthinking restriction. As we've seen, many people who become opioid-dependent got that way because of prescriptions written by their doctor, appropriately or not, to treat pain. But if that source was shut off abruptly, some of those people found out how to get OxyContin or Vicodin or Percocet on the street. All narcotics produce tolerance, so that a person gets a smaller and smaller effect from the same dose and craves more and more, just to avoid withdrawal. (Money can have the same effect on other people, though the neurotransmitter involved there appears to be dopamine.) Unfortunately, the doses, not to mention quality control, of street drugs are dangerously unpredictable: a common cause of overdose death is ingestion of a far higher dose of a street drug than one is expecting to get, especially now that fentanyl is ubiquitous, along with other drugs like xylazine. Also high on the list of addiction-related illness and death is the scarcity of clean needles and syringes leading to needle sharing, which often means disease-sharing.

Opioid molecules don't cause AIDS or hepatitis C, another disease that has ravaged intravenous drug users. Nor do they cause bacterial endocarditis, a blood-borne infection easily transmitted by shared needles that can chew up heart valves and render them useless. For that condition, the only treatment may be a costly and often-invasive procedure to repair or replace the valve. And yet we use opioids in the hospital in far greater doses than occurs on the street with hardly any occurrence of these problems or of fatal overdoses, so it's not all about the drug molecules. No, these outcomes are caused by the way society interacts with opioids, restricting their use in so many millions of people to unreliable supplies and illicit intravenous access, along with all the heightened risks of infection and inadvertent overdose. That's why many people advocate for clean needle exchange programs, supervised safe injection sites, easy access to the nasal spray naloxone (Narcan) to reverse overdose, and medically administered narcotics to help those who have become addicted to opioids. Providing users with test strips that can detect fentanyl and xylazine in what they're injecting can also help reduce fatal overdoses. Other countries have implemented such programs, usually with good results. But our insistence on seeing opioid use as a moral failure has slowed the adoption of these lifesaving approaches.

A Better Treatment

Over the years we've come to understand the neurochemistry of opioid dependence more clearly. That research has revealed that one effective way to manage the problem is by prescribing medications to fix the problem at the level of the synapse. Methadone has been employed for decades as an opioid that can be administered as a liquid in a carefully monitored setting to satisfy a patient's cravings and have its dose reduced under supervision—or kept at a manageable level. The routine of a daily check-in and just having someplace to go and get supportive care probably play an important role as well for many people; for patients who can cooperate with this regimen it can be an effective tool. However, methadone maintenance centers are few and far between, and not always easy to get to. But we also have a drug, buprenorphine, that attaches itself to opioid receptors in the brain and blocks the effect of abusable drugs. When all goes well, once a patient is taking it they stop craving other opioids and don't get high from them. Brilliant pharmacology followed by carefully conducted clinical trials gave patients and health-care practitioners a potentially great tool to wield against the curse of narcotic dependence. Could our health-care system mess everything up despite this? Absolutely.

After the discovery of buprenorphine, the federal government decided that it would be too dangerous to put this tool in the hands of all licensed physicians—even though it's much milder and less abusable than most of the potentially lethal opioids that any of us are allowed to prescribe. Instead, for many years doctors had to obtain a special additional license from the Drug Enforcement Administration just for its use, ominously named an X-waiver. Such extra licenses are extremely uncommon in medicine. I don't need one to give patients morphine, fentanyl, oxycodone, or other opioids. Nor would I need a special license to prescribe cancer chemotherapy that could save a patient's life or shut down their bone marrow, or an antibiotic that can kill their kidneys, or an antipsychotic medication that can reduce a patient to a drooling clump of protoplasm and—if the patient is elderly—increase their risk of death. No problem,

I'm a doctor. But if I want to treat a patient who has a crippling opioid-use disorder by giving them a safe and effective drug like buprenorphine, until recently I couldn't do so unless I got special permission from the DEA. A doctor was required to take eight additional hours of training (twenty-four hours for nurses and pharmacists) and fill out additional paperwork for every prescription written. There might also be periodic surprise visits by DEA agents to do spot audits of that paperwork. And for all that, when people got their first X-waiver licenses, they were allowed to use it to treat a maximum of thirty patients. All these extra requirements left doctors with the (mistaken) belief that "bupe" is somehow dangerous in its own right, or extremely difficult to use. Those restrictions were eased a bit during the Covid pandemic; that relaxation wasn't made permanent until 2024.

Why would the federal government take this potentially lifesaving treatment and make it harder to get than nearly every other prescription drug we use, including narcotics? The answers vary. "These drugs can be addictive in themselves," goes one response, though it fails to explain why the FDA and DEA have not applied similar restrictions to prescriptions for oxycodone or fentanyl, even in its super-addictive spray form of Subsys. Others wonder whether the puritanical approach came from a belief that buprenorphine might make opioid addiction safer, which in the eyes of some could be a problem. (Those are the same people who oppose wider availability of the overdose-reversing drug Narcan on the grounds that making opioid use less lethal might encourage addiction.) Whatever the reason, between the lack of adequate training in medical school about drug dependence, the failure of many clinicians to recognize it when they see it, the stigma of caring for such patients as if they were morally inferior to people with diabetes or hemophilia, and—until recently—the hassle of extra licensing and government surveillance, there is still a striking underuse of buprenorphine even as we are learning more about how helpful it can be for patients whose synapses have been deformed by excessive opioid use.

Our continuing struggle with opioids isn't just about prescribing the wrong drugs or not prescribing the right treatments to address it. We also need to recall Rudolf Virchow's observation that medicine is at its heart a social science. Along the same lines, the nineteenth-century physician John Snow performed careful epidemiological fieldwork to figure out that a severe cholera outbreak ravaging part of London was being caused by the sewage being dumped into the Thames upstream of the city, which was the source of the city's water supply. To fix the problem, it's said that he pulled the handle off the water pump in one badly afflicted neighborhood to stop transmission of the disease.

I appreciate the fact that both Virchow and Snow were also frontline clinical practitioners—the latter was the personal physician to Queen Victoria. We could use their mastery of these dual perspectives to help us think better about dealing with the opioid epidemic. That kind of upstream thinking can help us understand more about the other causes of our highest-in-the-world rate of opioid deaths. Yes, some of it was the result of the uniquely homegrown avarice of greedy opioid manufacturers, as well as gullible or venal doctors and overly demanding patients. Much of it was the FDA's failure to demand solid evidence of effectiveness and safety before it approved the wide use of these risky drugs long-term. We can also blame the way governments and health systems and companies that didn't track the ways that dangerous products were actually being used until millions of people became addicted or overdosed. But if we're looking for root causes, we need to go even further upstream and ask why so many Americans seek solace from potentially lethal chemicals.

As with Snow, we can learn a lot from the epidemiology of our opioid crisis—the microgeography of this disease of the soul. It began by hitting hardest at the heartland of America, among white working-class men with just a high school education who thought that showing up every day and doing hard work at the plant over several decades would guarantee them and their families success and security. Then the neoliberal agenda for global commerce moved their jobs to countries with lower wages and fewer protections for the environment, workers, or child labor. These are the parts of the country that were hardest hit by the opioid crisis as well as by alcoholism and suicide. Desperation leads to desperate measures, whether they are simplistic neurochemical solutions or simplistic authoritarian ones.

It's good that we're learning more each year about how to treat physical pain without addicting patients, and that we're getting better at spotting and helping people who have already fallen into that devastating neurochemical trap. But we need to also focus on how we got here. Humans have cultivated poppies and extracted opioids from them for thousands of years. Until the last several decades most cultures lived in some sort of equilibrium with these chemicals. Then something happened in the late twentieth century to shred our societal fabric and upset that equilibrium—more so in the U.S. than elsewhere. It's not just opioids: stimulant abuse is gaining ground, as are novel compounds like the animal tranquilizer xylazine; after that, people will undoubtedly turn to other new chemicals to dull their psychic pain. Trying to control such problems by limiting the supply of drugs has never worked well, as we should have learned from the terrible failure of Prohibition in the last century. We can't ban our way out of the problem that some people feel so miserable that they'll ingest any kind of mind-numbing substance they can get, even (especially, in some cases) if it might kill them. And whatever the poison of the moment, it will take root most fiercely in a social setting that makes the risk of self-destruction more appealing than normal life. It's an ongoing struggle that keeps reminding us that the molecules are important, but it's not just about the molecules.

In 2024, London health authorities reported new disease outbreaks they attributed to impurities in the city's water supply, caused by upstream contamination of the Thames. We're still trying to figure out how to rip the handle off the pump.

– PART SIX –

Empowering the Patient

CHAPTER 21

You Can't Get Your Medicines If You Can't Get Health Care

We can't think clearly about the use of medications without grappling with how the health-care system helps people access them or prevents them from doing so: that's where all therapeutics begins, or where it doesn't get off the ground. Obviously, a patient has to be able to see a medical professional who diagnoses the problem and writes the 'scrip. Then except for the cheapest drugs, most people need help paying for them. You can't rethink medication use without considering the health-care system any more than you can understand fish without considering water.

In the late 1990s, the U.S. remained an outlier among wealthy countries, since it was the only one that failed to guarantee access to medical care and prescription drugs to all its citizens. That took a toll on many of our patients, and we primary care doctors felt it particularly deeply. Medicare didn't yet pay for medications, and many of our patients under sixty-five also had enormous gaps in their medical coverage. Some worked for employers that offered health insurance, but many did not; the insurance may have covered prescription drugs, but often didn't. And if they lost their job, they lost their ability to pay for care. So what good did it do if we brilliantly diagnosed a problem and wrote a well-thought-out prescription if our patients couldn't fill it?

The poorest Americans might be able to enroll in a state-based Medicaid program, but states varied widely in how tough it was to qualify for those programs. More than once someone would tell me they couldn't keep taking the medicines I had prescribed because they no longer had their employer-provided insurance, or they took a new job that didn't come with health coverage. Or they were kicked off the Medicaid rolls because their child was no longer an eligible minor. Or their combination of low-wage jobs pushed them a bit above Medicaid's allowed income limit: they were still poor, but not quite poor enough to stay in the program.

As the century came to an end, the tightening vise of constrained coverage for medications and medical care also began to affect employed patients with health insurance. Through several quirks of history, after World War II the U.S. chose employer-based health insurance over the universal coverage that many other nations adopted. By the late 1990s, its costs were rising uncontrollably and were having more and more impact on corporations' personnel costs. Economists calculated that for each car coming off the assembly line, American automakers were spending more on medical coverage for the workers who built it than on the steel it contained. One quipped that General Motors could be thought of as an enormous health insurance company that also made cars.

Prescription drugs were part of the problem, but hospital care and physician services were the biggest drivers of those runaway expenditures. To address this, many employers turned to health maintenance organizations (HMOs) to contain costs. In its most innocent depiction, the HMO idea seemed appealing: flip the incentives so that the companies and insurers could do better financially by keeping people healthy rather than by paying for medical services that could be prevented. An employer could pay a fixed amount per patient per year: profits could be made by spending as little as possible on actual medical goods and services.

This might have worked if it had been embedded in a system of evidence-based clinical decision-making that was free of the imperative to turn a profit: along with clean living, the rational use of medications was the best way to maintain someone's health. But many HMOs, or managed care organizations, were run as profit-making cost-containment machines: they could make a lot more money by limiting the use of costly drugs, procedures, and hospital stays than they could from proactive patient-centered prescribing. Nonprofit health insurers had to compete for employers' business by out-containing the competition. It wasn't just financial incentives that were turned on their heads; so were the values of clinical care. The idea of rewarding insurers to help people maintain their health mutated into its evil twin: paying out as little as possible for medical care and costly drugs. The golems were taking over.

We physicians were caught in the middle, since our utilization decisions drove every dollar of those expenditures: Was there a cheaper medication that could be used rather than the expensive new one? Did that person with chronic headaches really need a CAT scan? Couldn't this patient recovering from a heart attack be sent home from the hospital a few days earlier? Our new generation of primary care doctors had thought we'd be the broadly educated and respected quarterbacks of the health-care team, coordinating and guiding all parts of the patient's medical experience. But the rise of managed care organizations was transforming us from quarterbacks to switchboard operators, and then to gatekeepers and finally, enforcers of rationing.

Our discomfort was more than ideological: the clinical recommendations we made were increasingly second-guessed by insurers or denied outright. Requirements were increasing for prior authorization of expensive prescriptions or referrals: we had to seek permission from an insurance company employee, often with no clinical training, at the other end of a phone line. Often the answer was no. We referred to those as 1-800-EAT-SHIT calls.

In addition, the ascent of managed care and HMOs was a major cause of our present widely despised system of direct-to-consumer drug ads. Pharmaceutical companies had traditionally avoided the costly arena of marketing to the public; their traditional sales model relied on promoting drugs to us doctors, since our prescribing decisions drove the entire pharmaceutical marketplace. But as HMOs began to step in and constrain our drug choices (a task later taken up by prescription benefit managers as well), drug companies became willing to dive into the costly arena of consumer advertising. The goal would be to get patients to demand specific medications from their physicians in order to combat insurers' efforts to push those choices in other directions.

With new pressures from patients and growing pushback from the HMOs, my clinical colleagues and I were getting increasingly frustrated that we had spent so many years learning exactly which drugs to prescribe in what circumstances, and which patients needed a complex procedure, or when they needed to be admitted to the hospital—only to find our choices overruled by a faceless insurance company employee whose main job was to reduce expenditures. Other patients simply fell through the thinning fabric of coverage; the new market-based logic left many without adequate help paying for drugs, clinical visits, or hospital care. The late twentieth century was an impressive period of discoveries in medications, diagnostic studies, and curative procedures unprecedented in human history, but doctors and patients were in an increasingly sour mood about health care.

As the millennium was coming to a close, that anger was about to boil over. In 1997 several of us, mostly doctors from Harvard's teaching hospitals, came together to try and create a movement that would guarantee medical care and drug coverage to everyone in Massachusetts. In the end, we generated momentum that many observers saw as laying the foundation for Obamacare years later; its story has not been told before in detail.

Our state was one of the wealthiest in the country; it had some of the world's best hospitals and medical schools, and spent an eye-watering amount on health care per capita. But we also had intolerably large numbers of people with no medical coverage at all; they had trouble getting to see us, and even if they did, they often couldn't afford the prescriptions we wrote for them. Even our patients with insurance faced growing restrictions on the drugs they could take.

A Call to Action

The opening salvo of the revolution that we planned appeared in the last weeks of 1997 in the *Journal of the American Medical Association.* It was a manifesto we titled "For Our Patients, Not for Profits: A Call to Action." Our movement was spearheaded by several of us who had trained or worked at the Cambridge City Hospital, the "safety net" Harvard hospital that attracted many of us concerned about the care of underserved populations. The group included several Cambridge-trained primary care internists, including Drs. Steffie Woolhandler, Susan Bennett, David Himmelstein, and me, along with many like-minded clinicians. We found a political and spiritual leader in Dr. Bernard Lown, who was more than a generation older than the rest of us. Born in Lithuania in 1921, he fled the Nazis in 1935 and taught himself English by memorizing the pages of a dictionary, eventually receiving an MD degree from Johns Hopkins University in 1945. Bernard went on to train in cardiology and spent virtually all his career at Harvard, mostly based at the Brigham. His pathbreaking research led to the use of medications to treat heart rhythm disorders, the invention of the defibrillator, and creation of the first coronary care unit—that unit at the Brigham is still named after him.

The descendant of a rabbi, Bernard had a strong commitment to social justice from early in life. As a medical student at Hopkins, he was temporarily suspended when he purposely mislabeled the race on blood that was donated by Black and white donors. At the height of the Cold War, the threat of nuclear catastrophe troubled him deeply. With colleagues from the Brigham and the Harvard School of Public Health, he joined with cardiologists from the Soviet Union to form the International Physicians for the Prevention of Nuclear War, which pushed for disarmament in both countries. Its work won the Nobel Peace Prize. Bernard was also a committed bedside practitioner who wrote movingly about the degradation of the doctor-patient relationship in the new world of profit-driven medicine. For me, he was the perfect role model: a smart, respected clinician who was also a productive researcher and a socially committed activist.

We called our group the Ad Hoc Committee to Defend Health Care and took aim at the growing clout of corporations in medicine, arguing that marketplace incentives were at odds with our patients' needs and our values as clinicians. One anecdote of the time seemed to typify the problem: a Boston-area HMO was said to have hired a marketing consultant in the early 1980s to find the demographic groups least likely to need medical services or expensive drugs. It clearly wasn't old people, or women of childbearing age or their families. According to the story, after months of analysis the consultant recommended that the HMO focus on marketing to young unmarried men—the demographic expected to be least likely to seek medical care or require costly medications. The HMO did so, and amassed a large concentration of people who later went on to contract AIDS.

Our *JAMA* Call to Action still resonates today with current concerns over the pharmaceutical industry and the growing corporate dominance of health care:

> Mounting shadows darken our calling and threaten to transform healing from a covenant into a business contract. Canons of commerce are displacing dictates of healing, trampling our professions' most sacred values. . . . Market medicine treats patients as profit centers. The time we are allowed to spend with the sick shrinks under the pressure to increase throughput, as though we were dealing with industrial commodities rather than afflicted human beings in need of compassion and caring.

By the time the statement ran in *JAMA*, we had obtained endorsements for it from hundreds of doctors and other health-care professionals. When published, that list consumed several pages of small-print names; the journal told us it was the longest list of people it had ever published with any article. But we wanted to do much more than just have an article in *JAMA*; we wanted to change the world.

Drawing on Bernard's roots in the Old Left of the 1930s and the background several of us had in the New Left of the 1960s, we created a series of events to draw attention to our cause. The day before the Call to Action was published, we went down to the harbor in our white coats and reenacted the Boston Tea Party aboard a replica of the ship from which American patriots had thrown crates of tea overboard to protest British commercial tyranny. One of our colleagues, Dr. Alice Rothchild, dressed as an overstuffed capitalist and hurled bags labeled with dollar signs into the harbor, symbolizing the billions she said HMOs spent each year on marketing, profits, shareholder dividends, and executive salaries. Others tossed out HMO corporate reports and wooden crates with phrases like "PROFIT-DRIVEN CARE" and "MD = GATEKEEPER" scrawled on their sides. To be ecologically responsible, we later retrieved all the stuff we had thrown into the harbor. No fish were harmed in the making of this protest; that damage had already been done by decades of severe pollution.

"You are seeing the beginning," Dr. Lown said from the ship's deck to the assembled crowd, in his light Eastern European accent. "When the original Boston Tea Party started, nobody predicted a revolution. Yet it happened." When Senator Bernie Sanders came to visit our PORTAL group a quarter century later to talk about controlling drug costs, he said just about the same thing.

After the Tea Party reenactment, we marched over to historic Faneuil Hall, the 1741 brick structure known as "the Cradle of Liberty" after the public meetings that colonists held there in the mid-1770s. Under the gaze of Founders staring down from huge oil paintings, we had decked out the stage with an arc of several dozen black balloons. In my opening comments, I reminded the audience that the balloons weren't there as a festive decoration: each one represented a million uninsured patients—people in the richest country on earth who had no protection in paying for their drugs or for any kind of medical care.

To address the fiscal issues before us we called on John Kenneth Galbraith, the eminent Harvard economist and former adviser to FDR, Truman, JFK, and Lyndon Johnson. He was a patient of Dr. Lown's and became an ally of our movement. Forty-five years earlier in his book *American Capitalism* he had warned that the rise of large corporations could put the necessary give-and-take of the American economy into jeopardy. Then in 1967, he had sounded an alarm that foreshadowed our concerns at Faneuil Hall that evening some thirty years later. The modern corporation, he wrote, "had readily at hand the means for controlling the prices at which it sells as well as those at which it buys. . . ." He wasn't writing about health care then, but he might as well have been. His comments had particular resonance for me in their direct applicability to the economics of medication use. Where human health and illness are concerned, how far should the reach of the marketplace extend? Could we stop the golems?

Galbraith moved his imposing six-foot-nine frame onto the ancient Faneuil Hall stage; it was uncanny hearing his comments on the origins of capitalism and of the nation's economy in the very room where those issues had been debated over 220 years earlier. Here is a portion of his comments:

> It is your questionable fortune tonight to have a lecture on the oldest subject in economic and political thought; that is, on the role of profit-motivated market forces, as opposed to that of the socially concerned community and government. . . .
>
> The modern discussion of the role of public and private enterprise began in 1776, more or less simultaneously with the birth of the American Republic. That was the year of publication of *Wealth of Nations* by Adam Smith. . . . He reserved important functions for the state, community and church; he was moved by practical and humane concerns and not by doctrine. Modern enthusiasts cite him as the ultimate advocate of market forces. In the Reagan years, the devout in Washington wore armbands inscribed with his name; it was perhaps unfortunate that they had not read him.
>
> Looking at the scene today, Adam Smith would be on your side and my side here tonight. He would not favor leaving health care and the larger institutional structure to private, profit-making enterprise. His, as ours, would be a humane and sensible judgment; I speak tonight in the best tradition of economic thought.

We also heard from Dr. Linda Peeno, an internist who had been medical director at the large health insurer Humana. She quit when she could no longer stand the responsibility of coming up with medical justifications for denying expensive but necessary treatments. "I can't view physicians and patients as operational problems," she said. Following her talk, patients and family members came onstage to describe what it was like having their insurer refuse to pay for a treatment their doctor recommended.

We veterans of the anti-war demonstrations of the 1960s knew that any movement worth the name needed a bit of theater, so some in the group created our own version of the 1979 Pink Floyd hit "Another Brick in the Wall":

We don't want perverse incentives,
We don't want your CEOs.
No accountants in exam rooms—
Wall Street, let our patients go!
[*With fists in air*] *HEY! WALL STREET! LET OUR PATIENTS GO!*
All in all, we're just another shop in their mall.
We won't be another shop in their mall!

The Faneuil Hall rally helped generate enthusiasm for our growing movement, and we sought to build on it and enlarge the numbers of our supporters. Our steering committee usually met in Dr. Lown's dining room in Newton, a Boston suburb inhabited by many academics from local universities, including many other Nobel Prize winners. His front foyer contained a photograph of a smiling, much younger Bernard standing with Fidel; memorabilia of his groundbreaking career in cardiology; and a framed copy of the 1987 treaty that reduced the size of U.S. and Soviet nuclear weapons stockpiles. It was signed by Mikhail Gorbachev with his thanks to Bernard for helping to make it possible.

Our little group went on to hold teach-ins and conferences at medical schools and hospitals throughout the state. But to what end? One option was to put a ballot initiative before the voters. In Massachusetts, these aren't just statements of citizen values: if one passes, it carries the force of law. We didn't have enough consensus in our group to demand a specific health-care delivery system; some were adamant advocates of a government-run single-payer system, others preferred a less centralized approach. But all of us on the steering committee agreed on one goal: making Massachusetts the first state to guarantee access to doctors, hospitals, and medications to all its residents.

As our numbers grew throughout 1998 and 1999, we needed to figure out how to transform our values and aspirations into concrete language for a petition we would try to put on the ballot in November 2000. It would have to be practical and actionable, compatible with existing laws, progressive enough to retain the respect and energy of our activist founders and sponsors, but not so far out on the political spectrum that we would lose centrist advocates. In addition, the language would have to survive a legal analysis by the office of the Secretary of State, and we'd have to collect thousands of verifiable signatures before July 7.

"We should hire one of those companies that collects signatures for this kind of thing," one of our group suggested.

"Pay some commercial company to get signatures?" a colleague objected. "No way! We have to go out there ourselves; this is a people's movement! We need to be on the streets with our fellow citizens to talk to them about the issues while we collect signatures. Those outside companies are whores; they'll work for anyone who pays them." However naive, that response fit well with our ideology and with our financial resources; we had plenty of the former and almost none of the latter. We fanned out across the state in our white coats to enlist supporters, stopping people on the street, at shopping centers, outside houses of worship. We got the required number of signatures.

Fundamentally, the issues we were grappling with were the same ones that define the debate about pharmaceuticals and health care to this day:

- What are the strengths and limits of the private sector and of profits in producing medical goods and services?
- What is the role of government in limiting what can be charged?
- Who's responsible for ensuring that patients have equitable access to medical care?
- When is it acceptable to limit a patient's choices (as for an expensive but overpriced new drug) to keep costs in control?
- How much of all this can be fixed by legislation?

We couldn't label the new ballot initiative "A Call to Action," the title of our *JAMA* piece. So we named it "An Act to Protect the Rights of Patients and to Promote Access to Quality Health Care for All Residents of the Commonwealth." As originally worded, it began:

> Be it enacted by the people, and by their authority, as follows:
>
> Whereas, Massachusetts residents are entitled to and desire a system of health care that has the needs of patients as its central purpose and priority;
>
> Whereas, the quality and availability of health care services and treatments is threatened by unreasonable restrictions on patient choice and interference with medical decision making;
>
> Whereas, the affordability of health care to residents is jeopardized by continued increases in health insurance costs and by reductions in health plan coverage, and many Massachusetts residents are uninsured or underinsured;
>
> Therefore, it is the purpose of this act to ensure that there will be access to health care for all Massachusetts residents, including strong patient protections and a bill of patient's rights.

Our grandest demand was the very first:

> There shall be established a patient-centered system of health care that will ensure comprehensive, high quality care and health coverage for all residents of the Commonwealth, to be in effect no later than July 1st, 2002.

If passed, this would be the first time a universal right to health-care access was guaranteed anywhere in the country. We deliberately chose the term "residents" rather than "citizens" to cover the many undocumented immigrants who needed such a guarantee, as many of us had learned firsthand in our work at the Cambridge City Hospital.

We went on to add the then-radical plan that no more than 10 percent of all payments to health insurance companies could be used for any nonmedical purpose such as profit, administrative costs, or executive salaries, thus preserving at least 90 percent of revenues to be devoted to patient care, public health, or training. We initially referred to that piece as the "care share." Sadly, that phrase has often been supplanted in the industry by the more cynical term "medical loss ratio" to refer to the proportion of premiums that actually goes to take care of people. We also sought to stop the conversion of nonprofit health care organizations to for-profit entities—a provision that would become even more important a quarter century later, as we will see.

A Vigorous Reaction

"Shitstorm" is a term too mild to describe the response to our draft initiative. We had started out as a group of physicians worried about the corporatization of medicine and the growing primacy of profit in health care. But we realized we had taken on some of the most entrenched forces in the state. The most powerful among these included its enormous insurance industry. This shouldn't have surprised us, since limiting costly care and treatments had become an important part of the business model for many of them. (For my first several years in Boston, the only two skyscrapers in town were those of the Prudential and John Hancock insurance companies. That architectural observation should have been a warning of the quiet power of these commercial behemoths.) Employer groups also opposed our initiative; with health-care costs one of their fastest-rising personnel expenditures, they preferred to cast their lot with the HMOs that promised to contain those costs rather than focusing on better access to care for their employees. But the state's unions said they'd be our natural allies in the coming struggle. The *Boston Globe* said our plan was "as sweeping as anything produced on Beacon Hill in a generation."

In February of 2000, Dr. Lown received a letter from Stuart Altman, an influential health economist at Brandeis University, and John McDonough, a former state legislator who had joined the faculty there. It posed fifty-six questions about our initiative, and didn't come across as particularly friendly. Altman and McDonough told Dr. Lown they wanted a written response to their questions, as well as a meeting with him to discuss their concerns.

Bernard was normally unflappable; his escape from Germany and decades of negotiating with world leaders probably helped with that. But these questions about health policy and legislation shook him a little. "Jerry, I want you with me when these people come to talk," he told me. In the years since, I've come to know Stuart and John better and found them to be smart, affable, and liberal people. But their demeanor that day in Bernard's office at his busy cardiology practice was anything but warm and fuzzy. Always candid, Stuart opened the meeting by smiling and explaining, "We have been sent here by your enemies to interrogate you." An economic analysis had been commissioned by a newly formed group of Massachusetts insurance companies and businesses calling itself the Coalition for Affordable Health Care Choices, and it didn't favor our cause.

The questioning from Altman and McDonough was politely confrontational. It quickly became clear that a main goal was to find out what it would take to get us to quiet down and withdraw the ballot initiative. We're all friends and colleagues here, let's not do anything rash, of course we all want everyone to have good health care at a reasonable price, it would be terrible if this wrecked the world-famous medical institutions of Massachusetts, what will it take to make you people go away? The policy analyses our opponents later cited implied that enactment of universal health-care coverage would lead to economic and clinical chaos in Massachusetts. Some of us expected the academic medical establishment to support our universal access plan, even though many of the medical schools had close ties to the local HMOs.

As the debate intensified the deans of all four medical schools in Massachusetts found themselves at the same public meeting—an event as rare as the perfect alignment of four planets. Somehow the topic of the ballot initiative came up, and all the deans agreed that it would be a bad idea.

At the Ad Hoc Committee, we brought on Jim Braude, an experienced community organizer who is still a progressive force in Massachusetts politics. We took our show on the road to meet with community and medical groups around Massachusetts. We reminded them that our state's annual per-person health-care expenditure was then $6,100, higher than any other state in the country and the highest per capita health-care cost in the entire world, even though many of our neighbors didn't have access to medical care. Those of us who were frontline primary care doctors spoke of the conflict we felt between wanting to focus on the needs of our patients versus the pressure from insurance companies and HMOs to reduce expenditures.

We worried that the legislature could try and undercut the movement by passing a much weaker "Patients' Bill of Rights" that offered few guarantees of anything, while the insurance industry would try to kill the ballot initiative with a massive and costly media campaign. Both worries proved prescient. As Election Day approached the state legislature—which had not really engaged with these issues before—roused itself into something designed to resemble action, in an attempt to preserve the status quo. If our opposition to being just "another brick in the wall" had been the theme of the early days of the Ad Hoc Committee, these last-minute proposals reminded us more of the Who's 1971 hit that ended with the memorable lyrics "Meet the new boss / Same as the old boss. . . ." Its chorus seemed particularly apt:

> I'll tip my hat to the new constitution
> Take a bow for the new revolution
> Smile and grin at the change all around
> Pick up my guitar and play, just like yesterday
> Then I'll get on my knees and pray
> We don't get fooled again.

As the deadline neared for us to get the signed petitions to the golden-domed Massachusetts statehouse in time to make it onto the November 2000 ballot, the normally passive lawmakers scrambled to do something to derail our momentum. On the deadline date, one of them told the *Boston Herald* that they were nearing an "agreement on a compromise that could mollify members of the Coalition for

Health Care." (That was the new name our group had adopted as the program gained traction, since "Ad Hoc" was starting to sound too, well, ad hoc.)

As the *Herald* article explained, "Faced with intense lobbying efforts to keep the initiative off the ballot, legislative leaders hammered away on several proposals in hopes of crafting a bill that would satisfy ballot measure supporters." They were talking about perhaps enacting some of the points we were demanding: universal health care for everyone in the state, a patients' Bill of Rights, and a ban on converting nonprofit institutions to for-profit ones. But it was just talk: by the initiative petition deadline of July 5, the legislature hadn't been able to get it done. (That's become an engrained tradition for our overwhelmingly Democrat state government, which has developed a record of being one of the most sluggish and nonproductive legislative bodies in the country.) We strapped the 110,000 signatures we had collected onto a stretcher, borrowed an ambulance, and with some fanfare had it driven down Beacon Street alongside the Boston Common, siren blaring and lights flashing, to deliver our "patient" to the Secretary of State's office. We got it there in time, ensuring that it would appear on every ballot in the state in the November election, to be officially named Question 5.

We had thrown down the gauntlet, and the reaction was immediate. "Opponents are gearing up," the *Herald* reported, "for a multimillion-dollar campaign to defeat the proposal they say would undermine managed care, even if lawmakers reach a compromise." In a front-page article in late September, the *Boston Business Journal* described the campaign mounted by one of the area's university-affiliated health maintenance organizations: "Tufts HMO Gives $430 K to Battle Referendum," in addition to its prior commitment of $105,000. The health insurer Aetna donated an additional $73,000 beyond its previous contribution of over $100,000. Other insurance industry titans eventually contributed millions of dollars to combat the initiative, including Blue Cross Blue Shield of Massachusetts and Harvard Pilgrim Health Care. Ironically, Blue Cross, Tufts Health Plan, and Harvard Pilgrim were ostensibly nonprofit organizations, but they managed to behave with similar entrepreneurial aggressiveness to protect what they saw as their organizations' needs. The chair of the coalition opposing us was president of an association representing the state's largest businesses.

The hastily organized industry-funded opposition quickly raised more than $1.2 million, according to the *Business Journal*. The paper contrasted that with our group's raising $11,735 at that point, almost all of it coming from health-care practitioners. One political consultant observed, "There is a fundamental flaw when the system allows [insurance company executives] to pool not their personal assets but money that comes from subscribers [patients] into a campaign that takes a position that advocates against subscribers' long-term interests." A public relations consultant hired by one HMO justified the expenditure by explaining that our group had "filed a ballot question that would essentially destroy the state's health care system. They've left it to others to save the system and educate everyone how bad the passage of the ballot question would be." The "No on Question 5" groups paid $156,500 to a California consulting firm specializing in defeating ballot initiatives, a lucrative cottage industry in that state, and $52,000 to a local polling company to gauge public opinion to shape and track their messaging—something we hadn't thought of doing. "By comparison," the *Boston Business Journal* noted, "the Yes on 5 Committee in the last month spent $1,970 on bumper stickers and $250 on campaign supplies."

The battle intensified throughout the summer of 2000. On September 17, the *Boston Globe* noted that the ballot initiative "dwelled in the shadow of the presidential contest," but would nonetheless restructure health care in Massachusetts "more dramatically than any proposal by [presidential candidates] George W. Bush or Al Gore." It predicted that in the run-up to the election, the "well-funded opposition campaign by HMOs will saturate Boston airwaves in the coming weeks." Our opponents argued that passing Question 5 would "throw Massachusetts healthcare into chaos." But privately, the article went on, "they worry that Question 5's innocuous wording, combined with voters' antipathy toward managed care, will result in its passage despite their deep-pocketed opposition." The No on 5 group persuaded several key professional groups we had expected to be our allies to come out against the measure, including the state's medical society and its powerful teaching hospitals.

Faced with the growing concern that our initiative petition still stood a good chance of winning, by September the legislature eventually passed a weak "Patients' Bill of Rights" and an HMO care bill that had been stalled in committee for three years. Our opponents said these would address many of the problems we identified, making the ballot question superfluous. But their halfway measure didn't mandate universal coverage or cap insurers' spending on administration, marketing, or profit. Still, it was good enough to peel off some of the groups that had been supporting us, including the unions. In letting us know about their defection, our labor colleagues explained they had to pick their battles, and that universal access to health care would not be one of them. Most union members, they explained, already had health coverage.

As Election Day neared, some polls were suggesting we were poised to win. This had turned into one of the costliest ballot question debates the state had ever seen, at least in terms of spending by the other side. The No on 5 forces ran frequent commercials on radio and television and carpet-bombed homes throughout the state with slick mailings describing how our plan would reduce the much-respected Massachusetts health-care system to rubble. Their website was much flashier and more professional than anything we put together. By contrast, we had been relying on rallies and on-the-ground outreach. By the end of the campaign, the No on 5 group was estimated to have spent about $5 million—nearly twenty times as much as we had raised. The race tightened throughout October and early November, as the din of the Bush vs. Gore presidential contest attracted increasing attention.

Election night started off strong for Question 5, but as the evening wore on our lead dwindled. (I assume Al Gore was having a similar experience that night, on a much larger scale.) As the sun came up, we realized that the costly campaign by the insurance and HMO industries, along with the feckless claims by the state legislature that it was really dealing with these issues effectively, had taken their toll. In the end, we lost by a narrow margin: 45 percent of voters supported our measure and 48 percent voted no. Among the people who voted that year, 7 percent, or 178,264, left Question 5 blank. If a little more than half of them had voted yes, we would have won. As we saw it, the patients, doctors, and nurses had been defeated by the golems of the medical-industrial complex. As a result, tens of thousands of our patients and neighbors would be unable to pay for the medicines, doctor visits, and procedures that they needed.

One important statistic went unnoticed at the time: in some of the state's larger cities like Cambridge, Boston, and Amherst, we had won with 60 to 70 percent of the vote. One of the movement's cofounders, Dr. Susan Bennett, remained doggedly optimistic. She told a local paper after the election, "If [nearly half] of the public could resist the pamphlets, the inserts, the advertisements, you know this is the will of the people."

Sometimes, losing can be a kind of winning, as we've seen from larger-scale failed movements that laid the groundwork for later victories. Our ragtag campaign of committed doctors, nurses, patients, and advocates paved the way for the idea that a substantial proportion of the public was ready for—and might soon demand—a health-care system that would guarantee medical services to everyone. If a small group of naive, idealistic political amateurs with hardly any financial support could build a citizen-based initiative that came so close to overcoming a well-funded corporate opposition, who knows what could happen the next time?

Before the Ad Hoc Committee and Question 5, there wasn't much discussion in public, at dinner tables, in hospitals, and in boardrooms about the dark path the health-care system was on. Little attention was being paid to the moral travesty of the uninsured whose ranks were growing daily, or to the appealing idea that government should provide coverage for medications and other forms of health care to all its citizens. People had doubted that voters could do anything about it without bringing the whole health-care system crashing down; we helped change that view.

Perhaps our activism around Question 5 shone a new light on what might be possible. Or maybe those who held power in Massachusetts health care had a "Fire next time" revelation that if the issues we raised weren't addressed adequately, those crazy lefties might do something to change the status quo in ways they might like even less. Whatever the explanation, our agenda resurfaced in Massachusetts in 2006. A still-chastened state legislature, with the acquiescence of centrist Republican governor Mitt Romney, passed the nation's first system of universal health-care access—one that looked a lot like what Question 5 proposed. Through a combination of employer mandates and subsidized or free care, the new system covered 98 percent of the state's residents, a national first. The plan embodied many of the values and principles we had put forward as the Ad Hoc Committee; it came to be known as "Romneycare," a term the ex-governor initially backed away from as he prepared for his failed presidential run, but later embraced. Two years later in 2008, when presidential candidate Barack Obama made health care one of his main policy priorities, he and his advisers looked to our state's experience as a model. Once he was elected, his legislation for the Affordable Care Act, soon called Obamacare, implemented many of the elements of the old Question 5 ballot initiative, including near-universal coverage for clinical care and medications, and the concept that 90 percent of insurers' premiums had to be devoted to paying for medical services. It passed both houses of Congress in 2010, ensuring for the first time that nearly all Americans would be able to get the care and prescriptions they need. The nation had finally implemented the vision that animated all those late-night debates we had in Dr. Lown's dining room in the late nineties.

So maybe we didn't lose after all.

The Empire Strikes Back

One key goal of Question 5 was to block the privatization of nonprofit health-care facilities in Massachusetts, a state whose hospitals had been relatively free of corporate ownership. We had argued that the incentives and hurly-burly of the commercial setting were ill-suited to providing care to vulnerable patients who lacked the expertise and flexibility needed to succeed in the combat of marketplace transactions. This insight seemed to prevail for several years after the Question 5 movement, the advent of Romneycare in Massachusetts, and then Obamacare nationally.

But as the new millennium wore on, that understanding began to fray. Each of Boston's three medical schools (Boston University, Tufts, and Harvard) wanted to maintain its own teaching hospitals, so that the city had more inpatient beds than it might have needed; institutions caring for poorer patients were the most vulnerable. The Brigham and the Mass General were in the strongest financial shape, but rumors of possible insolvency periodically swept through some of the city's other hospitals.

> Bertolt Brecht's play *The Good Woman of Szechwan* tells the story of a kindly girl who has trouble turning away anyone in need. Before long her small shop is taken over by freeloaders and crooks; she has to invent a fierce male cousin, whose identity she takes on as needed to rout the hangers-on and restore order to her life. Before long she is forced to assume the cousin's identity more and more often to protect herself from those trying to take advantage of her. In a climactic scene, as the girl's appearances in her shop become less and less frequent, the "cousin" is accused of having murdered her. He responds by berating the gods for having created a world in which they expect people to live a good life, though they refuse to intervene to make that possible.

Most everyone is familiar with the term "fiduciary," used to refer to the responsibility to further the economic or legal goals of an organization or person. But you hardly ever come across the term "eleemosynary," which describes charitable activity; it comes from the same root as "alms." You could even say it's gone out of style. Around 2010 a group of Massachusetts nonprofit Catholic hospitals called Caritas Christi ("Charity of Christ") found itself in worsening financial straits. The group's CEO, Ralph de la Torre, decided that a good solution would be to get a big infusion of cash by selling the hospitals and their land to a New York private equity firm called Cerberus Capital Management. Bizarrely, the company seems to have been named after the dog in Greek mythology that guards the gates of hell to prevent the dead from escaping. Etymologists suggest the dog's name was in turn derived from the words for "flesh-devouring" or "evil of the pit." An odd choice. Cerberus then sold most of its stake in the hospitals and land to a physician group led by de la Torre for about $350 million, creating a corporation with the altruistic-sounding name of Steward Health, ostensibly based on the idea that the new company would serve as stewards of the Church's original values.

In 2016, as detailed in extensive reporting by the *Boston Globe*, Steward and Cerberus sold off the hospitals' buildings and the land on which they stood for $1.25 billion to a real estate firm, Medical Properties Trust, based in Alabama. This sale-leaseback arrangement created an obligation for Steward to rent its facilities from MPT for the foreseeable future at over $100 million per year, a rate that would increase annually. In 2021 MPT sold a 50 percent share of these leases to the Australia-based Macquarie Infrastructure Partners for $1.8 billion. The same year Steward's management issued about $111 million in bonuses to its executives, with the largest share going to Dr. de la Torre. The company moved its corporate base from Massachusetts to the less-regulated state of Texas, and used part of the proceeds from the sale of its institutions to MPT to buy up struggling hospitals around the country, making it for a time the largest for-profit owner of hospitals in the nation.

Steward eventually began to have trouble paying the rent MPT demanded for use of its own hospitals. One of them suffered major damage in a flood, but was never rebuilt because contractors feared Steward wouldn't compensate them for their work; the hospital has remained closed for years. St. Elizabeth's, the group's flagship institution known in Boston as Saint E's, was originally named after a thirteenth-century Hungarian princess who abandoned her court life to give her wealth to those in need and live in poverty. In a modern-day reversal, under Steward's stewardship St. E's stiffed many of those it did business with: a company that produced an intravascular coil used to stop bleeding in obstetric emergencies repossessed its device because Steward never paid for it. In 2023, a pregnant woman who required it bled to death because it wasn't available.

Steward declared bankruptcy in May 2024, constituting one of the largest hospital bankruptcies in U.S. history. According to the *Boston Globe*, papers submitted to the court in connection with the proceedings revealed that as it was running out of money to fund its operations, Steward did manage to find $7 million to pay a surveillance company to spy on its critics, and $1.2 million for Dr. de la Torre's salary in the year before its bankruptcy filing. Patients, nurses, and doctors in the affected hospitals were left unsure what they'd do if their institutions, which served hundreds of thousands of people each year, had to close. Two did, including the Carney Hospital in the poor neighborhood of Dorchester, which had to station ambulances at the shuttered doors of its emergency room to transport patients who showed up and bring them to a still-functioning hospital. Others, including Saint Elizabeth's and the poignantly named Good Samaritan Hospital, were handed off to various other health systems in New England. (You can almost hear St. E spinning in her crypt.) Another giant private equity firm, Apollo Global Management, with more than half a trillion dollars under management, had loaned the drowning venture $920 million, effectively making it the hospitals' de facto landlord. Elected officials predicted that the state itself would have to find $700 million more to bail out the hospital chain. We've seen this before: the privatization of gain, the socialization of risk. Later in the summer, Steward sold the 5,000-doctor physician group it owned to a separate private equity firm—a surprising development for those of us who didn't understand that doctors could be bought and sold like widgets.

The companies based in Texas (Steward), Alabama (MPT), Australia (MPT's financial partner), and New York (Apollo) seemed mostly beyond reach. People in Massachusetts called for repossessing de la Torre's $40 million, 190-foot yacht, and/or his $15 million, 90-foot fishing boat, or the company's corporate jets, used frequently for vacation junkets. Dr. de la Torre apparently didn't understand the old maxim that people are to be loved and things are to be used, not the other way around.

A Larger Trend

This privatization of health care was worse than anything we had anticipated in the activist days of the Ad Hoc Committee to Defend Health Care. A quarter century on, for-profit companies continue to acquire hospitals and medical practices, especially in lucrative specialty care; many health insurers still find that denying claims is one of the best ways to increase shareholder returns. Growing public outrage explains the surprising outpouring of sympathy for the young man who assassinated the CEO of UnitedHealthcare—a company whose business model apparently led it to reject about a third of the claims it received.

Patients want access to generalists, but the nation's pay scale dramatically disadvantages such physicians. That isn't surprising, because the pay scales established by programs like Medicare, which often sets the pace for other insurers, are created by a federal panel that underrepresents primary care doctors and overrepresents specialists. We have yet to fully embrace the idea that physicians should be embedded in coordinated primary care teams along with nurse practitioners, physician assistants, social workers, pharmacists, and other clinical professionals. But health systems themselves prefer to emphasize lucrative procedures like joint replacement and pacemaker insertion over day-to-day frontline care, which is far more professionally demanding, in both personal and cognitive terms. When I talk to medical students about their career plans, they often refer to "the ROAD to happiness"—that is, high-paying, lower-stress jobs in Radiology, Ophthalmology, Anesthesiology, or Dermatology.

Massachusetts has a well-intentioned Health Policy Commission mandated to address such imbalances, but it is often politically outgunned. The hapless state legislature recently tried to weigh in on this problem. As the *Globe* noted in an editorial,

> The bill would shrink the Health Policy Commission from 11 to nine members, adding two representatives of the health care industry—a hospital representative and an "innovation" representative from the pharmaceutical, biotech, or medical device field—while eliminating a primary care doctor, nurse, mental health expert, and business representative.

And people wonder why it's so hard to find a primary care provider in a city that has more medical schools per capita than nearly anyplace else on earth.

As I look back over four decades of studies on how to make the health-care system more evidence-based, equitable, and affordable, I take pride in the work my colleagues and I conduct in PORTAL and the Division of Pharmacoepidemiology, along with others throughout the country who perform such research. Our efforts are based on the idea that in medicine, careful inquiry will yield findings that can be used to improve patient outcomes. That seems to work well for our friends who do traditional biomedical research. But our work? It depends.

I sometimes imagine two collections of scholars working separately in a verdant valley. One group comprises basic medical scientists; the other team of researchers do the sort of population-based epidemiologic and policy studies that we do in DoPE and its PORTAL unit. Each of my imagined groups works intensively in its own domains, the former performing meticulous studies of the genetic basis of disease, or the mechanism of action of new drugs, or the molecular biology of cancer. The other group looks at how well those findings are put into action in the "last mile" of direct patient care: what doctors prescribe and whether patients can afford it, how to optimize implementation of new findings throughout the health-care system. Both teams create delicate capsules of new knowledge, precious Fabergé egg–like creations that take years to develop. Within each team, its members excitedly discuss what they've found or built, display their work proudly, have meetings to present their discoveries to one another.

In my fantasy, the two groups in the valley then put their little Fabergé eggs of new knowledge onto two separate conveyor belts that lead up a mountain and down the other side, out of sight. When the scientists' packets of knowledge arrive in the next valley, they are eagerly taken up by other teams that process them further. They combine their jewel-like productions with one another, building vast, sparkling new towers of discovery. They transform that information into new medications, or novel kinds of imaging studies, or innovative tools to diagnose disease; sometimes a packet of new information will be moved directly into a Brink's truck and sped off to a factory for mass production. But when the conveyor belt carrying the intricate hard-won discoveries of the health policy and population-based researchers arrives on the other side of the mountain, on bad days my fantasy envisions its contents getting scooped up by large bulldozers and dumped into a landfill.

Over the decades, we've made several important advances in equitable health-care delivery policy, though a cynic might note this brings the organization of our system to about where Great Britain was in 1950. Yet the mismatch between marketplace incentives and patient-centered medicine grows each year; with almost $5 trillion changing hands annually for health care in the U.S., increasing commercialization has proven heard to stop. Even nonprofit systems like teaching hospitals that retain that tax designation find themselves focusing more and more on enhancing revenue and avoiding populations that represent a "problematic payer mix" (i.e., poor people).

In his 1961 farewell speech, President Eisenhower cautioned the nation about the development of what he termed a new "military-industrial complex" whose motivations and priorities threatened to skew America's foreign policy. Nearly twenty years later, Dr. Arnold Relman, then the editor of the *New England Journal of Medicine*, modified the term to describe the growing influence of what he called the "medical-industrial complex." Both men were well-positioned to issue their warnings—one a wartime hero, the other a leader of the scientific medical enterprise. And both were prescient. Despite the policy victories we've won in health care since 2000, inexorable pressures persist.

The golems don't sleep, the jungle grows back, the invisible hand continues to pleasure itself. The work continues.

> In the end of *The Good Woman,* Brecht has an actor break the theater's fourth wall by stepping out of character and apologizing to the audience because the play doesn't have a satisfactory conclusion. "It is for you to find a way my friends, to help good men find happy ends," he declares, to figure out how goodness can prevail in a world that is inherently not good. "*You* write the happy ending of the play!"
>
> I guess that means us.

EPILOGUE

Healing the Wounds

Let's end at the very beginning. I attended my first medical school lecture while still an undergraduate. Columbia's College of Physicians and Surgeons had been founded in 1767 before the U.S. was a country; it granted the first MD degree in North America a few years later. (It's now officially called the Vagelos College of Physicians and Surgeons, renamed for a former CEO of Merck after he made a $250 million gift; he added another $400 million in 2024, making him the largest donor ever in the 270-year history of the entire university. No pressure.) Back in 1967, to commemorate the medical school's two hundredth anniversary it sponsored a symposium on the medical aspects of wound healing—a fit topic for the fractured times of both then and now. As one of the only pre-meds on the staff of the *Columbia Daily Spectator*, I was assigned to cover the event. Distinguished speakers discussed a range of subjects related to the main theme: operative incisions, military injuries (the Vietnam War was producing these at an appalling rate), other traumatic wounds. Their intertwined talks cut across disciplines from biochemistry to pharmacology to surgery. One presentation particularly captured my interest—a basic science lecture on how wounds somehow know how to repair themselves after a body is sliced into, either therapeutically or aggressively. This was the first time I heard of cytokines, the chemical messengers released in response to injury, infection, or inflammation. When all goes well, these proteins generate a signal that increases the production of certain cells, including those that make the connective tissue needed to repair wounds, and then turns them on and gets them to migrate to the affected site. Cytokines also tune the inflammatory process up or down, amplifying it to fight infection or reducing its activity if things get too hot. Sometimes cytokines create too much inflammation, which itself produces disease. Back then, this was an exciting new field of research: the first cytokine, interferon alpha, had been discovered just ten years before the symposium.

Breakthrough studies going on at that time were elucidating how these clever little messengers knew when and where to show up, and what signals they need to send to which target cells. I thought of *The Wisdom of the Body*, written in 1932 by Harvard physiologist Walter B. Cannon. In it, he had detailed how organisms somehow know which chemicals to secrete to restore balance in the face of disorder, including the fight-or-flight response, which he also discovered. He named the restoration of that balance "homeostasis." *The body knows what it needs to do to get back to equilibrium.*

The following year I was back on the main undergrad campus covering and participating in another kind of inflammation, the student demonstrations in opposition to the Vietnam War and in support of the rights of Columbia's Black neighbors in nearby Harlem. A few years later I found myself at Spring Grove State Hospital in Maryland as a medical student, witnessing another kind of boundary-busting activity in which dyring people given a different kind of chemical messenger realized that they were specks in a universe into which they'd soon remerge. Then several decades later came the reflections about herring, the Alosa-genus fish with an inborn drive and savvy that compel them to swim against the current to find the streams in which they were born. Each seemed to be an example of self-correcting systems that by their very natures strove to end up where they needed to be.

But there were also the golems arrayed against those well-intentioned, wise systems and instincts—much simpler forces answering only to crude, mindless, one-dimensional drives. The golems may have been programmed with plausible-seeming instructions at first, but lacking the right feedback loops or anything resembling human values, they could wreak powerful havoc, whatever the original intentions of their creators might have been.

The rightward shift of the U.S. government following the 2024 elections will create a challenging environment in which to consider these issues in the context of medicine. As we rethink medications and health care overall, the herrings and the golems may both be instructive models. The former might represent the urge to find one's origins, restore balance, struggle against the currents, and nurture life—motivations that guide so many of the clinicians and scientists I've been fortunate to work with. The latter are driven by automatized force endowed with intense motivation and power, but less modulation or judgment. Cytokines, too, can act in both ways: they can signal which parts of a damaged body need repair, or they can bring about a destructive immune overreaction that can lead to death. In a way, this book might be like a cytokine in well-behaved mode; its goal is to send out a signal to enable healing of a wounded system, without creating a counterproductive state of excessive inflammation.

There is still some reason for hope as we try to figure out how best to use the impressive arsenal of medicines that decades of great science and hard work have given us. The Talmud tells us that Adam was the world's first golem, created from dust. But with the help of a good woman, he got himself some knowledge and became human, even if his rule-breaking got him into trouble. Our creation and use of medications—in fact, the whole health-care enterprise—faces some tough choices that have recently gotten tougher. Is it all just about a collection of competing businesses, each one driven by the idea that if we all simply push ahead to maximize our own self-interest, somehow everyone will benefit? Until now, we've relied on governments and universities to provide a check on that golem-drive. Now it's less clear how that will work. The nation's rightward swing and the norm-busting values of its latest leadership make this a hard time to think about what each of us can do to bring about a more science-based and compassionate approach to medications. It can feel like a David vs. Goliath sort of struggle, but we need to remember who won that one. Governments come and go, but core values and the realities of science can be even more durable.

Nearly two thousand years ago, Rabbi Tarfon said, "It is not your responsibility to finish the work, but you are also not free to avoid it." It's time for medicine to rediscover its own unique imperative—following the instincts that drew many of us into the field, doing what we can to help people who are suffering without constantly asking what's in it for us. Getting that rethinking right will shape the future of our medicines, and of our health.

APPENDIX A

Resources for Consumers

Individual consumers can build on the issues we've considered to help rethink their own approach to the medications they take: Does it work? Is it safe? Can I afford it? What's the truth? Action is possible at two levels: the *personal*—to take a more active role in decisions about one's own medicines, and the *political*—to reshape the policies that govern these domains. The resources below (and more, as they are updated on the companion website, www.RethinkMeds.info) can be helpful in learning a bit more about specific drugs you've been prescribed—their safety, effectiveness, cost, and alternatives.

Your Own Medication Use

Most of us are in a state of at least mild anxiety when we go to see our doctor; I know I am. Things move fast during increasingly rushed visits, and many practitioners spew out terms and recommendations that may as well be in Latin. We physicians often make assumptions that our patients will know how to take their prescriptions to maximize benefit and reduce harm, but that sometimes presumes more medical knowledge than it's fair to expect most patients to have. For example, the "right" way to take a medicine may well differ across classes of drugs:

- take this only as long as you feel you need it (e.g., anti-inflammatory drugs for acute pain);

- you'll probably have to take this for the rest of your life (e.g., drugs for high blood pressure, diabetes, elevated cholesterol, glaucoma, etc.);

• the pill container says "Take one at bedtime for sleep" and contains thirty tablets as a one-month supply, but that *doesn't* mean you should take one every night (e.g., drugs like Ambien);

• take this for the full course of therapy; don't stop even if you feel better (e.g., antibiotics);

• use as little of this as possible and stop it as soon as you can (e.g., opioids).

Nuances are often not conveyed adequately on the label printed on the container; it may simply say "Take as directed." The printed material provided by the drugstore may be of unpredictable quality (see below), and the pharmacist, potentially an expert on these matters, may be hard to reach or too rushed to talk much, especially in chain stores. But patients can still take action to maximize the effectiveness, safety, and cost of what you're prescribed:

- For each medication, make sure you find out from the prescriber:
  - what this is for (to treat a particular condition, or to prevent an illness);
  - what is the goal of treatment (to achieve blood pressure of X, or to relieve a symptom);
  - how you will know when that goal is reached;
  - what are the most important side effects.

• Take notes during the clinical visit; people often forget details of instructions after they leave the office. Get your health-care professional to repeat things or spell them out; a good clinician won't think less of you for asking.

• Make sure you and your practitioner agree about what you're currently taking, including all over-the-counter and herbal remedies. Many of those can have relevant interactions with prescriptions, or important side effects of their own; consumers don't often think of them as "real drugs," even though they can sometimes act like them, even if their effectiveness isn't so real.

• "Brown bagging": Some of the most useful time I've spend with patients occurred when I asked them to bring in a bag full of *everything* they were taking, including over-the-counter treatments or "supplements." I resorted to the bag technique after discovering problems stemming from patients' commonly taking unknown pills I hadn't prescribed. ("You wanted me to tell you about the drugs I got from the *other doctors* also? And my OTC medicines?")

• Drug names can be so obscure that the same drug can have several names (the generic name plus one or more brand names), making for much confusion. I've had patients whose brown bag exercise revealed they were taking potentially dangerous doses of duplicative medicines, sometimes provided by different doctors who may not have been aware of the others' prescriptions: naproxen for low back pain, Motrin for arthritis of the knee, aspirin to prevent a second heart attack, over-the-counter ibuprofen for a sprained ankle, and the occasional Advil for headaches. All of these are NSAIDs, and some are the very same drug. Their cumulative effects can produce gastrointestinal bleeding and cardiovascular problems, but the names alone may not be enough to make that clear.

• Ideally, the brown bag exercise will result in a single list for each patient showing not just what you're taking, but also what each treatment is for and how to use it. Some primary care practices employ a pharmacist to do this review periodically for each patient. It's well worth it, though most insurers don't reimburse for this vital service.

If you want to look into specific medications that you're taking to learn more about the evidence for their effectiveness, or safety concerns, or more affordable alternatives, you have several options.

Artificial Intelligence and Drug Information

It might seem at first that AI would be a natural answer to the medication-related needs of both patients and health-care professionals. In principle, the argument goes, large language models like ChatGPT can scan the vast volumes of all known information about medications and determine which ones work the best, are the safest, and offer the best economic value. Then they'd present the summary findings in cogent, easy-to-read paragraphs that can be written at any level of sophistication desired.

Not so fast. First are all the complexities of those drug studies that we try so hard to teach our medical students and physician-trainees to consider, and that we obsess over at Alosa when we're developing recommendations about specific medication categories: Was the comparison group appropriate? Were all the drug outcomes tracked adequately? Was the difference clinically meaningful? (For a good discussion of all this, see the free Evidence-Based Medicine link under DynaMed.com on page 442.) Some of the smartest people I know spend their lifetimes trying to understand these nuances; many doctors, professors, and even medical journals sometimes get them wrong. Perhaps one day a ChatGPT10 will be able to read the medical literature with great insight and grasp these issues that still elude many of my colleagues, but that is still a few years away.

These concerns are separate from the ethical issues involved in AI companies' harvesting the internet for its content with little regard for the rights of those who produced or published it. At present, this seems like an apt analogy: Imagine a dining service that offers to provide you with any meal you request, delivered to your doorstep any time of the day or night, at no charge. Sounds appealing, right? But what if it turned out that the service gets these meals by stealing them from the kitchens of neighborhood restaurants on the grounds that this is "fair use," or going through the dumpsters behind them, or sometimes snapping up ceramic display models of the foods on offer because it thinks they're real? Unfortunately, since medications are even more complex than cuisine, this is often the state of the art for some AI drug information programs.

When researchers have asked AI programs some straightforward drug-use questions, the output can sometimes—and unpredictably—be remarkably obtuse. And then there are the striking anecdotes, as when Google's vaunted new Overview feature stated that UC Berkeley recommended that people eat "at least one small rock a day," explaining that "Eating the right rocks can be good for you because they contain minerals that are important for your body's health." This was presented by

Google in showcasing its new state-of-the-art product in 2024; it wasn't some hacker or random computer science grad student. (Apparently its program scraped the "eat rocks" advice from the satirical publication *The Onion*, but didn't understand it was a parody.) AI can behave like its own kind of golem, forging blindly ahead with enormous power, but sometimes with very poor judgment. (One advanced approach is called Generative Large Language Multimodal Models—GLLMMs—sometimes fittingly referred to as Gollem AI.) Google's new AI-driven "Overview" format is actually a step backward; its conventional searches at least provide links to specific sites, making it possible to see where a given fact came from (*JAMA*? *The Onion*?) and to go directly to that article to see the evidence firsthand. That's more work than being spoon-fed a predigested link-free summary, but it's worth it and much better than chewing on pebbles.

The reliability of AI-generated drug information might well improve with time, or it could degrade further in coming years with the growth of AIO, or artificial intelligence optimization. That is a growing trend akin to search engine optimization: a new sub-industry of clever programming that can increase the prominence of a given "fact" as large language models scrape the internet, whether it's true or not.

In addition, the phenomenon of "hallucinations" in AI systems is now well established: the programs sometimes just make stuff up, and no one can tell where it came from. Problems ensued when a lawyer had ChatGPT prepare a brief for a case he was litigating. To do so, the program simply invented several nonexistent precedents to defend his argument; the judge was not impressed. That may seem humorous to us non-lawyers, but hallucinations like that can infect clinical recommendations as well, which would not be funny at all.

Still, patients' relationships with human pharmacists have become so degraded by the assembly-line nature of chain drugstores that a well-programmed bot will soon be more accessible than a real professional. How should we deal with this?

> *Positives:* If the informational content is based rigorously and simply on well-established human-vetted evidence, it might be all right to have an immediately accessible friendly voice to con-

nect with at any hour of the day or night to answer some basic questions like:

- Is it okay to take this medicine with this other prescription I'm using?
- Should it make me drowsy or confused?
- I broke out in hives after my first dose; what should I do?

Negatives: The inability to know the provenance of drug-related statements that come from AI and the current inevitability of hallucinations presently make any but the simplest recommendations risky. Large language models aren't fully ready for prime time in this arena, yet.

If you prefer not to eat rocks or plastic cheeseburgers, you have several options. Unfortunately, some of the most obvious sources are the worst; they're described later. Here are some of the better alternatives:

• Standard search engines: Web browsers will often present paid drug-maker sites at the top of the list of links for any medication you look up; ignore these. However, Google often places a more balanced description taken directly from Wikipedia to the right of those ads. That's good, but, of course, you could always search Wikipedia first on your own (see below).

• Wikipedia usually does a pretty good job of summarizing the evidence about many widely used drugs. Because its entries are constantly monitored and edited by a worldwide community of volunteers, skewed promotional statements are usually reined in reasonably well, and the site generally covers the major points about a medication fairly accurately, with references to the underlying papers.

• The NIH's National Library of Medicine offers **MedlinePlus.gov** for patients; it's a current, comprehensive overview of many illnesses and their treatments written in lay language; it also provides useful links to additional sources of information.

• Professional societies like the American Heart Association or the American Diabetes Association periodically issue guidelines summarizing the latest evidence on recommended medications for the conditions their specialists treat.

Positives: Often but not always, professional society information sites are carefully based on evidence from well-conducted studies. Some of them offer their recommendations in a version accessible to laypeople as well.

Negatives: Price is usually not considered in these recommendations. In addition, a few professional groups receive funding from drug companies, which can color their recommendations. And many offer their clinical reviews in turgid prose graced by algorithms that are sometimes unreadable tangles of boxes and arrows that resemble a map of Middle Earth.

• Websites offered by the Cleveland Clinic, Johns Hopkins, Mayo, or other distinguished academic medical centers present solid, free online overviews of many clinical conditions, including recommendations about the medications used to treat them. My own institution sells the *Harvard Health Letter*, but unlike the others its information is not free and sometimes comes with hokey add-ons like "Best Diets for Cognitive Fitness."

Positives: The first three sites above are usually evidence-based and current, produced by experts.

Negatives: The drug ads that sometimes adorn these online sites can be distracting.

• **UpToDate.com** is a constantly renewed encyclopedia of the latest evidence and recommendations for every disease. Each of its hundreds of sections are prepared by respected experts in a given clinical area, peer-reviewed, and updated frequently. Most topics include separate sections for laypeople, which doctors can print out for their patients at the end of a visit. (The cost of medications and other treatments is usually not addressed.) Such intensive high-class information comes at a cost: a subscription to UpToDate costs $60 per month. Patients can also get a one-week subscription for $20, for a quick binge of data on drug options.

• Our own **AlosaHealth.org** nonprofit academic detailing program posts free reviews of the best medications to use for selected conditions and provides cost information as well; the site includes illustrated brochures, longer heavily referenced evidence documents, and materials for patients. The information is clear, comprehensive, and bias-free. A separate Canadian academic detailing site is at **RxFiles.ca**. Its listings are also comprehensive, but are often extremely dense visually, and not free.

• **DynaMed.com** provides detailed and current information about medications, but it is aimed at health-care professionals and is costly. However, the "EBM" tab on its home page links to an excellent and accessible overview of how evidence-based evaluations are conducted, and it's free.

• ***The Medical Letter* (medicalletter.org):** Since 1959, this newsletter has been publishing reviews of new drugs and medication categories from a perspective that tilts toward the plausibly skeptical. Directed at professional audiences, it costs $150 per year and is also available as an app.

• ***Worst Pills, Best Pills* (worstpills.org)** has been published since 1971 by the Health Research Group component of Ralph Nader's Public Citizen organization, and is written for laypeople. It covers specific drugs, FDA decisions, and medication-related health policy, offering a bracing contrarian view of medicines and policy. Overviews of some medication issues are provided at no cost; a subscription is $15 per year.

• The Center for Science in the Public Interest is an excellent nonprofit dedicated to presenting rigorous, impartial information about food and health. It publishes ***Nutrition Action*** magazine **(cspinet.org/page/nutrition-action)**, an excellent source of curated peer-reviewed findings that's particularly strong on debunking the claims of "dietary supplement" nostrums. A digital subscription is $25 a year; print plus digital is $35.

• **PubMed.gov** is a public site maintained by the National Library of Medicine that contains nearly every peer-reviewed paper published in the biomedical literature (about a million new papers are added each year, or two per minute). Most of them have their main findings summarized in a short abstract; these are usually available online for free. While it can be challenging for someone who isn't a health-care professional to dive into the raw medical literature, the site offers screening features that make it possible to look only at review articles, or clinical trials in humans, or just the last *x* years, and so on. It's the most fundamental source of medical evidence, but not for the fainthearted.

• **ClinicalTrials.gov** is the federal repository of all clinical trials conducted for specific drugs.

Positives: It contains basic information on virtually every medication study that is ongoing, imminent, or completed, including its design, size, endpoints measured, and dates.

Negatives: It is daunting in its complexity, and the actual study results are often not reported promptly or fully.

• Advocacy groups for particular conditions such as Alzheimer's disease, ALS, or multiple sclerosis often present patient-oriented updates on medications for their target conditions. Some of these are useful, but many such groups are heavily funded by the manufacturers of the drugs involved, and this can distort the messages that some of them present.

Some other information resources ought to be helpful, but aren't:

• **FDA.gov**: This is the official website for the Food and Drug Administration and could be a leading contender for the most user-unfriendly site in the country. Besides drugs, the FDA is also responsible for regulating the nation's food, tobacco, vaccines, blood, biologic products, cosmetics, medical devices, veterinary products, and radiation-emitting devices. As a result its home page, like its mission, is way overburdened. But even if you click on the site's "Drugs" tab (or go there directly via Drugs@FDA—which looks like an email address, but isn't), you'll be hit with a blizzard of random-seeming announcements and self-congratulatory notices declaring what a great job the agency is doing. Want to look up a specific medication you're taking? Good luck. You can put its name in the search field, but you won't see an overview of its uses or its risks. Instead, you'll see a long list of meeting notices, minutes, announcements, Freedom of Information requests, and any random documents that happen to contain that drug name. This is sometimes a treasure trove for obsessive researchers like my colleagues and me, but it's nearly useless for actual patients trying to look up their medicines.

• The "Information for Patients" papers you get with your pills when you fill a prescription: These vary greatly in quality, from good to utterly unhelpful. Some are useful but many others focus on listing all possible side effects, and read like a "Don't say we didn't warn you" document designed by lawyers rather than doctors, created more to manage litigation than to help patients. Sometimes patients decide not to take the prescription they've just filled because of this written cavalcade of horrors. The content of these messages is not standardized or subject to regulation; some drugstores dispense very useful ones, others prefer more legalistic doomsday CYA inserts.

• The drug's official "label": As we've seen, this is sometimes referred to as a "patient package insert," even though it's not written for patients and usually isn't inserted in the package. Instead, it's the lengthy and dense official language that sets forth a drug's official uses and warnings in highly technical terminology and very small type. This official labeling is written by the drugmaker and approved by the FDA, often after contentious back-and-forth negotiation. The resulting lengthy document is too dense to be of much use to patients.

• Consultation from your friendly neighborhood pharmacist: Retail pharmacists' work in the U.S. has achieved what may be the biggest mismatch in any profession between the training and acumen of its practitioners (high), and their opportunity to use that knowledge in their everyday patient encounters (low). Chain pharmacies prioritize rapid processing and sales of prescriptions over allowing pharmacists to interact a great deal with patients about the drugs they're giving them, compromising this once highly valued relationship. Most conversations you'll have aren't with actual pharmacists anymore, but with pharm techs, who have less training. On several occasions, my colleagues and I have proposed programs to chain drugstores in which pharmacists would talk more with patients about their prescriptions to encourage them to take them as directed, given the very high level of non-adherence; other ideas we proposed were to "upskill" the pharmacists about important medication issues. In each case, we were told that doing so could slow down the assembly line too much, and wasn't in the company's interest to support. That form you're asked to sign at the drugstore before picking up your pills? It's not to acknowledge receiving them, as many people think. Read it more closely: you're agreeing that consultation with a pharmacist is available, but you consent not to receive it. If you try hard enough and manage to connect with a pharmacist, you will probably get a useful result. Better not to try this by phone if it's a chain store; the voicemail runaround and delays may require you to ask your doctor to add an anti-anxiety drug to your prescriptions. This problem is less pervasive in the smaller independent "mom-and-pop" pharmacies that still place a premium on pharmacist-patient contact, but they're a threatened species.

- Direct-to-consumer ads: Ignore them. We've seen that virtually no other country on earth allows them, since relevant information about a medication can't possibly be communicated adequately in a magazine ad or sixty-second commercial. Only the most expensive (and often overpriced) drugs warrant the enormous expense it takes to create and place such commercials; it's simply not economically plausible for a company to go to that expense to promote inexpensive generics or biosimilars that may work just as well.

- The FDA Adverse Event Reporting System (FAERS): This is the collection of spontaneous reports sent to the FDA by patients, pharmacists, doctors, and drug companies noting one-off adverse events that occurred in patients while taking a given drug. Most of us in the field of pharmacoepidemiology see it as unreliable, given the randomness of reporting and the absence of reliable numerators and denominators. It's not a useful source of information for consumers.

Affording Your Medications

Co-payments for prescriptions sometimes seem to be based on the same logic that auto insurers use to discourage people from claiming reimbursement for repairing minor car dents: put up a financial barrier so people don't file for payment on every little thing. That may make sense for automotive body damage, but it's not what we want for human body damage. If a medication reduces the likelihood of a heart attack or stroke or hip fracture, the last thing we ought to do is put up *any* barrier to discourage its use.

Consumers can employ some common principles to come out as well as possible on their drug expenses. For very costly drugs, you can ask your health-care professional whether there's a more affordable generic or biosimilar version available. Most states require substitution of an identical generic drug if one is available, but this isn't always the case for biosimilars, the generic-like lower-priced versions of complex, costly drugs classified as biologics. For both kinds of drugs, even if a generic or biosimilar doesn't exist, sometimes a doctor can change the prescription from a still-branded costly drug to a different one that works just as well.

The system of reimbursement has become so unbearably complicated, and the extra complications imposed by prescription benefit management companies so daunting that for many generic drugs it's often cheaper not to use your health insurance at all, and simply pay out of pocket at a low-price pharmacy such as Cost Plus Drugs, the game-changing company established by Mark Cuban.

Because of all these complexities, when a health-care professional writes a prescription it can be hard for anyone to know what it will cost the patient, even if they are well-insured. Payers and prescription benefit managers vary widely in which drugs they include on their preferred lists, what co-payments they will impose, and what offsets to that charge they may accept (such as manufacturer-provided coupons). Your doctor is likely to care for people with dozens of different kinds of coverage, and can't know this for each patient-drug combination. For a given person the charge may also vary over the course of a year depending on where you are in spending down your annual deductible. I've tried to explain this strange system to colleagues from other countries, whose eyes usually glaze over. "I just prescribe the medicine I think the patient needs, and it gets covered," one European commented. "End of story." That's not the case here, but consumers can access several resources to wend their way through the affordability maze:

- **GoodRx.com** tracks the prices of nearly all commonly used drugs in pharmacies around the country, and also offers coupons to provide lower prices. Of course, it can't address specific circumstances like one's own insurance coverage, deductible status, etc.

- For people enrolled in Medicare, a dizzying array of information about its drug benefit (Part D) is provided at **medicare.gov/drug-coverage-part-d**. The patient is expected to shop around to find the private company (the "Part D administrator") that offers the best deal on the drugs they're taking at the moment. The government offers a program called Extra Help for low-income Medicare beneficiaries who struggle to pay their drug bills. The Inflation Reduction Act expanded eligibility for this program.

- Drug company "coupons": These are the inducements mentioned in the ubiquitous drug ads that say "If you're having trouble paying for your prescription, Company X can help," referring the patient to a website or 1-800 number. That help frequently comes in the form of a coupon you can present at the drugstore to reduce or eliminate the co-payment that private health insurance companies demand for covering a given costly prescription. The coupons were designed in reaction to these steep charges (sometimes hundreds or thousands of dollars a year) that insurers impose on patients to disincentivize them from asking their doctor for a particular branded medicine. If the drug company coupon covers most of that patient co-pay, the patient becomes an ally in advocating for use of the drug. But the insurers themselves hate these coupons, which might cover only a small fraction of the drug's cost (the patient's share), leaving the insurer on the hook for the rest, often for many thousands of dollars. Because of this unsavory part of the deal, federal and state governments don't allow such coupons to be used in Medicare or Medicaid programs.

• Other manufacturer patient assistance programs: Sometimes a drugmaker will provide direct assistance to a patient who can't afford to fill a prescription for one of their drugs; these are often means-tested. Or they may just tell you to apply for Medicaid. A roster of such programs is maintained by the nonprofit groups **NeedyMeds.org** and **RxAssist.org**.

• "Coverage Search" is the name of a smartphone app that attempts the daunting task of determining which medications are reimbursable on the approved formularies of each insurer. It's a constantly changing array, but can sometimes form a good starting point for discussions with a prescriber.

• Direct-to-consumer pharmacy sites such as Amazon, Walmart, Costco, or Cost Plus Drugs often offer generic drugs at a lower price than the co-pay charge imposed by many insurance plans.

Finding Out More about Medication Policy

Several groups actively engage with medication policy issues that ultimately affect individual patients. Some address drug affordability, while others work on other issues including FDA decisions. Each organization hosts a website with links to ongoing issues, relevant background, and areas for action. Some of the best ones are listed below.

• **STAT (statnews.com)** is a news service that provides some of the smartest coverage of medications and health care in general. It's owned by the *Boston Globe*, but is independent of the newspaper.

• **PORTALresearch.org** lists all the papers published by our division's Program On Regulation, Therapeutics, And Law, led by Aaron Kesselheim—one of the most active groups in the country on medication policy issues.

• **The Institute for Clinical and Economic Review (icer.org)** is the respected Boston-based nonprofit that publishes comprehensive expert overviews of the effectiveness and cost of new medications.

- **DrugEpi.org** is the overall website of our Division of Pharmacoepidemiology and Pharmacoeconomics (DoPE), based in the Department of Medicine of the Brigham and Women's Hospital and Harvard Medical School. It provides access to the sites for all our division's component units and their research on topics such as medications in pregnancy, diabetes drugs, and cancer treatments, among others.

- **The National Academy for State Health Policy (nashp.org)** serves as a resource for improving state-level approaches to health care in general, and medications in particular.

- **Patients for Affordable Drugs (patientsforaffordabledrugs.org)** is a national nonprofit working to contain the costs people pay for their medications.

- **The Initiative for Medicines, Access, and Knowledge (i-mak.org)** is an activist public-interest research group that studies patenting and pricing that limit access to medications around the world, and how they can be addressed.

- **Open Secrets (opensecrets.org)** is supported by the nonprofit Center for Responsive Politics, founded in 1983. It monitors all payments from industry to politicians as well as tracking lobbyist activity and revolving-door job changes between federal positions and commercial ones. The site can be searched by industry (pharma is at the top) as well as by your local congressperson.

- **Open Payments (openpaymentsdata.cms.gov)** is a federal dataset that began with Obamacare, and was originally called the Sunshine Act. It attempts to bring out of the shadows all the payments made to doctors and other health-care professionals by pharmaceutical companies and medical device makers, and is sometimes known colloquially as Dollars for Docs. Drug companies are required to report all such payments, from a free lunch to tens of thousands of dollars of consulting contracts. Often these are totally appropriate, sometimes less so. Reports for the most recent fiscal year are based on 14 million records comprising $12.6 billion in payments to doctors. A user-friendly search function makes it easy to look up your own physician.

- **Knowledge Ecology International (keionline.org)** explores the connection between publicly funded research, drug ownership, patents, and prescription prices.

- **NaRCAD.org** is the federally funded National Resource Center for Academic Detailing that our group established; it offers information and training on educational outreach programs to improve prescribing.

Connecting with others: Everything we've covered—from drug approval, safety, and cost to those damn TV commercials—are the products of specific policy decisions made over the years in our democracy. If policy lies downstream from politics, and politics lies downstream from culture, this book is a small attempt to change that culture. Lend it to colleagues and friends or get them their own copies, and talk about these issues. The future of our medications, and of our health-care system, is ours to rethink.

APPENDIX B

A Note to Health-Care Professionals and Trainees

Doctors, nurses, and pharmacists are at the front lines of medication decisions, but we often haven't had enough training in these areas. Beyond that, many of us lack ready access to the resources and connections we need to make optimal choices or even to talk about these issues with each other. One of my goals for *Rethinking Medications* is to encourage discussion about these topics among health-care professionals and students: there is a lot we can do to educate one another. Lend this book to your colleagues, or get them their own copies. The website RethinkMeds.info will offer additional resources such as follow-up research, news, and updates on the issues covered here, as well as corrections and additional ways to find more information about these topics.

Beyond that, DoPE, PORTAL, and Alosa are always looking for smart health-care professionals or students to join us as trainees or as colleagues; the website can be a point of access for that as well. Finally, the site will serve as a connecting point for practitioners and health professional students who want to find one another in their own institutions or cities for occasional discussions of these topics and get-togethers in person or by teleconference.

—JA

Acknowledgments

This book owes its existence to Karen Tucker, my best friend of fifty-six years and my wife of fifty-two years. Over the decades of my upstream career, Karen provided vital sanity-sustaining support, counsel, and loving encouragement as I sought them in vain elsewhere. Professionally, much of the work on medication policy I've described here was done with Aaron Kesselheim, the internist-lawyer-protege-researcher-friend who leads the Program On Regulation, Therapeutics, And Law (PORTAL) in my division at Harvard and the Brigham and Women's Hospital. Over many years of collaboration, he and his colleagues have generated countless valuable insights into the regulation and economics of prescription drugs, and taught me a great deal. The innovative population perspectives presented here owe much to the epidemiologists in our program, led by Sebastian Schneeweiss. My colleagues at Alosa Health and the National Resource Center for Academic Detailing have led the effort to bring the best prescription drug information to practitioners throughout the country.

Our research program is totally dependent on external grant support; through their foundation, John and Laura Arnold provided the vital funding needed to do much of the policy-related work I've described; additional support came from the Commonwealth Fund, the Kaiser Permanente Institute for Health Policy, the Engelberg Foundation, and several federal agencies, including the FDA and the Agency for Health Care Research and Quality. In 1997 Victor Dzau, then chair of Medicine at Brigham and Women's Hospital and Harvard Medical School, allowed me to create our Division of Pharmacoepidemiology and Pharmacoeconomics, the first such program in an academic department of medicine; I hope our success since then has justified his long-shot gamble.

Michael Carlisle connected me with Simon & Schuster, for which I'm grateful. My first editor at the company was Robert Bender; on his retirement, that role was taken on with alacrity by Ian Straus.

I acknowledge with respect the hard and often brilliant work of the front-line scientists in universities, academic medical centers, and, yes, pharmaceutical and biotech firms whose efforts help create the awesome medicines we currently have. The implementation of that research is utterly dependent on the hard work of the beleaguered clinicians who do their best every day to deploy them to meet patients' needs. Gratitude is also due to the unsung heroes who staff a number of federal agencies, trying to ensure that our medicines are safe, effective, and affordable.

I would also like to thank a large number of teachers and mentors who took me under their wing during my fifty-six years at Harvard Medical School and its teaching hospitals, reassuring me throughout that time that my atypical interests were indeed worthwhile, encouraging and helping me in my work. Sadly, I can't.

Notes

A note about the notes: What follows is a small fraction of the references relevant to each of the issues discussed; when applicable, I've focused on papers published by our group in DoPE, using links that are publicly available whenever possible. Readers who work at a university or academic medical center will have ready access to journal articles through the citations provided. For others, federally funded projects are required to provide public access through the government's PubMed Central; when that's the case, clicking on the PMC "Free Content" box should send you there. A companion website, RethinkMeds.info, will provide active hyperlinks for all citations that have them, along with updates and corrections that are likely to be necessary in a book that takes on as many issues as this one does.

INTRODUCTION: A FRIEND OF THE COURT

2 *the doctor who prescribed it*: Increasingly, prescriptions are also written by nurses, pharmacists, physician assistants, and other health-care professionals. The latter phrase is cumbersome, and the term "provider" is unpleasant. The use of "doctor" in the text should be seen as including these other colleagues as well.

3 *my last book*: Jerry Avorn, *Powerful Medicines: The Benefits, Risk, and Costs of Prescription Drugs* (New York: Knopf, 2004).

9 *book on the 1968 student movement at Columbia*: Jerry Avorn et al., *Up Against the Ivy Wall: A History of the Columbia Crisis* (New York: Atheneum, 1968). It is available on Amazom.com and for free at the Internet Archive: https://archive.org/details/upagainstivywall00avor.

10 *Some of the most important questions we've tackled*: For example, I saw that older patients given antipsychotic medication to manage their behavior were sometimes brought in by family members to evaluate their "new Parkinson's disease." Our group was able to show that this is a common and often misdiagnosed side effect of those drugs: J. Avorn et al., "Neuroleptic Drug Exposure and Treatment of Parkinsonism in the Elderly: A Case-Control Study," *American Journal of Medicine* 99, no. 1 (July 1995): 48–54, doi: 10.1016/s0002-9343(99)80104-1, PMID: 7598142, https://pubmed.ncbi.nlm.nih.gov/7598142/.

10 *the Division of Pharmacoepidemiology and Pharmacoeconomics*: See www.DrugEpi.org for an overview of DoPE's work.

10 *harvest such data on a very large scale*: S. Schneeweiss and J. Avorn, "A Review of Uses of Health Care Utilization Databases for Epidemiologic Research on Ther-

apeutics," *Journal of Clinical Epidemiology* 58, no. 4 (April 2005): 323–37, doi: 10.1016/j.jclinepi.2004.10.012, PMID: 15862718, https://pubmed.ncbi.nlm.nih.gov/15862718/.

11 *among the most highly cited researchers in the country*: Jerry Avorn: https://www.adscientificindex.com/scientist/jerry-avorn/4512570; Aaron Kesselheim: https://www.adscientificindex.com/scientist/aaron-kesselheim/4511833; Sebastian Schneeweiss: https://www.adscientificindex.com/scientist/sebastian-schneeweiss/1388992.

11 *spin-off nonprofit organization*: Alosa Health, www.AlosaHealth.org.

CHAPTER 1: HOW DO WE KNOW?

21 *book about the Soviet Union*: Peter Pomerantsev, *This Is Not Propaganda: Adventures in the War against Reality* (New York: Public Affairs, 2019).

22 *"Americanitis Elixir"*: Greg Daugherty, "A Brief History of 'Americanitis,'" *Smithsonian*, March 25, 2015, https://www.smithsonianmag.com/history/brief-history-americanitis-180954739/.

23 *attempt at drug regulation*: The most comprehensive history of the FDA's development is Daniel Carpenter, *Reputation and Power: Organizational Image and Pharmaceutical Regulation at the FDA* (Princeton, NJ: Princeton University Press, 2010). Another account is Philip J. Hilts, *Protecting America's Health: The FDA, Business, and One Hundred Years of Regulation* (New York: Knopf, 2003).

24 *medication effectiveness*: In optimal usage, "efficacy" describes how well a drug works in the formal setting of a randomized controlled trial, while "effectiveness" describes how well it performs in routine use. However, these terms are often used interchangeably—a problem made worse by the fact that much of the FDA's enabling legislation uses "effectiveness" when it means "efficacy."

28 *over a thousand furious AIDS protesters*: "Seize Control of the FDA," ACT UP Oral History Project, https://www.actuporalhistory.org/actions/seize-control-of-the-fda.

30 *Accelerated Approval*: J. J. Darrow, J. Avorn, and A. S. Kesselheim, "FDA Approval and Regulation of Pharmaceuticals, 1983–2018," *JAMA* 323, no. 2 (2020): 164–76, doi: 10.1001/jama.2019.20288, https://jamanetwork.com/journals/jama/article-abstract/2758605.

31 *surrogate measure-accelerated approval system*: M. Mitra-Majumdar et al., "Analysis of Supportive Evidence for US Food and Drug Administration Approvals of Novel Drugs in 2020," *JAMA Network Open* 5, no. 5 (2022): e2212454, doi: 10.1001/jamanetworkopen.2022.12454, https://jamanetwork.com/journals/jamanetworkopen/fullarticle/2792372.

31 *PORTAL*: See www.PORTALresearch.org for a full list of this program's activities.

31 *"21st Century Cures Act"*: J. Avorn and A. S. Kesselheim, "The 21st Century Cures Act—Will It Take Us Back in Time?" *New England Journal of Medicine* 372, no. 26 (June 2015): 2473–475, doi: 10.1056/NEJMp1506964, Epub June 3, 2015, PMID: 26039522, https://pubmed.ncbi.nlm.nih.gov/26039522/.

31 *marinating in funds from the pharmaceutical lobby*: Open Secrets is a Washing-

ton, D.C.–based nonprofit that tracks political contributions. It notes that pharmaceutical companies "have been among the biggest political spenders for years," and backs that up with data broken down by party and specific recipients. Here is the link to the summary for the industry as a whole: https://www.opensecrets.org/industries/indus?cycle=2024&ind=H4300. Additional tabs there break down contributions by company, lobbying activity, and specific recipients.

31 *expedited pathways*: A. S. Kesselheim et al., "Trends in Utilization of FDA Expedited Drug Development and Approval Programs, 1987–2014: Cohort Study," *BMJ* 351 (2015): h4633, doi: 10.1136/bmj.h4633, https://www.bmj.com/content/351/bmj.h4633.

31 *lower standards of evidence*: J. J. Darrow, J. Avorn, and A. S. Kesselheim, "FDA Approval and Regulation of Pharmaceuticals, 1983–2018," *JAMA* 323, no. 2 (2020): 164–76, doi: 10.1001/jama.2019.20288; J. M. Sharfstein, "Reform at the FDA—in Need of Reform," *JAMA* 323, no. 2 (2020): 123–24, doi: 10.1001/jama.2019.20538.

33 *Goodhart's law*: Michael F. Stumborg et al., "Goodhart's Law: Recognizing and Mitigating the Manipulation of Measures in Analysis," CNA, September 1, 2022, https://www.cna.org/reports/2022/09/goodharts-law.

33 Counting: Deborah Stone, *Counting: How We Use Numbers to Decide What Matters* (New York: Liveright, 2020).

33 *write a commentary*: J. Avorn, "Surrogate Measures of Drug Efficacy—A Finger Pointing at the Moon," *JAMA Network Open* 6, no. 4 (2023): e238835, doi: 10.1001/jamanetworkopen.2023.8835, https://jamanetwork.com/journals/jamanetworkopen/fullarticle/2804265.

34 *2024 paper in* JAMA: I. T. T. Liu, A. S. Kesselheim, and E. R. S. Cliff, "Clinical Benefit and Regulatory Outcomes of Cancer Drugs Receiving Accelerated Approval," *JAMA* 331, no. 17 (May 2024): 1471–79, doi: 10.1001/jama.2024.2396, PMID: 38583175, PMCID: PMC11000139, https://pubmed.ncbi.nlm.nih.gov/38583175/.

34 *effectiveness of parachutes*: G. C. S. Smith and J. P. Pell, "Parachute Use to Prevent Death and Major Trauma Related to Gravitational Challenge: Systematic Review of Randomised Controlled Trials," *BMJ* 327 (2003): 1459, doi: 10.1136/bmj.327.7429.1459, PMID: 14684649, PMCID: PMC300808 https://pubmed.ncbi.nlm.nih.gov/14684649/.

35 *evidence-based medicine*: The Dynamed platform offers a good, free review of the principles behind evidence-based medicine: "EBM Fundamentals," DynaMed, 2023, https://resources.ebsco.zone/mfe-container/assets/documents/EBM_Fundamentals.pdf.

35 *such a controlled trial*: R. W. Yeh et al., "Parachute Use to Prevent Death and Major Trauma When Jumping from Aircraft: Randomized Controlled Trial," *BMJ* 363 (December 13, 2018): k5094, doi: 10.1136/bmj.k5094, PMID: 30545967, PMCID: PMC6298200. https://pubmed.ncbi.nlm.nih.gov /30545967/. Erratum in *BMJ* 363 (December 18, 2018): k5343, doi: 10.1136/bmj.k5343.

36 *2012 opinion piece*: Scott Gottlieb, "Changing the FDA's Culture," *National Affairs*, Summer 2012, https://www.nationalaffairs.com/publications/detail/changing-the-fdas-culture%20.

36 *led by Kesselheim*: K. N. Vokinger et al., "Regulatory Review Duration and Differences in Submission Times of Drugs in the United States and Europe, 2011 to 2020," *Annals of Internal Medicine* 176 (2023): 1413–18, doi: 10.7326/M23-0623, https://www.acpjournals.org/doi/10.7326/M23-0623.

36 *Joe Ross, and his colleagues*: N. S. Downing, A. D. Zhang, and J. S. Ross, "Regulatory Review of New Therapeutic Agents—FDA versus EMA, 2011–2015," *New England Journal of Medicine* 376 (2017): 1386–87, doi: 10.1056/NEJMc1700103, PMID: 28379798, https://www.nejm.org/doi/full/10.1056/NEJMc1700103.

38 *analysis of this issue*: E. H. Turner et al., "Selective Publication of Antidepressant Trials and Its Influence on Apparent Efficacy," *New England Journal of Medicine* 358, no. 3 (January 17, 2008): 252–60, doi: 10.1056/NEJMsa065779, PMID: 18199864, https://pubmed.ncbi.nlm.nih.gov/18199864/.

40 *the magic of the marketplace*: Andrew von Eschenbach, "Medical Innovation: How the U.S. Can Retain Its Lead. The FDA should approve drugs based on safety and leave efficacy testing for post-market studies." *Wall Street Journal*, February 14, 2012, https://www.wsj.com/articles/SB10001424052970203646004577215403399350874.

40 *"expanded access"*: J. J. Darrow et al., "Practical, Legal, and Ethical Issues in Expanded Access to Investigational Drugs," *New England Journal of Medicine* 372, no. 3 (January 15, 2015): 279–86, doi: 10.1056/NEJMhle1409465, PMID: 25587952, https://pubmed.ncbi.nlm.nih.gov/25587952/.

41 *geriatric conditions*: C. M. Quinlan, "When the Epidemic Ends, Our Work Begins: The Pharmacoepidemiology of HIV Primary Care," *Journal of the American Geriatrics Society*, March 11, 2024, doi: 10.1111/jgs.18873, PMID: 38465775, https://agsjournals.onlinelibrary.wiley.com/doi/10.1111/jgs.18873.

41 *65 percent of new drugs*: "New Drug Therapy Approvals 2022: Advancing Health through Innovation," FDA, January 2023, https://www.fda.gov/drugs/novel-drug-approvals-fda/new-drug-therapy-approvals-2022.

41 *turn out not to work well*: Liu, Kesselheim, and Cliff, "Clinical Benefit and Regulatory Outcomes of Cancer Drugs Receiving Accelerated Approval."

41 *more careful scrutiny*: H. Naci, K. R. Smalley, and A. S. Kesselheim, "Characteristics of Preapproval and Postapproval Studies for Drugs Granted Accelerated Approval by the US Food and Drug Administration," *JAMA* 318, no. 7 (August 15, 2017): 626–36, doi: 10.1001/jama.2017.9415, PMID: 28810023, PMCID: PMC5817559, https://pubmed.ncbi.nlm.nih.gov/28810023/.

41 *only a fifth of new cancer drugs*: B. Gyawali, S. P. Hey, and A. S. Kesselheim, "Assessment of the Clinical Benefit of Cancer Drugs Receiving Accelerated Approval," *JAMA Internal Medicine* 179, no. 1 (July 1, 2019): 906–13, doi: 10.1001/jamainternmed.2019.0462, PMID: 31135808, PMCID: PMC6547118, https://pubmed.ncbi.nlm.nih.gov/31135808/.

42 *inspector general*: "Delays in Confirmatory Trials for Drug Applications Granted FDA's Accelerated Approval Raise Concerns," Office of the Inspector General of the Department of Health and Human Services, Washington, D.C., 2022.

42 *FDA announced new policies*: Sydney Lupkin, "FDA Has New Leverage over Com-

panies Looking for a Quicker Drug Approval," NPR, March 3, 2023, https://www.npr.org/sections/health-shots/2023/03/03/1160702899/fda-enforcement-drug-approval-manufacturer-promises.

CHAPTER 2: DECISION-MAKING AND DEMENTIA

43 *The Ethics of Belief*: William K. Clifford in *Contemporary Review*, 1877; reprinted in *Lectures and Essays* (London: Macmillan, 1901); cited by Thomas Friedman, *New York Times*, April 18, 2024.

46 *A team of investigative reporters*: Adam Feuerstein, Matthew Herper, and Damian Garde, "Inside 'Project Onyx': How Biogen Used an FDA Back Channel to Win Approval of Its Polarizing Alzheimer's Drug," STAT, June 29, 2021, https://www.statnews.com/2021/06/29/biogen-fda-alzheimers-drug-approval-aduhelm-project-onyx/.

48 *As the STAT team reported*: Matthew Herper, Damian Garde, and Adam Feuerstein, "Newly Disclosed FDA Documents Reveal Agency's Unprecedented Path to Approving Aduhelm," STAT, June 22, 2021, https://www.statnews.com/2021/06/22/documents-reveal-fda-unprecedented-aduhelm-decision/.

50 *quit the advisory committee*: Bill Chappell, "3 Experts Have Resigned from an FDA Committee over Alzheimer's Drug Approval," NPR, June 11, 2021, https://www.npr.org/2021/06/11/1005567149/3-experts-have-resigned-from-an-fda-committee-over-alzheimers-drug-approval.

50 *an op-ed in the* New York Times: Aaron S. Kesselheim and Jerry Avorn, "The FDA Has Reached a New Low," *New York Times*, June 15, 2021.

51 *"accelerated withdrawal"*: P. Whitehouse et al., "Making the Case for Accelerated Withdrawal of Aducanumab," *Journal of Alzheimer's Disease* 87, no. 3 (2022): 1003–7, doi: 10.3233/JAD-220262, PMID: 35404287, https://pubmed.ncbi.nlm.nih.gov/35404287/.

52 *retracting the paper*: Charles Piller, "Researchers Plan to Retract Landmark Alzheimer's Paper Containing Doctored Images," *Science*, June 4, 2024, https://www.science.org/content/article/researchers-plan-retract-landmark-alzheimers-paper-containing-doctored-images.

52 *problems with the FDA's approval*: J. Lenzer and S. Brownlee, "Donanemab: Conflicts of Interest Found in FDA Committee That Approved New Alzheimer's Drug," *BMJ* 3864 (September 25, 2024): q2010, doi: 10.1136/bmj.q2010, https://www.bmj.com/content/386/bmj.q2010.

56 *"yes" over 80 percent of the time*: Alexandra Pecci, "FDA's 2022 Drug Approvals Fall Short of Recent Norms," PharmaVoice, January 19, 2023, https://www.pharmavoice.com/news/FDA-2022-drug-approvals-fell-by-the-numbers/640690/.

56 *large randomized clinical trial*: C. H. van Dyck et al., "Lecanemab in Early Alzheimer's Disease," *New England Journal of Medicine* 388, no. 1 (January 5, 2023): 9–21, doi: 10.1056/NEJMoa2212948, PMID: 36449413, https://pubmed.ncbi.nlm.nih.gov/36449413/.

57 *an op-ed for the* Washington Post: Jerry Avorn, "New Alzheimer's Drug Is a Prob-

lem for FDA's Pass-Fail Approach," *Washington Post*, June 15, 2023, https://www.washingtonpost.com/opinions/2023/06/15/fda-conditional-approval-alzheimers-drug-leqembi/.

58 *educational materials for prescribers and patients about the drug*: See https://alosahealth.org/clinical-modules/dementia/.

59 *a genetic trait*: Walt Bogdanich and Carson Kessler, a version of this article appears in print on October 24, 2024, section A, page 1 of the New York edition with the headline, "Drugmakers Had a Secret in Alzheimer's Trials," *New York Times*, October 24, 2024.

61 *The inspector general concluded*: "Delays in Confirmatory Trials for Drug Applications Granted FDA's Accelerated Approval Raise Concerns," Office of the Inspector General of the Department of Health and Human Services, Washington, D.C., September 29, 2022, https://oig.hhs.gov/reports-and-publications/all-reports-and-publications/delays-in-confirmatory-trials-for-drug-applications-granted-fdas-accelerated-approval-raise-concerns/.

61 *a congressional investigation*: "Maloney and Pallone Release Staff Report on Review, Approval, and Pricing of Biogen's Alzheimer's Drug Aduhelm," House Committee on Oversight and Accountability (Democrats), December 29, 2022, https://oversightdemocrats.house.gov/news/press-releases/maloney-and-pallone-release-staff-report-on-review-approval-and-pricing-of.

62 *FDORA*: Sydney Lupkin, "FDA Has New Leverage over Companies Looking for a Quicker Drug Approval," NPR, March 2,2023, https://www.npr.org/sections/health-shots/2023/03/03/1160702899/fda-enforcement-drug-approval-manufacturer-promises.

62 *follow-up OIG report*: "How FDA Used Its Accelerated Approval Pathway Raised Concerns in 3 of 24 Drugs Reviewed," Office of the Inspector General of the Department of Health and Human Services, Washington, D.C., January 14, 2025, https://oig.hhs.gov/reports/all/2025/how-fda-used-its-accelerated-approval-pathway-raised-concerns-in-3-of-24-drugs-reviewed/.

62 *exit interview with STAT*: Sarah Owermohle, "FDA's Woodcock Reflects on More Than 30 Years at Agency—and Hints at What's Next," STAT, January 30, 2024, https://www.statnews.com/2024/01/30/janet-woodcock-fda-next-chapter/.

CHAPTER 3: LOWERING THE BAR

65 *Its public session in April 2016*: Andrew Pollack, "Advisers to FDA. Vote against Duchenne Muscular Dystrophy Drug," *New York Times*, April 25, 2016, https://www.nytimes.com/2016/04/26/business/muscular-dystrophy-drug-fda-sarepta-eteplirsen.html; Food and Drug Administration, Center for Drug Evaluation and Research, "Summary Minutes of the Peripheral and Central Nervous System Drugs Advisory Committee Meeting," April 25, 2016, https://public4.pagefreezer.com/content/FDA/25-12-2021T00:45/https://www.fda.gov/media/121640/download.

66 *parents said it would be heartless*: Rita Rubin, "Patients' and Parents' Pleas Couldn't Trump Data Concerns at FDA Meeting on Muscular Dystrophy Drug," *Forbes*, April 16, 2016, https://www.forbes.com/sites/ritarubin/2016/04/26/patients-and

-parents-pleas-couldnt-trump-data-concerns-at-fda-meeting-on-muscular-dystrophy-drug/?sh=380b54395bde.

68 *Sarepta "needed to be capitalized"*: Ben Adams, "No Storm for Sarepta, but Has the FDA Created Its Own Tempest?" Fierce Biotech, September 19, 2016, https://www.fiercebiotech.com/biotech/no-winter-storm-time-for-sarepta-but-has-fda-created-its-own-tempest.

68 *net revenue of $1.1 billion*: "Sarepta Therapeutics Announces Fourth Quarter and Full-Year 2023 Financial Results and Recent Corporate Developments," Sarepta Therapeutics, February 28, 2024, https://investorrelations.sarepta.com/news-releases/news-release-details/sarepta-therapeutics-announces-fourth-quarter-and-full-year-2023.

69 *FDA has had no power*: There is hope that following the inspector general's scathing review of how the FDA has managed its accelerated approval program, new legislation will give it more authority to withdraw medications that fail to confirm their initial promise. But at present this is just aspirational.

69 *a series of papers from PORTAL*: L. Bendicksen et al., "The Regulatory Repercussions of Approving Muscular Dystrophy Medications on the Basis of Limited Evidence," *Annals of Internal Medicine* 176, no. 9 (September 2023): 1251–56, doi: 10.7326/M23-1073, Epub August 22, 2023, PMID: 37603868, https://pubmed.ncbi.nlm.nih.gov/37603868/; D. Hong et al., "Characteristics of Patients Receiving Novel Muscular Dystrophy Drugs in Trials vs. Routine Care," *JAMA Network Open* 7, no. 1 (January 2, 2024): e2353094, doi: 0.1001/jamanetworkopen.2023.53094, PMID: 38265797, PMCID: PMC10809016, https://pubmed.ncbi.nlm.nih.gov/38265797/; L. Bendicksen, A. S. Kesselheim, and B. N. Rome, "Spending on Targeted Therapies for Duchenne Muscular Dystrophy," *JAMA* 331, no. 13 (April 2, 2024): 1151–53, doi: 10.1001/jama.2024.2776, PMID: 38466271, PMCID: PMC10928534, https://pubmed.ncbi.nlm.nih.gov/38466271/.

69 *The Japanese company*: "Viltolarsen (NS-065/NCNP-01) for the Treatment of Duchenne Muscular Dystrophy: Preliminary Results of the Analysis of the Phase III Trial (RACER53 Study)," Nippon Shinyaku, May 27, 2024, https://www.nippon-shinyaku.co.jp/file/download.php?file_id=7613.

73 *My PORTAL colleagues wrote a compelling op-ed*: Liam Bendicksen, Edward Cliff, and Aaron S. Kesselheim, "This Gene Therapy May Not Work. So Why Did the FDA Fully Approve It? The Agency Has Repeatedly Neglected Its Obligation to Ensure That Drugs Are Effective," *Washington Post*, July 22, 2024, https://www.washingtonpost.com/opinions/2024/07/22/fda-gene-therapy-elevidys/.

73 *"Peter Marks makes a mockery of scientific reasoning"*: Jason Mast and Matthew Herper, "Top FDA Official Peter Marks Overruled Staff, Review Team to Approve Sarepta Gene Therapy," STAT, June 20, 2024, https://www.statnews.com/2024/06/20/sarepta-duchenne-elevidys-fda-approval-peter-marks-overruled-staff/

74 *as reported by STAT*: Adam Feuerstein, "Edited Video Stirs Questions over Financial Ties," *Boston Globe*, July 31, 2024, https://www.statnews.com/2024/07/29/sarepta-duchenne-parent-project-muscular-dystrophy/.

75 *used the same surrogate measure*: Liu et al., "Clinical Benefit and Regulatory Outcomes of Cancer Drugs Receiving Accelerated Approval."

76 *five of the FDA's own scientists*: M. Merino et al., "Irreconcilable Differences: The Divorce between Response Rates, Progression-Free Survival, and Overall Survival," *Journal of Clinical Oncology* 41, no. 15 (March 17, 2023): 2706–12, doi: 10.1200/JCO.23.00225, https://ascopubs.org/doi/10.1200/JCO.23.00225.

76 *quality of life*: B. Kovic et al., "Evaluating Progression-Free Survival as a Surrogate Outcome for Health-Related Quality of Life in Oncology: A Systematic Review and Quantitative Analysis," *JAMA Internal Medicine* 178, no. 12 (2018): 1586–96, doi: 10.1001/jamainternmed.2018.4710, https://jamanetwork.com/journals/jamainternalmedicine/fullarticle/2705082.

77 *80 to 90 percent of new drug submissions were approved*: There is great variability in how the numerator and denominator are defined here, but this is a good approximation. See "Summary of NDA Approvals and Receipts, 1938 to the Present," FDA, January 31, 2018, https://www.fda.gov/about-fda/histories-fda-regulated-products/summary-nda-approvals-receipts-1938-present.

80 *decisions that were made right up against the deadline*: D. Carpenter, E. J. Zucker, and J. Avorn, "Drug-Review Deadlines and Safety Problems," *New England Journal of Medicine* 358, no. 13 (March 27, 2008): 1354–61, doi: 10.1056/NEJMsa0706341, PMID: 18367738, https://pubmed.ncbi.nlm.nih.gov/18367738/.

80 *drugs for rare diseases were being approved*: A. S. Kesselheim, J. A. Myers, and J. Avorn, "Characteristics of Clinical Trials to Support Approval of Orphan vs. Nonorphan Drugs for Cancer," *JAMA* 305, no. 22 (June 8, 2011): 2320–26, doi: 10.1001/jama.2011.769, PMID: 21642684, https://pubmed.ncbi.nlm.nih.gov/21642684/.

83 The Constitution of Knowledge: Jonathan Rauch, *The Constitution of Knowledge: A Defense of Truth* (Washington, D.C., Brookings Institution Press, 2021).

CHAPTER 4: STANDARDS THAT MATTER TO PATIENTS

88 *the Oxford researchers:* https://www.ox.ac.uk/news/2020-06-16-low-cost-dexamethasone-reduces-death-one-third-hospitalised-patients-severe; RECOVERY Collaborative Group, P. Horby et al., "Dexamethasone in Hospitalized Patients with Covid-19," *New England Journal of Medicine* 384, no. 8 (February 25, 2021): 693–704, doi: 10.1056/NEJMoa2021436, Epub July 17, 2020, PMID: 32678530, PMCID: PMC7383595, https://pubmed.ncbi.nlm.nih.gov/32678530/.

90 *releasing some of those vital data*: See this paper from PORTAL, which presents a different perspective: C. J. R. Daval and A. S. Kesselheim, "The Origins of 'Confidential Commercial Information' at the FDA," *JAMA* 332, no. 7 (August 20, 2024), doi: 10.1001/jama.2024.9639, PMID: 39037797, https://pubmed.ncbi.nlm.nih.gov/39037797/.

92 *Alzheimer's drug Leqembi*: Jerry Avorn and Alexander Chaitoff, "Registry Enrollment for Alzheimer's Drug Coverage Won't Help Much—A Minimalist Policy for a Minimalist Treatment," MedPage Today, July 11, 2023, https://www.medpagetoday.com/opinion/second-opinions/105427.

93 *survey of a random sample*: S. S. Dhruva et al., "Physicians' Perspectives on FDA

Regulation of Drugs and Medical Devices: A National Survey," *Health Affairs* 43, no. 1 (January 2024): 27–35, doi: 10.1377/hlthaff.2023.00466, PMID: 38190596, https://pubmed.ncbi.nlm.nih.gov/38190596/.

93 *"a basketball that's probably going to stay inflated"*: Richard Morin, "Remembering Deflategate: What Really Happened? Did Tom Brady Cheat with New England Patriots?" *USA Today*, January 29, 2022, https://www.usatoday.com/story/sports/nfl/2022/01/29/deflategate-explained-did-tom-brady-cheat-new-england-patriots/9274248002/.

CHAPTER 5: HOW DO WE FIND OUT ABOUT DRUG RISKS?

100 *"Epidemiology in Plato's Cave: Claims Data and Clinical Reality"*: J. Avorn, "Epidemiology in Plato's Cave: Claims Data and Clinical Reality," *Journal of Clinical Epidemiology* 44, no. 9 (1991): 867–69, doi: 10.1016/0895-4356(91)90046-c, PMID: 1890429, https://pubmed.ncbi.nlm.nih.gov/1890429/. A related paper from this early period is: J. Avorn, "Medicaid-Based Pharmacoepidemiology: Claims and Counterclaims," *Epidemiology* 1, no. 2 (March 1990): 98–100, PMID: 2073512, https://pubmed.ncbi.nlm.nih.gov/2073512/.

101 *well described in an FDA publication:* Carol Ballentine, "Taste of Raspberries, Taste of Death: The 1937 Elixir Sulfanilamide Incident," *FDA Consumer*, June 1981, https://www.fda.gov/about-fda/histories-product-regulation/sulfanilamide-disaster.

104 *Dr. Kelsey was declared a hero*: J. Avorn, "Two Centuries of Assessing Drug Risks," *New England Journal of Medicine* 367, no. 3 (July 19, 2012): 193–97, doi: 10.1056/NEJMp1206652, PMID: 22808954, https://pubmed.ncbi.nlm.nih.gov/22808954/.

111 JAMA *published a striking paper*: F. E. Silverstein et al., "Gastrointestinal Toxicity with Celecoxib vs. Nonsteroidal Anti-Inflammatory Drugs for Osteoarthritis and Rheumatoid Arthritis: The CLASS Study: A Randomized Controlled Trial. Celecoxib Long-Term Arthritis Safety Study," *JAMA* 284, no. 10 (September 13, 2000): 1247–55, doi: 10.1001/jama.284.10.1247, PMID: 10979111, https://pubmed.ncbi.nlm.nih.gov/10979111/.

111 *selective inhibition of the study's findings*: J. M. Wright et al., "Reporting of 6-Month vs. 12-Month Data in a Clinical Trial of Celecoxib," *JAMA* 286, no. 19 (November 21, 2001): 2398–400, PMID: 11712925, https://pubmed.ncbi.nlm.nih.gov/11712925/.

111 *coauthored a statement*: F. Davidoff et al., "Sponsorship, Authorship, and Accountability," *New England Journal of Medicine* 345, no. 11 (September 13, 2001): 825–26, discussion 826–27, doi: 10.1056/NEJMed010093, PMID: 11556304, https://pubmed.ncbi.nlm.nih.gov/11556304/.

112 *published the VIGOR trial*: C. Bombardier et al., "Comparison of Upper Gastrointestinal Toxicity of Rofecoxib and Naproxen in Patients with Rheumatoid Arthritis," *New England Journal of Medicine* 343, no. 21 (November 23, 2000): 1520–28, 2 p following 1528, doi: 10.1056/NEJM200011233432103, PMID: 11087881, https://pubmed.ncbi.nlm.nih.gov/11087881/.

114 *poisons the well of trust*: A. S. Kesselheim et al., "A Randomized Study of How Phy-

sicians Interpret Research Funding Disclosures," *New England Journal of Medicine* 367, no. 12 (September 20, 2012): 1119–27, doi: 10.1056/NEJMsa1202397, PMID: 22992075, PMCID: PMC3538846, https://pubmed.ncbi.nlm.nih.gov/22992075/.

118 *The DSMB was led*: Snigdha Prakash and Vikki Valentine, "Timeline: The Rise and Fall of Vioxx," NPR, November 10, 2007, https://www.npr.org/2007/11/10/5470430/timeline-the-rise-and-fall-of-vioxx.

118 *But it didn't correct the paper*: G. D. Curfman, S. Morrissey, and J. M. Drazen, "Expression of Concern Reaffirmed," *New England Journal of Medicine* 354, no. 11 (March 16, 2006): 1193, doi: 10.1056/NEJMe068054, PMID: 16495386, https://pubmed.ncbi.nlm.nih.gov/16495386/.

118 *cardiologists from the Cleveland Clinic*: D. Mukherjee, S. E. Nissen and E. J. Topol, "Risk of Cardiovascular Events Associated with Selective COX-2 Inhibitors," *JAMA* 268, no. 8 (August 22–29, 2001): 954–59, doi: 10.1001/jama.286.8.954, PMID: 11509060, https://pubmed.ncbi.nlm.nih.gov/11509060/.

119 *"Expressions of Concern"*: G. D. Curfman, S. Morrissey, and J. M. Drazen, "Expression of Concern: Bombardier et al., 'Comparison of Upper Gastrointestinal Toxicity of Rofecoxib and Naproxen in Patients with Rheumatoid Arthritis,' N Engl J Med 2000;343:1520-8," *New England Journal of Medicine* 353, no. 26 (December 29, 2005): 2813–14, doi: 10.1056/NEJMe058314, Epub December 8, 2005, PMID: 16339408, https://pubmed.ncbi.nlm.nih.gov/16339408/.

CHAPTER 6: DOWNFALL OF A GIANT

120 *Here is how the approach works*: J. Avorn, "Systematic Detection of Adverse Drug Events," ch. 12, in *Principles of Pharmacology: The Pathophysiologic Basis of Drug Therapy*, 5th ed., ed. D. Golan (Philadelphia: Lippincott Williams & Wilkins, 2025); see also S. Schneeweiss and J. Avorn, "A Review of Uses of Health Care Utilization Databases for Epidemiologic Research on Therapeutics."

121 *adjust for those differences*: S. Schneeweiss et al., "High-Dimensional Propensity Score Adjustment in Studies of Treatment Effects Using Health Care Claims Data," *Epidemiology* 20, no. 4 (July 2009): 512–22, doi: 10.1097/EDE.0b013e3181a663cc. Erratum in *Epidemiology* 29, no. 6 (November 2018): e63–e64, doi: 10.1097/EDE.0000000000000886, PMID: 19487948, PMCID: PMC3077219.

122 *our growing field of pharmacoepidemiology*: For a good overview, see A. Abbasi et al., "Post-Approval Evidence Generation: A Shared Responsibility for Healthcare," *Nature Medicine* 30, no. 11 (September 13, 2024): 3046–49, doi: 10.1038//41591-024-03241-x, PMID: 39271845.

122 *that research in our program*: A summary of our division's work in this area is at www.harvardpreg.org.

128 *Singh said that Dr. Lou Sherwood*: These facts later came to light in sworn Senate testimony: "FDA, Merck, and Vioxx: Putting Patient Safety First?," U.S. Senate Committee on Finance, November 18, 2004, https://www.finance.senate.gov/hearings/fda-merck-and-vioxx-putting-patient-safety-firstd.

129 Circulation . . . *accepted the paper*: D. H. Solomon et al., "Relationship between Selective Cyclooxygenase-2 Inhibitors and Acute Myocardial Infarction in

Older Adults," *Circulation* 109, no. 17 (May 4, 2004): 2068–73, doi: 10.1161/01.CIR.0000127578.21885.3E, Epub April 19, 2004, PMID: 15096449, https://pubmed.ncbi.nlm.nih.gov/15096449/.

130 *an article on the front page of the paper's business section*: Thomas M. Burton, "Merck Takes Author's Name off Vioxx Study," *Wall Street Journal*, May 18, 2004, https://www.wsj.com/articles/SB108482794030613720.

132 *APPROVe*: R. S. Bresalier et al., "Cardiovascular Events Associated with Rofecoxib in a Colorectal Adenoma Chemoprevention Trial," *New England Journal of Medicine* 352, no. 11 (March 17, 2005). 1092–102, doi: 10.1056/NEJMoa050493, Epub February 15, 2005. PMID: 15713943, https://pubmed.ncbi.nlm.nih.gov/15713943/. Erratum in *New England Journal of Medicine* 355, no. 2 (July 13, 2006): 221.

132 *they had to take the drug off the market*: Terence Neilan, "Merck Pulls Vioxx Painkiller from Market, and Stock Plunges," *New York Times*, September 30, 2004, https://www.nytimes.com/2004/09/30/business/merck-pulls-vioxx-painkiller-from-market-and-stock-plunges.html.

135 *paper I wrote with Aaron Kesselheim*: A. S. Kesselheim and J. Avorn, "The Role of Litigation in Defining Drug Risks," *JAMA* 297, no. 3 (January 17, 2007): 308–11, doi: 10.1001/jama.297.3.308, PMID: 17227983, https://pubmed.ncbi.nlm.nih.gov/17227983/.

CHAPTER 7: TEXAS HOLD'EM

138 *Mark Lanier*: See https://www.lanierlawfirm.com/attorneys/w-mark-lanier/.

140 *What Did They Warn*: For a book-length description of the Humeston trial, see Snigdha Prakash, *All the Justice Money Can Buy* (Berkshire, UK: Kaplan, 2011).

141 *the company had conducted a trial*: The statements that follow are taken from internal memos discovered by plaintiffs' attorneys through the Vioxx litigation.

144 *FDA-approved drug labels*: W. Shrank et al., "Effect of Content and Format of Prescription Drug Labels on Readability, Understanding, and Medication Use: A Systematic Review," *Annals of Pharmacotherapy* 41, no. 5 (May 2007): 783–801, doi: 10.1345/aph.1H582, Epub April 10, 2007, PMID: 17426075, https://pubmed.ncbi.nlm.nih.gov/17426075/.

146 *The jury agreed with our side of the case*: "$47.5 Million Payout in N.J. Vioxx Case," NBC News, March 12, 2007, https://www.nbcnews.com/id/wbna17580006; Associated Press, "In Big Penalty, Jury Reverses a Vioxx Verdict," *New York Times*, March 13, 2007, https://www.nytimes.com/2007/03/13/business/13vioxx.html. See also J. H. Tanne, "Merck Appeals Rofecoxib Verdict," *BMJ* 334, no. 7594 (March 24, 2007): 607, doi: 10.1136/bmj.39157.476910.DB, PMID: 17379897, PMCID: PMC1832024, https://www.ncbi.nlm.nih.gov/pmc/articles/PMC1832024/.

146 *"an extreme deviation from reasonable standards of conduct"*: The University of California San Francisco maintains a remarkable archive of documents related to a wide range of litigation about drugs and other topics of public interest. There is a trove of material on the Humeston case and other Vioxx case–related materials at https://www.industrydocuments.ucsf.edu/drug/collections/vioxx-litigation-documents/. Additional material about Merck's marketing of Vioxx

is archived at https://www.industrydocuments.ucsf.edu/drug/collections/vioxx-marketing-collection/.

149 *We published our paper*: D. Madigan et al., "Under-Reporting of Cardiovascular Events in the Rofecoxib Alzheimer Disease Studies," *American Heart Journal* 164, no. 2 (August 2012): 186–93, doi: 10.1016/j.ahj.2012.05.002, Epub July 3, 2012, PMID: 22877803, https://pubmed.ncbi.nlm.nih.gov/22877803/.

150 *Those results were reported*: F. K. Chan et al., "Celecoxib versus Diclofenac and Omeprazole in Reducing the Risk of Recurrent Ulcer Bleeding in Patients with Arthritis," *New England Journal of Medicine* 347, no. 26 (December 26, 2002): 21041–10, doi: 10.1056/NEJMoa021907, PMID: 12501222, https://pubmed.ncbi.nlm.nih.gov/12501222/.

CHAPTER 8: THE LABEL AS PROTECTIVE TALISMAN

154 *extra-strength narcotic painkiller*: Y. Olsen and J. M. Sharfstein, "Chronic Pain, Addiction, and Zohydro," *New England Journal of Medicine* 370, no. 22 (May 29, 2014): 2061–63, doi: 10.1056/NEJMp1404181, Epub April 23, 2014, PMID: 24758596, https://pubmed.ncbi.nlm.nih.gov/24758596/.

154 *the high court didn't see it that way*: "*Wyeth v. Levine*," Cornell Law School Legal Information Institute, https://www.law.cornell.edu/supct/html/06-1249.ZS.html; see also S. David and S. Rosenbaum, "*Wyeth v. Levine*: Implications for Public Health Policy and Practice," *Public Health Reports* 125, no. 3 (May–June 2010): 494–97, doi: 10.1177/003335491012500319, PMID: 20433045, PMCID: PMC2848278, https://www.ncbi.nlm.nih.gov/pmc/articles/PMC2848278/.

157 *reject the anti-abortion doctors' case*: Mark Sherman, "Unanimous Supreme Court Preserves Access to Widely Used Abortion Medication," Associated Press, June 13, 2024, https://apnews.com/article/supreme-court-abortion-mifepristone-fda-4073b9a7b1cbb1c3641025290c22be2a.

158 "*dangerous controlled substances*": Carl Nasman, "Louisiana Designates Abortion Pills as Controlled Substances," BBC News, May 23, 2024, https://www.bbc.com/news/articles/c722llz5dz3o.

CHAPTER 9: A NEW ERA OF REFORM

161 *Project 2025*: Project 2025 Presidential Transition Project, https://www.project2025.org/about/about-project-2025/.

163 *Senate Finance Committee held hearings*: "FDA, Merck, and Vioxx: Putting Patient Safety First?," U.S. Senate Committee on Finance.

164 *test the comparative effectiveness and safety of drugs*: J. Avorn, "Debate about Funding Comparative-Effectiveness Research," *New England Journal of Medicine* 360, no. 19 (May 7, 2009): 1927–29, doi: 10.1056/NEJMp0902427, PMID: 19420361, https://pubmed.ncbi.nlm.nih.gov/19420361/.

167 *FDAAA*: J. Avorn, A. Kesselheim, and A. A. Sarpatwari, "The FDA Amendments Act of 2007—Assessing Its Effects a Decade Later," *New England Journal of Medicine* 379, no. 12 (September 20, 2018): 1097–99, doi: 10.1056/NEJMp1803910, PMID: 30231220, https://pubmed.ncbi.nlm.nih.gov/30231220/.

168 *an editorial in* Circulation: J. Avorn, "Evaluating Drug Effects in the Post-Vioxx World: There Must Be a Better Way," *Circulation* 113, no. 18 (May 9, 2006): 2173–76, doi: 10.1161/CIRCULATIONAHA.106.625749, PMID: 16684873, https://pubmed.ncbi.nlm.nih.gov/16684873/.

168 *build a nationwide system*: See https://www.sentinelinitiative.org/about and https://www.sentinelinitiative.org/.

169 *The foundation's website*: See https://reaganudall.org/programs/research/post-market-research.

170 *reanalyzed . . . Avandia*: S. E. Nissen and K. Wolski, "Effect of Rosiglitazone on the Risk of Myocardial Infarction and Death from Cardiovascular Causes," *New England Journal of Medicine* 356, no. 24 (June 14, 2007): 2457–71, doi: 10.1056/NEJMoa072761, Epub May 21, 2007. PMID: 17517853, https://pubmed.ncbi.nlm.nih.gov/17517853/. Erratum in *New England Journal of Medicine* 357, no. 1 (July 5, 2007): 100.

172 *FDAAA changed that*: See https://www.clinicaltrials.gov/about-site/selected-publications.

172 *still very incomplete*: J. T. Nelson et al., "Comparison of Availability of Trial Results in ClinicalTrials.gov and PubMed by Data Source and Funder Type," *JAMA* 329, no. 16 (April 25, 2023): 1404–6, doi: 10.1001/jama.2023.2351, PMID: 36995689, PMCID: PMC10064282, https://pubmed.ncbi.nlm.nih.gov/36995689/. See also: N. J. DeVito, S. Bacon, and B. Goldacre, "Compliance with Legal Requirement to Report Clinical Trial Results on ClinicalTrials.gov: A Cohort Study," *Lancet* 395, no. 10221 (February 1, 2020): 361–69, doi: 10.1016/S0140-6736(19)33220-9, Epub: January 17, 2020, PMID: 31958402, https://pubmed.ncbi.nlm.nih.gov/31958402/.

174 *under-completion of such vital studies:* B. L. Brown et al., "Fulfillment of Postmarket Commitments and Requirements for New Drugs Approved by the FDA, 2013–2016," *JAMA Internal Medicine* 182, no. 11 (2022): 1223–26, doi:10.1001/jamainternmed.2022.4226, https://jamanetwork.com/journals/jamainternalmedicine/fullarticle/2797103.

CHAPTER 10: THE PRICE OF A WONDER DRUG

179 *I couldn't afford that:* See https://patientsforaffordabledrugs.org/.

180 *The U.S. spends about 17 percent*: Emma Wagner et al., "How Does Health Spending in the U.S. Compare to Other Countries?," Peterson-KFF Health System Tracker, January 23, 2024, https://www.healthsystemtracker.org/chart-collection/health-spending-u-s-compare-countries/#Per%20capita%20health%20expenditures,%20U.S.%20dollars,%20PPP%20adjusted,%202021%20and%202022%C2%A0.

180 *health outcomes don't lead the pack globally*: David Blumenthal et al., "Mirror, Mirror 2024: A Portrait of the Failing U.S. Health System—Comparing Performance in 10 Nations," Commonwealth Fund, September 2024, https://www.commonwealthfund.org/publications/fund-reports/2024/sep/mirror-mirror-2024.

181 *trouble paying for the prescriptions*: Lunna Lopes et al., "Americans' Challenges

with Health Care Costs," KFF, March 1, 2024, https://www.kff.org/health-costs/issue-brief/americans-challenges-with-health-care-costs/.

182 Wonder Drug: Amie Kendall, "*Wonder Drug*: A Comedy about Cystic Fibrosis," Fringe Review, August 20, 2023, http://fringereview.co.uk/review/edinburgh-fringe/2023/wonder-drug-a-comedy-about-cystic-fibrosis/.

185 *the gene that caused cystic fibrosis*: L. C. Tsui and R. Dorfman, "The Cystic Fibrosis Gene: A Molecular Genetic Perspective," *Cold Spring Harbor Perspectives in Medicine* 3, no. 2 (February 1, 2013): a009472, doi: 10.1101/cshperspect.a009472, PMID: 23378595, PMCID: PMC3552342, https://www.ncbi.nlm.nih.gov/pmc/articles/PMC3552342/.

187 *"venture philanthropy"*: "Our Venture Philanthropy Model," Cystic Fibrosis Foundation, https://www.cff.org/about-us/our-venture-philanthropy-model.

187 *nearly $10 billion per year*: "Vertex Reports Third Quarter 2023 Financial Results," Securities and Exchange Commission, https://www.sec.gov/Archives/edgar/data/875320/000087532023000029/ex-991_q32023.htm; see also https://investors.vrtx.com/news-releases/news-release-details/vertex-reports-first-quarter-2024-financial-results.

188 *Aurora Biosciences*: Andrew Pollack, "Vertex Buys Biotechnology Rival for $592 Million," *New York Times*, May 1, 2001, https://www.nytimes.com/2001/05/01/business/technology-vertex-buys-biotechnology-rival-for-592-million.html.

188 *"Because I can"*: Zachary Folks, "'Pharma Bro' Martin Shkreli Still Banned for Life from Pharmaceutical Industry," *Forbes*, January 13, 2024, https://www.forbes.com/sites/zacharyfolk/2024/01/23/pharma-bro-martin-shkreli-still-banned-for-life-from-pharmaceutical-industry/.

189 Journal of Cystic Fibrosis: S. Seyoum et al., "Cost Burden among the CF Population in the United States: A Focus on Debt, Food Insecurity, Housing, and Health Services," *Journal of Cystic Fibrosis* 22, no. 3 (May 2023): 471–77, doi: 10.1016/j.jcf.2023.01.002, Epub January 27, 2023, PMID: 36710098, https://pubmed.ncbi.nlm.nih.gov/36710098/.

194 *$5,700 for a year's supply*: J. Guo et al., "Current Prices versus Minimum Costs of Production for CFTR Modulators," *Journal of Cystic Fibrosis* 21, no. 5 (September 2022): 866–72, doi: 10.1016/j.jcf.2022.04.007, Epub April 16, 2022, PMID: 35440408, https://pubmed.ncbi.nlm.nih.gov/35440408/.

195 *slash its patient assistance programs*: Ed Silverman, "'Caught in the Middle': A Battle between Vertex and Insurers Is Leaving Cystic Fibrosis Patients with Crushing Drug Costs," STAT, February 20, 2023, https://www.statnews.com/pharmalot/2023/02/20/cystic-fibrosis-drug-costs-copays-vertex/.

CHAPTER 11: GIVING IT ALL AWAY

199 *"a backwater office"*: Editorial Board, "Save America's Patent System," *New York Times*, April 16, 2022, https://www.nytimes.com/2022/04/16/opinion/patents-reform-drug-prices.html.

203 A JAMA *study from Yale*: A. S. Long et al., "Evaluation of Trials Comparing Single-Enantiomer Drugs to Their Racemic Precursors: A Systematic Re-

view," *JAMA Network Open* 4, no. 5 (2021): e215731, doi:10.1001/jamanetworkopen.2021.5731, https://jamanetwork.com/journals/jamanetworkopen/fullarticle/2779579.

204 *I-MAK (the Initiative for Medicines, Access, and Knowledge)*: https://www.i-mak.org.

204 *the productive group at Yale*: Yale Collaboration for Regulatory Rigor, Integrity, and Transparency (CRRIT), https://medicine.yale.edu/crrit/.

204 *helped establish the legal basis for the generic drug industry*: Alfred Engelberg, *Breaking the Medicine Monopolies: Reflections of a Generic Drug Pioneer* (Nashville, TN: Post Hill Press, 2025).

204 *the relationship between patents and medication access*: Robin Feldman, *Drugs, Money, and Secret Handshakes* (Cambridge, UK: Cambridge University Press, 2019).

205 *striking report*: "Overpatented, Overpriced: Curbing Patient Abuse: Tackling the Root of the Drug Pricing Crisis" (Lewes, DE: Initiative for Medicines, Access, and Knowledge, 2022).

210 *virtually no new drugs to address novel cellular targets since 1986*: William B. Feldman and Aaron S. Kesselheim, "How the Makers of Inhalers Keep Prices so High," *Washington Post*, June 1, 2023.

213 *A Sinister HIV Hop?*: Rebecca Rollins and Sheryl Gay Stolberg, "How a Drugmaker Profited by Slow-Walking a Promising HIV Therapy," *New York Times*, July 22, 2023, https://www.nytimes.com/2023/07/22/business/gilead-hiv-drug-tenofovir.html.

214 *Bayh-Dole Act*: Kevin J. Hickey and Emily G. Blevins, "March-In Rights under the Bayh-Dole Act: Draft Guidance," Congressional Research Service, Washington, D.C., 2024, https://crsreports.congress.gov. See also A. Sarpatwari, A. S. Kesselheim, and R. Cook-Deegan, "The Bayh-Dole Act at 40: Accomplishments, Challenges, and Possible Reforms," *Journal of Health Politics, Policy, and Law* 47, no. 6 (December 1, 2022): 879–95, doi: 10.1215/03616878-10041247. PMID: 35877952, https://pubmed.ncbi.nlm.nih.gov/35877952/.

214 *eminent domain*: A. S. Kesselheim and J. Avorn, "Biomedical Patents and the Public's Health: Is There a Role for Eminent Domain?," *JAMA* 295, no. 4 (2006): 434–37, doi: 10.1001/jama.295.4.434, https://jamanetwork.com/journals/jama/article-abstract/202235; see also Patrick McGeehan, "Pfizer to Leave City That Won Land-Use Case," *New York Times*, November 12, 2009, https://www.nytimes.com/2009/11/13/nyregion/13pfizer.html.

CHAPTER 12: A LICENSE TO PRINT MONEY

221 *forced to limit use of the drug*: S. Davey et al., "Changes in Use of Hepatitis C Direct-Acting Antivirals after Access Restrictions Were Eased by State Medicaid Programs," *JAMA Health Forum* 5, no. 4 (2024): e240302, doi: 10.1001/jamahealthforum.2024.0302, https://jamanetwork.com/journals/jama-health-forum/fullarticle/2817286.

221 *analysis by the Centers for Disease Control*: C. Wester et al., "Hepatitis C Virus Clearance Cascade—United States, 2013–2022," *Morbidity and Mortality Weekly*

Report 72, No. 26 (June 30, 2023): 716–20, http://dx.doi.org/10.15585/mmwr.mm7226a3, https://www.cdc.gov/mmwr/volumes/72/wr/mm7226a3.htm.

222 *ferreted out all the patents associated with Sovaldi*: R. E. Barenie et al., "Public Funding for Transformative Drugs: The Case of Sofosbuvir," *Drug Discovery Today* 26, no. 1 (January 2021): 273–81, doi: 10.1016/j.drudis.2020.09.024, Epub October 1 2020, PMID: 33011345, PMCID: PMC7528745, https://pubmed.ncbi.nlm.nih.gov/33011345/.

223 *The congressional hearings*: "The Price of Sovaldi and Its Impact on the U.S. Health Care System," U.S. Senate Committee on Finance, Washington, D.C., 2015, https://www.finance.senate.gov/imo/media/doc/1%20The%20Price%20of%20Sovaldi%20and%20Its%20Impact%20on%20the%20U.S.%20Health%20Care%20System%20(Full%20Report).pdf.

226 *$75 million in public support*: B. Gyawali et al., "Government Funding for the Development of Enzalutamide." *JAMA Oncol*, December 19, 2024. doi: 10.1001/jamaoncol.2024.5661. Epub ahead of print. PMID: 39699929. https://pubmed.ncbi.nlm.nih.gov/39699929/

229 *The situation on the ground*: Teddy Rosenbluth, "UCLA's Fight to Patent a Life-Saving Cancer Drug Could Make the Medicine Virtually Unobtainable in India," *Los Angeles Magazine*, January 7, 2020, https://lamag.com/featured/ucla-xtandi-india; see also Helen Santoro, "UCLA Benefits Handsomely from Xtandi Cancer Drug Royalties amid Controversy over Drug Pricing," *Los Angeles Magazine*, April 18, 2024, https://lamag.com/health/ucla-benefits-handsomely-from-xtandi-cancer-drug-royalties-amid-controversy-over-drug-pricing.

231 *a letter to the secretary of Health and Human Services*: Claire Cassedy, "Harvard Academics' Letter Supporting Use of U.S. Government Rights in Xtandi Patents to Remedy Price Discrimination against U.S. Residents," Knowledge Ecology International, February 3, 2022, https://www.keionline.org/37323; see also https://www.keionline.org/?s=xtandi.

231 *public funding was common*: R. K. Nayak, J. Avorn, and A. S. Kesselheim, "Public Sector Financial Support for Late Stage Discovery of New Drugs in the United States: Cohort Study," *BMJ* 367 (October 23, 2019): l5766, doi: 10.1136/bmj.l5766, PMID: 31645328, PMCID: PMC6812612, https://pubmed.ncbi.nlm.nih.gov/31645328/.

233 *"Trade Public Risk for Private Reward"*: J. Avorn and A. S. Kesselheim, "The NIH Translational Research Center Might Trade Public Risk for Private Reward," *Nature Medicine* 17, no. 10 (October 11, 2011): 1176, doi: 10.1038/nm1011-1176, PMID: 21988983, https://pubmed.ncbi.nlm.nih.gov/21988983/.

234 *"Fewer Cures for Patients"*: Richard Payerchin, "House Republicans Rip Prospect of Medicare Drug Price Negotiations," *Medical Economics*, September 21, 2023, https://www.medicaleconomics.com/view/house-republicans-rip-prospect-of-medicare-drug-price-negotiations.

235 *an erroneous industry-funded number*: J. Avorn, "The $2.6 Billion Pill—Methodologic and Policy Considerations," *New England Journal of Medicine* 372, no. 20 (May 14, 2015): 1877–79, doi: 10.1056/NEJMp1500848, PMID: 25970049, https://pubmed.ncbi.nlm.nih.gov/25970049/.

235 *plow back only 10 to 15 percent of their revenues into research*: The most recent estimate of this is: A. Sertkaya et al., "Costs of Drug Development and Research and Development Intensity in the U.S., 2000–2018, *JAMA Network Open* 7, no. 6 (2024): e2415445, doi: 10.1001/jamanetworkopen.2024.15445, https://jamanetwork.com/journals/jamanetworkopen/fullarticle/2820562. This paper also provides a comprehensive estimate of the cost of developing a new drug—including the cost of failures—that is only about a third of industry estimates.

236 *Tauzin announced he would retire from Congress*: Olga Pierce, "Medicare Drug Planners Now Lobbyists, with Billions at Stake," ProPublica, October 20, 2009, https://www.propublica.org/article/medicare-drug-planners-now-lobbyists-with-billions-at-stake-1020.

237 *the* chutzpah *underlying the largesse*: Victoria Knight, Rachana Pradhan, and Elizabeth Lucas, "Pharma Campaign Cash Delivered to Key Lawmakers with Surgical Precision," KFF Health News, October 27, 2021, https://kffhealthnews.org/news/article/pharma-campaign-cash-delivered-to-key-lawmakers-with-surgical-precision/; see also Isaiah Poritz, "Pharmaceutical Industry Backs Democratic Holdouts on Drug Pricing Plan," OpenSecrets, September 17, 2021, https://www.opensecrets.org/news/2021/09/pharmaceutical-industry-backs-democratic-holdouts-on-drug-pricing-plan/.

244 *quality-adjusted life-year*: S. D. Pearson, "Why the Coming Debate over the QALY and Disability Will Be Different," *Journal of Law, Medicine & Ethics* 47, no. 2 (June 2019): 304–7, doi: 10.1177/1073110519857286, PMID: 31298099, https://icer.org/wp-content/uploads/2020/10/Pearson-ASLME-article-on-QALY-and-disability.pdf.

248 *"value flower"*: P. J. Neumann, L. P. Garrison, and R. J. Willke, "The History and Future of the 'ISPOR Value Flower': Addressing Limitations of Conventional Cost-Effectiveness Analysis," *Value Health* 25, no. 4 (April 2022): 558–65, doi: 10.1016/j.jval.2022.01.010, Epub March 9, 2022, PMID: 35279370, https://pubmed.ncbi.nlm.nih.gov/35279370/.

249 *an ongoing process of comparative effectiveness research*: J. Avorn, "Debate about Funding Comparative-Effectiveness Research."

250 *"Legislating against Use of Cost-Effectiveness Information"*: P. J. Neumann and M. C. Weinstein, "Legislating against Use of Cost-Effectiveness Information," *New England Journal of Medicine* 363, no. 16 (October 14, 2010): 1495–97, doi: 10.1056/NEJMp1007168, PMID: 20942664, https://pubmed.ncbi.nlm.nih.gov/20942664/.

251 *the National Academy for State Health Policy*: https://nashp.org/.

252 *PIPC played the race card*: "Issue Brief: Traditional Value Assessment Methods Fail Communities of Color and Exacerbate Health Inequities," Partnership to Improve Patient Care, September 28, 2020, https://www.pipcpatients.org/resources/issue-brief-traditional-value-assessment-methods-fail-communities-of-color-and-exacerbate-health-inequities.

253 *the Colorado State Prescription Drug Affordability Board*: Andrew Perez, "Colorado Is Trying to Cap a Drug's Price. Big Pharma Has Other Plans," *Rolling*

Stone, February 28, 2024, https://www.rollingstone.com/politics/politics-features/colorado-drug-price-enbrel-pharma-1234977554/.

254 *A local network affiliate*: https://www.cbsnews.com/colorado/video/patients-doctors-worry-miracle-drug-may-no-longer-be-available-in-colorado/.

255 *the NHS announced that it would back down*: Tristan Manalac, "Vertex Finally Reaches Pricing Deal with England's NHS for Cystic Fibrosis Drugs," BioSpace, June 21, 2024, https://www.biospace.com/vertex-reaches-pricing-deal-with-england-s-nhs-for-cystic-fibrosis-drug; see also National Institute for Health and Care Excellence, *Final Draft Guidance: Ivacaftor–Tezacaftor–Elexacaftor, Tezacaftor–Ivacaftor, and Lumacaftor–Ivacaftor for Treating Cystic Fibrosis* (London: NICE, 2024), https://www.nice.org.uk/guidance/ta988/documents/674.

CHAPTER 14: CONFLICTED INTERESTS

258 *series by the* Boston Globe: Liz Kowalczyk et al., "Boston's Hospital Chiefs Moonlight on Corporate Boards at Rates Far beyond the National Level," *Boston Globe*, April 3, 2021, https://www.bostonglobe.com/2021/04/03/metro/bostons-hospital-chiefs-moonlight-corporate-boards-rates-far-beyond-national-rate/?event=event12.

260 *the paper did a 2024 follow-up analysis*: Liz Kowalczyk, "Boston's Hospital Chiefs Have Turned Away from Sitting on Outside Boards," *Boston Globe*, January 31, 2024, https://www.bostonglobe.com/2024/01/31/metro/boston-hospital-chiefs-outside-boards/.

261 *part-time service on the corporate boards of two drug companies*: Elizabeth Koh, "Corporate Compensation for Harvard's New Interim President Stands Out among Ivy League Peers," *Boston Globe*, January 5, 2024, https://www.bostonglobe.com/2024/01/05/metro/alan-garber-harvard-interim-president/.

262 *a remarkably generous donor*: "Len Blavatnik," Wikipedia, https://en.wikipedia.org/wiki/Len_Blavatnik; see also https://otd.harvard.edu/accelerators/blavatnik-biomedical-accelerator/.

265 *a book of solid recommendations*: Institute of Medicine (U.S.) Committee on Standards for Developing Trustworthy Clinical Practice Guidelines, *Clinical Practice Guidelines We Can Trust*, eds. R. Graham et al. (Washington, D.C.: National Academies Press, 2011), PMID: 24983061, https://pubmed.ncbi.nlm.nih.gov/24983061/.

266 *measured how long each disclosure slide was shown*: S. Martin and D. P. J. Hunt, "Assessment of Comprehensibility of Industry Conflicts of Interest and Disclosures by Multiple Sclerosis Researchers at Medical Conferences," *JAMA Network Open* 4, no. 4 (2021): e212167, doi: 10.1001/jamanetworkopen.2021.2167, https://jamanetwork.com/journals/jamanetworkopen/fullarticle/2778147

CHAPTER 15: MAKING MEDICINES AFFORDABLE

268 *devote far more resources to lobbying*: O. J. Wouters, "Lobbying Expenditures and Campaign Contributions by the Pharmaceutical and Health Product Industry in the United States, 1999–2018," *JAMA Internal Medicine* 180, no. 5 (2020): 688–97, doi: 10.1001/jamainternmed.2020.0146, https://jamanetwork.com

/journals/jamainternalmedicine/fullarticle/2762509. See also "Pharmaceutical Manufacturing Lobbying," OpenSecrets, https://www.opensecrets.org/industries/lobbying?ind=H4300. See also Statista Research Department, "Leading Lobbying Industries in the U.S. 2023," Statista, July 5, 2024, https://www.statista.com/statistics/257364/top-lobbying-industries-in-the-us/.

268 *DoPE*: See www.DrugEpi.org; *Kesselheim's PORTAL*: See www.PORTALresearch.org.

269 *their eponymous foundation*: https://www.arnoldventures.org/.

270 *errors in defining the end date*: S. S. Tu et al., "The Cost of Drug Patent Expiration Date Errors," *Nature Biotechnology* 42, no. 7 (July 2024): 1024–25, doi: 10.1038/s41587-024-02298-w, PMID: 39020202, https://pubmed.ncbi.nlm.nih.gov/39020202/

272 *recent court filing*: "Brief of 14 Professors of Medicine and Law as Amicus Curiae in Support of Defendants-Appelles" in *Teva Branded Pharm. Prods. R&D v. Amneal Pharm. of N.Y.*, Civil Action 23-20964 (SRC), (D.N.J. September 6, 2024).

272 *colleagues at I-MAK*: See Initiative for Medicines, Access, and Knowledge, www.I-MAK.org

273 *legal strategies the executive branch could use*: A. B. Engelberg, J. Avorn, and A. S. Kesselheim, "A New Way to Contain Unaffordable Medication Costs—Exercising the Government's Existing Rights," *New England Journal of Medicine* 386, no. 12 (March 24, 2022): 1104–6, doi: 10.1056/NEJMp2117102, Epub February 9, 2022, PMID: 35139270, https://pubmed.ncbi.nlm.nih.gov/35139270/.

276 *VA drug expenditures*: B. Venker, K. B. Stephenson, and W. F. Gellad, "Assessment of Spending in Medicare Part D if Medication Prices from the Department of Veterans Affairs Were Used," *JAMA Internal Medicine* 179, no. 3 (March 1, 2019): 431–33, doi: 10.1001/jamainternmed.2018.5874, PMID: 30640367, PMCID: PMC6439699, https://www.ncbi.nlm.nih.gov/pmc/articles/PMC6439699/.

277 *We don't have to start from scratch on this*: Thomas Waldrop, "Value-Based Pricing of Prescription Drugs Benefits Patients and Promotes Innovation," Center for American Progress, September 13, 2021, https://www.americanprogress.org/article/value-based-pricing-prescription-drugs-benefits-patients-promotes-innovation/. See also Richard G. Frank, Jerry Avorn, and Aaron S. Kesselheim, "What Do High Drug Prices Buy Us?" *Health Affairs*, April 29, 2020, https://www.healthaffairs.org/content/forefront/do-high-drug-prices-buy-us.

278 *a not-for-profit generic drug company*: https://civicarx.org/.

279 *bring down the cost of creating such new gene therapy*: https://innovativegenomics.org/.

279 *nonprofit on the far edge of innovative treatments*: https://odylia.org/.

280 *the 340B designation*: I. T. T. Liu et al., "Commercial Markups on Pediatric Oncology Drugs at 340B Pediatric Hospitals," *Pediatric Blood & Cancer* 71, no. 9 (2024): e31158, https://doi.org/10.1002/pbc.31158.

282 *scathing reports about the often-overlooked industry*: "FTC Releases Interim Staff Report on Prescription Drug Middlemen," Federal Trade Commission, July 9, 2024, https://www.ftc.gov/news-events/news/press-releases/2024/07/ftc-releases

-interim-staff-report-prescription-drug-middlemen-staff-report.pdf. See also "Hearing Wrap-Up: Oversight Committee Exposes How PBMs Undermine Patient Health and Increase Drug Costs," House Committee on Oversight and Accountability, July 23, 2024, https://oversight.house.gov/release/hearing-wrap-up-oversight-committee-exposes-how-pbms-undermine-patient-health-and-increase-drug-costs/. See also "Prescription Drugs: Selected States' Regulation of Pharmacy Benefit Managers," U.S. Government Accountability Office, April 15, 2024, https://www.gao.gov/products/gao-24-106898.

282 *Cost Plus Drugs*: https://costplusdrugs.com/.

282 *could have spent $3.6 billion less* each year: H. S. Lalani, A. S. Kesselheim, and B. N. Rome, "Potential Medicare Part D Savings on Generic Drugs from the Mark Cuban Cost Plus Drug Company," *Annals of Internal Medicine* 175, no. 7 (July 2022): 1053–55, doi: 10.7326/M22-0756, https://pubmed.ncbi.nlm.nih.gov/35724381/.

283 *an investigative report*: Rebecca Robbins and Reed Abelson, "The Opaque Industry Secretly Inflating Prices for Prescription Drugs," *New York Times*, June 21, 2024, https://www.nytimes.com/2024/06/21/business/prescription-drug-costs-pbm.html. See also "Specialty Generic Drugs: A Growing Profit Center for Vertically Integrated Pharmacy Benefit Managers," Federal Trade Commission Second Interim Staff Report, January 2025, https:/www.ftc.gov/system/files/ftc_gov/pdf/PBM-6b-Second-Interim-Staff-Report.pdf.

286 *two astonishing accounts*: Jeffrey Flier, "How Pfizer Ended Up Passing on My GLP-1 Work Back in the Early '90s," STAT, September 9, 2024, https://www.statnews.com/2024/09/09/glp-1-history-pfizer-john-baxter-jeffrey-flier-calbio-metabio/; Jeffrey S. Flier, "Drug Development Failure: How GLP-1 Development Was Abandoned in 1990," *Perspectives in Biology and Medicine* 67, no. 3 (Summer 2024): 325–36, https://dx.doi.org/10.1353/pbm.2024.a936213, https://muse.jhu.edu/article/936213.

290 *an angry op-ed in* USA Today: Joe Biden and Bernie Sanders, "Novo Nordisk, Eli Lilly Must Stop Ripping Off Americans with High Drug Prices," *USA Today*, July 2, 2024, https://www.usatoday.com/story/opinion/2024/07/02/biden-sanders-prescription-drug-cost-ozempic-wegovy/74232827007/.

CHAPTER 16: A FAILURE TO COMMUNICATE

297 *$50 billion annual promotion budget*: L. M. Schwartz and S. Woloshin, "Medical Marketing in the United States, 1997–2016," *JAMA* 321, no. 1 (January 1, 2019): 80–96, doi: 10.1001/jama.2018.19320, PMID: 30620375, https://pubmed.ncbi.nlm.nih.gov/30620375/.

302 *in a surprise decision*: Katie Thomas, "Ruling Is Victory for Drug Companies in Promoting Medicine for Other Uses," *New York Times*, December 3, 2012, https://www.nytimes.com/2012/12/04/business/ruling-backs-drug-industry-on-off-label-marketing.html. See also A. S. Kesselheim, M. M. Mello, and J. Avorn, "FDA Regulation of Off-Label Drug Promotion under Attack," *JAMA* 309, no. 5 (February 6, 2013): 445–46, doi: 10.1001/jama.2012.207972, PMID: 23385267, https://pubmed.ncbi.nlm.nih.gov/23385267/.

303 *its title summed up the situation neatly*: J. Avorn, A. Sarpatwari, and A. S. Kesselheim, "Forbidden and Permitted Statements about Medications—Loosening the Rules," *New England Journal of Medicine* 373, no. 10 (September 3, 2015): 967–73, doi: 10.1056/NEJMhle1506365, PMID: 26332553, https://pubmed.ncbi.nlm.nih.gov/26332553/.

304 *The frontispiece of the 1651 edition*: https://devonandexeterinstitution.org/wp-content/uploads/2021/02/2.jpg&tbnid=FJV9gwH3KkZDpM&vet=1&imgrefurl=https://devonandexeterinstitution.org/the-frontispiece-as-a-threshold-of-interpretation-thomas-hobbes-leviathan-1651/&docid=eZvQOmNhJe_uLM&w=1619&h=1355&source=sh/x/im/m1/1&kgs=6a22f55c9bc5ef4d&shem=abme,trie.

304 *an article in the* Annals of Internal Medicine: J. Avorn, "In Opposition to Liberty: We Need a 'Sovereign' to Govern Drug Claims," *Annals of Internal Medicine* 163, no. 3 (August 4, 2015): 229–30, doi: 10.7326/M15-1429, PMID: 26121615, https://pubmed.ncbi.nlm.nih.gov/26121615/.

306 *FDA actions against drugmakers*: S. Liu, M. M. Mello, and A. S. Kesselheim, "Prospects for Enforcing Prohibitions on Off-Label Drug Promotion after *United States v. Caronia*: An Analysis of Litigated Cases," *Journal of Health Politics, Policy, and Law* 46, no. 3 (June 1, 2021): 487–504, doi: 10.1215/03616878-8893571, PMID: 33647951, https://pubmed.ncbi.nlm.nih.gov/33647951/.

307 *requiring a company to make certain statements*: J. Avorn, "Wedding Websites, Free Speech, and Adverse Drug Effects," *New England Journal of Medicine* 389, no. 16 (October 19, 2023): 1447–49, doi: 10.1056/NEJMp2307908, Epub October 14, 2023, PMID: 37843109, https://pubmed.ncbi.nlm.nih.gov/37843109/.

CHAPTER 17: SHAPING THE PRESCRIBERS OF TOMORROW

311 The Doctor *by Sir Luke Fildes*: A. C. Kao, "What Is Represented 'Worthily' in Luke Fildes' *The Doctor*?," *AMA Journal of Ethics* 24, no. 7 (July 1, 2022): e697–E713, doi: 10.1001/amajethics.2022.697, PMID: 35838401, https://pubmed.ncbi.nlm.nih.gov/35838401/; https://journalofethics.ama-assn.org/gallery/what-represented-worthily-luke-fildes-doctor.

CHAPTER 18: BETTER SIGNALS

334 *test it in a randomized controlled trial*: J. Avorn and S. B. Soumerai, "Improving Drug-Therapy Decisions through Educational Outreach. A Randomized Controlled Trial of Academically Based 'Detailing,'" *New England Journal of Medicine* 308, no. 24 (June 16, 1983): 1457–63, doi: 10.1056/NEJM198306163082406, PMID: 6406886, https://pubmed.ncbi.nlm.nih.gov/6406886/.

334 *Good Evidence Doesn't Disseminate Itself*: This is Avorn's Tenth Law. I'm not sure what the first nine are.

334 *using population-based data from health-care systems*: Jerry Avorn, "Interventional Pharmacoepidemiology: Origins, Current Status, and Future Possibilities," *American Journal of Epidemiology* (October 10, 2024), https://academic.oup.com/aje/advance-article/doi/10.1093/aje/kwae383/7817814.

335 *randomized trial in nursing homes:* J. Avorn et al., "A Randomized Trial of a Program to Reduce the Use of Psychoactive Drugs in Nursing Homes," *New England Journal of Medicine* 327, no. 3 (July 16, 1992): 168–73, doi: 10.1056/NEJM199207163270306, PMID: 1608408, https://pubmed.ncbi.nlm.nih.gov/1608408/.

335 *systematic reviews*: M. A. O'Brien et al., "Educational Outreach Visits: Effects on Professional Practice and Health Care Outcomes," *Cochrane Database of Systematic Reviews* 2007, no. 4 (October 17, 2007): CD000409, doi: 10.1002/14651858.CD000409.pub2, PMID: 17943742, PMCID: PMC7032679, https://pubmed.ncbi.nlm.nih.gov/17943742/. See also B.N. Rome et al., "Academic Detailing Interventions and Evidence-Based Prescribing: A Systematic Review," *JAMA Netw Open*. January 2, 2025, 8(1):e2453684, doi: 10.1001/jamanetworkopen.2024.53684. PMID: 39775805, https://pubmed.ncbi.nlm.nih.gov/39775805/.

336 *Veterans Affairs health systems*: https://www.pbm.va.gov/PBM/academicdetailingservice/AboutUs.asp.

337 *our new counter-current nonprofit*: See www.AlosaHealth.org.

338 *a front-page story*: Scott Hensley, "As Drug Bill Soars, Some Doctors Get an 'Unsales' Pitch: Harvard Professor Helps Team in Pennsylvania Publicize Alternatives to Pricey Pills," *Wall Street Journal*, March 13, 2006, https://www.wsj.com/articles/SB114221796975796288. See also Avorn, "Interventional Pharmacoepidemiology."

339 *evidence-based practical recommendations*: https://alosahealth.org/clinical-modules/.

CHAPTER 19: ACID REDUX: THE DEATH AND REBIRTH OF PSYCHEDELICS

356 *Treatment sessions at Spring Grove*: Jerry Avorn, "Beyond Dying," *Harper's*, March 1973, https://harpers.org/archive/1973/03/beyond-dying/.

363 *the Multidisciplinary Association for Psychedelic Studies*: https://maps.org/about-maps/.

364 *Boston Psychedelic Research Group*: https://www.bostonpsychedelicresearchgroup.com/.

373 *journal* Nature Medicine *in September 2023*: J. M. Mitchell et al., "MDMA-Assisted Therapy for Moderate to Severe PTSD: A Randomized, Placebo-Controlled Phase 3 Trial," *Nature Medicine* 29, no. 10 (October 2023): 2473–80, doi: 10.1038/s41591-023-02565-4, Epub September 14, 2023, PMID: 37709999, PMCID: PMC10579091, https://pubmed.ncbi.nlm.nih.gov/37709999/.

374 *"substantial concerns about the validity of the results"*: R. A. Mustafa et al., *Midomafetamine-Assisted Psychotherapy for Post-Traumatic Stress Disorder: Final Evidence Report* (Institute for Clinical and Economic Review, June 27, 2024), https://icer.org/assessment/ptsd-2024/#overview; https://icer.org/wp-content/uploads/2024/06/PTSD_Final-Report_For-Publication_06272024.pdf.

374 *citizen petition*: Neșe Devenot et al., "Citizen Petition to FDA Commissioner," Regulations.gov, April 28, 2024, https://www.regulations.gov/document/FDA-2024-P-2148-0001.

375 *the FDA advisory committee met in early June*: Kai Kupferschmidt, "In a Setback for Psychedelic Therapy, FDA Advisers Vote against Medical Use of Ecstasy," *Science*, June 5, 2024, https://www.science.org/content/article/fda-advisory-panel-rejects-mdma-ptsd-treatment.

376 *The FDA did indeed follow that advice:* Kai Kupferschmidt, "FDA Rejected MDMA-Assisted PTSD Therapy. Other Psychedelics Firms Intend to Avoid That Fate," *Science*, August 12, 2024, https://www.science.org/content/article/fda-rejected-mdma-assisted-ptsd-therapy-other-psychedelics-firms-intend-avoid-fate.

376 *"changing the goalposts"*: Meghana Keshavan, "Rick Doblin, 'Unleashed,' Blasts FDA over Lykos Drug Rejection and Turns to Global Push for MDMA Therapy," STAT, August 17, 2024, https://www.statnews.com/2024/08/17/mdma-psychedelics-rick-doblin-lykos-exit/.

379 *the city of Denver*: Gregory Ferenstein, "A Glimpse into Colorado's Emerging Legal Psychedelics Scene," *Reason* magazine, July 10, 2024, https://reason.org/commentary/a-glimpse-into-colorados-emerging-legal-psychedelics-scene/.

379 *the Dutch Committee on MDMA*: Mari Eccles, "Dutch Committee Recommends MDMA for Post-Traumatic Stress Disorder," Politico, June 6, 2024, https://www.politico.eu/article/dutch-panel-recommends-mdma-ecstasy-post-traumatic-stress-disorder/. See also Wim van den Brink, "Report of the Dutch State Committee on MDMA: A Summary of Findings and Recommendations," Drug Science, June 19, 2024, https://www.drugscience.org.uk/mdma-netherlands-report.

CHAPTER 20: PAIN, KILLERS

383 *FDA laid the groundwork:* Bill Whitaker, "Did the FDA Ignite the Opioid Epidemic?," *60 Minutes*, February 24, 2019, https://www.cbsnews.com/news/opioid-epidemic-did-the-fda-ignite-the-crisis-60-minutes/. See also Gerald Posner, "FDA's Janet Woodcock Failed to Stop the Opioid Epidemic," *USA Today*, February 3, 2021, https://www.usatoday.com/story/opinion/2021/02/03/janet-woodcocks-failure-fda-opioid-epidemic-column/4352787001/.

384 *the SPACE trial*: E. E. Krebs et al., "Effect of Opioid vs. Nonopioid Medications on Pain-Related Function in Patients with Chronic Back Pain or Hip or Knee Osteoarthritis Pain: The SPACE Randomized Clinical Trial," *JAMA* 319, no. 9 (March 6, 2018): 872–82, doi: 10.1001/jama.2018.0899, PMID: 29509867, PMCID: PMC5885909, https://pubmed.ncbi.nlm.nih.gov/29509867/.

387 *"the Jick paper"*: https://www.nejm.org/doi/pdf/10.1056/NEJM198001103020221.

388 *A follow-up letter to the* NEJM *in 2017*: P. T. M. Leung et al., "A 1980 Letter on the Risk of Opioid Addiction," *New England Journal of Medicine* 376, no. 22 (June 1, 2017): 2194–95, doi: 10.1056/NEJMc1700150, PMID: 28564561, https://pubmed.ncbi.nlm.nih.gov/28564561/.

389 *a high-flying Arizona start-up*: *Frontline*, season 2020, episode 15, "Opioids, Inc.," produced by Tom Jennings, Annie Wong, and Nick Verbitsky, aired June 23, 2021, on PBS, https://www.pbs.org/wgbh/frontline/documentary/opioids-inc/.

390 *scathing* JAMA *paper*: J. E. Rollman et al., "Assessment of the FDA Risk Eval-

uation and Mitigation Strategy for Transmucosal Immediate-Release Fentanyl Products," *JAMA* 321, no. 7 (2019): 676–85, doi: 10.1001/jama.2019.0235, https://pmc.ncbi.nlm.nih.gov/articles/PMC6439622/.

CHAPTER 21: YOU CAN'T GET YOUR MEDICINES IF YOU CAN'T GET HEALTH CARE

408 *The opening salvo of the revolution*: J. Agretelis et al., "For Our Patients, Not for Profits: A Call to Action," *JAMA* 278, no. 21 (1997): 1733–38, doi: 10.1001/jama.1997.03550210031020, https://jamanetwork.com/journals/jama/article-abstract/419060; https://pubmed.ncbi.nlm.nih.gov/9388138/.

409 *degradation of the doctor-patient relationship*: Bernard Lown, *The Lost Art of Healing: Practicing Compassion in Medicine* (New York: Random House, 1999).

425 *extensive reporting by the* Boston Globe: Elizabeth Koh, Chris Serres, Jessica Bartlett, and Mark Arsenault, "Timeline: Steward Health Care Kept Expanding, Even as the Situation Turned Dire," *Boston Globe*, September 6, 2024, https://apps.bostonglobe.com/metro/investigations/spotlight/2024/09/steward-hospitals/timeline/.

425 *Steward and Cerberus*: Robert Weisman, "Cerberus Says Its Investment in Steward Hospitals Yielded an $800 Million Profit," *Boston Globe*, April 2, 2024, https://www.bostonglobe.com/2024/04/02/business/cerberus-capital-management-steward-health-care/. See also Robert Kuttner, "Steward Health Care Should Face a Full-Scale Criminal Investigation," *Boston Globe*, February 29, 2024, https://www.bostonglobe.com/2024/02/29/opinion/steward-health-care-criminal-investigation/.

426 *the company's corporate jets*: Excellent coverage of the Steward fiasco has been provided by the Spotlight Team of the *Boston Globe*. See, for example, Hanna Krueger, Yoohyun Jung, and Brendan McCarty, "For Steward CEO: Jet Travel, Yacht Adventures," *Boston Globe*, September 19, 2024, https://apps.bostonglobe.com/metro/investigations/spotlight/2024/09/steward-hospitals/flights/.

428 *hard to find a primary care provider*: "A Dire Diagnosis: The Declining Health of Primary Care in Massachusetts and the Urgent Need for Action," Massachusetts Health Policy Commission, January 2025, https://masshpc.gov/sites/default/files/HPC Chartpack_A Dire Diagnosis - The Declining Health of Primary Care in MA_0.pdf.

429 *growing influence*: A. S. Relman, "The New Medical-Industrial Complex," *New England Journal of Medicine* 303, no. 17 (October 23, 1980): 963–70, doi: 10.1056/NEJM198010233031703, PMID: 7412851, https://pubmed.ncbi.nlm.nih.gov/7412851/.

APPENDIX A: RESOURCES FOR CONSUMERS

446 *Affording your medications*: See H.S. Lalani et al., "Strategies to Help Patients Navigate High Prescription Drug Costs," *JAMA* 332, no. 20 (November 26, 2024): 1741–49, doi: 10.1001/jama.2024.17275, PMID: 39432312, https://pubmed.ncbi.nlm.nih.gov/39432312/. For patients: K.L. Walter, "Strategies to Help Patients Afford Their Medicines in the US." *JAMA*. 2024; 332, no. 20 (October 21, 2024): 1767–68, doi: 10.1001/jama.2024.21143. https://jamanetwork.com/journals/jama/fullarticle/2825161.

Index

About the Author

Jerry Avorn was raised in Queens, New York City, where he attended Far Rockaway High School. His undergraduate education was at Columbia University. Following the demonstrations there in 1968, he joined with other student editors of *The Columbia Daily Spectator* to write *Up Against the Ivy Wall: A History of the Columbia Crisis*, first published by Atheneum and now available at no cost on the Internet Archive. He began his career at Harvard Medical School in 1969 as an entering student and never left. After being awarded the MD degree in 1974, he completed his training in internal medicine at Harvard's teaching hospitals and then joined its faculty.

Dr. Avorn helped launch the field of pharmacoepidemiology, using computer-assisted analysis of detailed health-care data to study patterns of medication use and their clinical consequences. He also developed the approach of academic detailing—non-commercial educational outreach to doctors to promote the best information on effective prescribing; it is now in widespread use throughout the world. In 1997, he founded the Division of Pharmacoepidemiology and Pharmacoeconomics at Harvard and its teaching institution, Brigham and Women's Hospital. Over the next two decades, it became one of the nation's most respected programs of research on prescription drug use, cost, and outcomes.

A professor of medicine at Harvard, Dr. Avorn is one of the nation's most highly cited researchers and is the author or co-author of over six hundred papers in the medical literature. He wrote *Powerful Medicines: The Benefits, Risks, and Costs of Prescription Drugs* (Knopf), and numerous commentaries in the *New England Journal of Medicine*, the *New York Times*, and the *Washington Post*.